T0249608

Critical Care of the Solid Organ Transplant Patient
Part I: Heart and Lung
Part II: Liver, Kidney, and Small Bowel

Editors

KENNETH R. MCCURRY
ALI AL-KHAFAJI

CRITICAL CARE CLINICS

www.criticalcare.theclinics.com

Consulting Editor
JOHN A. KELLUM

January 2019 • Volume 35 • Number 1

ELSEVIER

1600 John F. Kennedy Boulevard • Suite 1800 • Philadelphia, Pennsylvania, 19103-2899

http://www.theclinics.com

CRITICAL CARE CLINICS Volume 35, Number 1
January 2019 ISSN 0749-0704, ISBN-13: 978-0-323-65463-0

Editor: Colleen Dietzler
Developmental Editor: Casey Potter

Critical Care Clinics (ISSN: 0749-0704) is published quarterly by Elsevier Inc., 360 Park Avenue South, New York, NY 10010-1710. Months of issue are January, April, July, and October. Business and Editorial Offices: 1600 John F. Kennedy Blvd., Suite 1800, Philadelphia, PA 19103-2899. Customer Service Office: 6277 Sea Harbor Drive, Orlando, FL 32887-4800. Periodicals postage paid at New York, NY and additional mailing offices. Subscription prices are $243.00 per year for US individuals, $650.00 per year for US institution, $100.00 per year for US students and residents, $285.00 per year for Canadian individuals, $815.00 per year for Canadian institutions, $315.00 per year for international individuals, $815.00 per year for international institutions and $150.00 per year for Canadian and foreign students/residents. To receive student/resident rate, orders must be accompanied by name of affiliated institution, date of term, and the signature of program/residency coordinator on institution letterhead. Orders will be billed at individual rate until proof of status is received. Foreign air speed delivery is included in all *Clinics* subscription prices. All prices are subject to change without notice. POSTMASTER: Send address changes to *Critical Care Clinics*, Elsevier Periodicals Customer Service, 11830 Westline Industrial Drive, St. Louis, MO 63146. **Customer Service: 1-800-654-2452 (US). From outside of the US, call 1-314-447-8871. Fax: 1-314-447-8029. E-mail: journalscustomerservice-usa@ elsevier.com (for print support) or journalsonlinesupport-usa@elsevier.com (for online support).**

Reprints. For copies of 100 or more of articles in this publication, please contact the Commercial Reprints Department, Elsevier Inc., 360 Park Avenue South, New York, NY 10010-1710. Tel.: 212-633-3874; Fax: 212-633-3820; E-mail: reprints@elsevier.com.

Critical Care Clinics is also published in Spanish by Editorial Inter-Medica, Junin 917, 1er A, 1113, Buenos Aires, Argentina.

Critical Care Clinics is covered in *MEDLINE/PubMed (Index Medicus)*, *EMBASE/Excerpta Medica*, *Current Concepts/ Clinical Medicine*, *ISI/BIOMED*, and *Chemical Abstracts*.

Contributors

CONSULTING EDITOR

JOHN A. KELLUM, MD, MCCM
Professor, Critical Care Medicine, Medicine, Bioengineering and Clinical & Translational Science, Director, Center for Critical Care Nephrology, Vice Chair for Research, Department of Critical Care Medicine, University of Pittsburgh School of Medicine, Pittsburgh, Pennsylvania, USA

EDITORS

KENNETH R. McCURRY, MD
Director, Lung and Heart-Lung Transplantation, Director, Respiratory ECMO Program, Co-Director, Organ Perfusion Center, Staff Cardiac Surgeon, Department of Thoracic and Cardiovascular Surgery, Heart and Vascular Institute and Lerner Research Institute, Cleveland Clinic, Cleveland, Ohio, USA

ALI AL-KHAFAJI, MD, MPH, FCCM
Professor, Department of Critical Care Medicine, Director, Transplant Intensive Care Unit, University of Pittsburgh School of Medicine, University of Pittsburgh Medical Center, The CRISMA (Clinical Research, Investigation and Systems Modeling of Acute Illness) Center, Pittsburgh, Pennsylvania, USA

AUTHORS

ALI AL-KHAFAJI, MD, MPH, FCCM
Professor, Department of Critical Care Medicine, Director, Transplant Intensive Care Unit, University of Pittsburgh School of Medicine, University of Pittsburgh Medical Center, The CRISMA (Clinical Research, Investigation and Systems Modeling of Acute Illness) Center, Pittsburgh, Pennsylvania, USA

MOHAMMED ALSAEED, MD
Clinical Fellow, Division of Infectious Diseases, Multi-Organ Transplant Program, Department of Medicine, University of Toronto, University Health Network, Toronto, Ontario, Canada; Senior Registrar, Division of Infectious Diseases, Department of Medicine, Prince Sultan Military Medical City, Riyadh, Saudi Arabia

BALARAM ANANDAMURTHY, MD
Clinical Assistant Professor of Anesthesiology, Department of Cardiothoracic Anesthesiology, Cleveland Clinic Lerner College of Medicine of Case Western Reserve University, Cleveland Clinic, Cleveland, Ohio, USA

JOSE F. BERNARDO, MD, MPH
Renal-Electrolyte Division, University of Pittsburgh Medical Center, Pittsburgh, Pennsylvania, USA

HANNELISA CALLISEN, PA-C
Physician Assistant, Department of Critical Care Medicine, Mayo Clinic, Phoenix, Arizona, USA

MANPREET S. CHADHA, MD, FACS
Surgical ICU Medical Director, Aurora Critical Care Service and Aurora Abdominal Transplant and Hepatobiliary Program, Advocate Aurora Health Care, Milwaukee, Wisconsin, USA

SUBHASIS CHATTERJEE, MD, FACS, FACC, FCCP
Assistant Professor of Surgery, Director, Thoracic Surgical ICU, ECMO Program, Michael E. DeBakey Department of Surgery, Division of Cardiothoracic Transplantation and Circulatory Support, Baylor College of Medicine, CHI Baylor St. Lukes, Neurosensory Center, Houston, Texas, USA

VICTOR DONG, MD
Division of Gastroenterology (Liver Unit), Department of Critical Care Medicine, University of Alberta, Edmonton, Canada

SARAH J. FROGGE, DNP, APNP
Director, Advanced Practice Clinicians (Hospital Based), Lead Nurse Practitioner, Aurora Critical Care Service, Advocate Aurora Health Care, Milwaukee, Wisconsin, USA

MARIYA GEUBE, MD
Assistant Professor of Anesthesiology, Department of Cardiothoracic Anesthesiology, Cleveland Clinic Lerner College of Medicine of Case Western Reserve University, Cleveland Clinic, Cleveland, Ohio, USA

ALEXIS GUENETTE, DO
Transplant Infectious Disease Fellow, Division of Infectious Disease, University Health Network, University of Toronto, Toronto, Ontario, Canada

ABHINAV HUMAR, MD, FRCSC
Department of Surgery, University of Pittsburgh Medical Center, Thomas E. Starzl Transplantation Institute, Pittsburgh, Pennsylvania, USA

SHAHID HUSAIN, MD, MS, FECMM, FRCP
Professor of Medicine, Staff Physician, Director of Transplant Infectious Disease, Division of Infectious Diseases, Multi-Organ Transplant Program, University Health Network, University of Toronto, Toronto, Ontario, Canada

DAVID J. KACZOROWSKI, MD
Assistant Professor, Department of Surgery, Division of Cardiac Surgery, University of Maryland School of Medicine, Baltimore, Maryland, USA

PREM A. KANDIAH, MD
Assistant Professor, Division of Neuro Critical Care & co appt. in 5E Surgical/Transplant Critical Care, Departments of Neurology and Neurosurgery, Emory University Hospital, Atlanta, Georgia, USA

CONSTANTINE J. KARVELLAS, MD, SM, FRCPC, FCCM
Associate Professor of Medicine, Division of Gastroenterology (Liver Unit), Department of Critical Care Medicine, University of Alberta, Edmonton, Canada

JOHN A. KELLUM, MD, MCCM
Professor, Critical Care Medicine, Medicine, Bioengineering and Clinical & Translational Science, Director, Center for Critical Care Nephrology, Vice Chair for Research, Department of Critical Care Medicine, University of Pittsburgh School of Medicine, Pittsburgh, Pennsylvania, USA

BEVERLEY KOK, MBBS
Division of Gastroenterology (Liver Unit), Department of Critical Care Medicine, University of Alberta, Edmonton, Canada

DAVID J. KRAMER, MD, FACP
System Medical Director, Aurora Critical Care Service, Advocate Aurora Health Care, Milwaukee, Wisconsin, USA; Clinical Professor of Medicine (Adjunct), University of Wisconsin-Madison School of Medicine and Public Health, Madison, Wisconsin, USA

KRISTINA LEMON, MD, FRCSC
Department of Surgery, University of Pittsburgh Medical Center, Thomas E. Starzl Transplantation Institute, Pittsburgh, Pennsylvania, USA

STACY LIBRICZ, PA-C
Physician Assistant, Department of Critical Care Medicine, Mayo Clinic, Phoenix, Arizona, USA

GABRIEL LOOR, MD
Associate Professor, Michael E. DeBakey Department of Surgery, Division of Cardiothoracic Transplantation and Circulatory Support, Texas Heart Institute, Surgical Director of Lung Transplantation, Co-Chief, Section of Adult Cardiac Surgery, Baylor St Luke's Medical Center, Baylor College of Medicine, Houston, Texas, USA

ALADDEIN MATTAR, MD
Assistant Professor, Michael E. DeBakey Department of Surgery, Division of Cardiothoracic Transplantation and Circulatory Support, Baylor College of Medicine, Houston, Texas, USA

KENNETH R. McCURRY, MD
Director, Lung and Heart-Lung Transplantation, Director, Respiratory ECMO Program, Co-Director, Organ Perfusion Center, Staff Cardiac Surgeon, Department of Thoracic and Cardiovascular Surgery, Heart and Vascular Institute and Lerner Research Institute, Cleveland Clinic, Cleveland, Ohio, USA

BHAVESH PATEL, MD
Consultant, Department of Critical Care Medicine, Mayo Clinic, Phoenix, Arizona, USA

CHETHAN M. PUTTARAJAPPA, MD, MS
Renal-Electrolyte Division, University of Pittsburgh Medical Center, Pittsburgh, Pennsylvania, USA

JOSEPH RABIN, MD, FACS
Assistant Professor, Department of Surgery, R Adams Cowley Shock Trauma Center, University of Maryland School of Medicine, Baltimore, Maryland, USA

AYAN SEN, MD, MSc, FCCM
Consultant, Department of Critical Care Medicine, Mayo Clinic, Phoenix, Arizona, USA

ERIC M. SIEGAL, MD
Intensivist, Aurora Critical Care Service, Advocate Aurora Health Care, Milwaukee, Wisconsin, USA; Clinical Professor of Medicine (Adjunct), University of Wisconsin-Madison School of Medicine and Public Health, Madison, Wisconsin, USA

RAM M. SUBRAMANIAN, MD
Associate Professor of Medicine and Surgery, Critical Care and Hepatology, Emory University, Atlanta, Georgia, USA

JEAN-PIERRE YARED, MD
Department of Cardiothoracic Anesthesiology, Cleveland Clinic, Cleveland, Ohio, USA

Contents

Section I: Heart & Lung

Kenneth R. McCurry

Lung transplantation, heart transplantation, and heart-lung transplantation are life-saving treatment options for patients with lung and/or cardiac failure. Evolution in these therapies over the past several decades has led to better outcomes with application to more patients. The complexity and severity of illness of patients in the pretransplant phase has steadily increased, making posttransplant intensive care unit management more difficult. Despite these factors and the pervasive complications of immunosuppressive therapy, outcomes continue to improve.

Aladdein Mattar, Subhasis Chatterjee, and Gabriel Loor

Lung transplantation is the gold standard for treating patients with end-stage lung disease. Such patients can present with severe illness on the waitlist and may deteriorate before a lung donor is available. Bridging strategies with extracorporeal membrane oxygenation (ECMO) are valuable for getting patients to transplant and provide a chance at survival. The current article describes the indications, contraindications, and techniques involved in bridging to lung transplantation with ECMO.

Mariya Geube, Balaram Anandamurthy, and Jean-Pierre Yared

Perioperative management of patients undergoing lung transplantation is one of the most complex in cardiothoracic surgery. Certain perioperative interventions, such as mechanical ventilation, fluid management and blood transfusions, use of extracorporeal mechanical support, and pain management, may have significant impact on the lung graft function and clinical outcome. This article provides a review of perioperative interventions that have been shown to impact the perioperative course after lung transplantation.

Joseph Rabin and David J. Kaczorowski

Management of the cardiac transplant recipient includes careful titration of inotropes and vasopressors. Recipient pulmonary hypertension and ventilatory status must be optimized to prevent allograft right ventricular failure.

Vasoplegia, coagulopathy, arrhythmias, and renal dysfunction also require careful management to achieve an optimal outcome. Primary graft dysfunction (PGD) can be an ominous problem after cardiac transplantation. Although mild degrees of PGD may be managed medically, mechanical circulatory support with extracorporeal membrane oxygenation or temporary ventricular assist devices may be required. Retransplantation may be necessary in some cases.

Chethan M. Puttarajappa, Jose F. Bernardo, and John A. Kellum

Renal complications are common following heart and/or lung transplantation and lead to increased morbidity and mortality. Renal dysfunction is also associated with increased mortality for patients on the transplant wait list. Dialysis dependence is a relative contraindication for heart or lung transplantation at most centers, and such patients are often listed for a simultaneous kidney transplant. Several factors contribute to the impaired renal function in patients undergoing heart and/or lung transplantation, including the interplay between cardiopulmonary and renal hemodynamics, complex perioperative issues, and exposure to nephrotoxic medications, mainly calcineurin inhibitors.

Mohammed Alsaeed and Shahid Husain

Infections in heart and lung transplant recipients are complex and heterogeneous. This article reviews the epidemiology, risk factors, specific clinical syndromes, and most frequent opportunistic infections in heart and/or lung transplant recipients that will be encountered in the intensive care unit and will provide a practical approach of empirical management.

Section II: Liver, Kidney, and Small Bowel

Ali Al-Khafaji

David J. Kramer, Eric M. Siegal, Sarah J. Frogge, and Manpreet S. Chadha

Perioperative management of the liver transplant recipient is a team effort that requires close collaboration between intensivist, surgeon, anesthesiologist, hepatologist, nephrologist, other specialists, and hospital staff before and after surgery. Transplant viability must be reassessed regularly and particularly with each donor organ. Regular discussions with patient and family facilitate realistic determinations of goals based on patient aspirations and clinical realities. Early attention to hemodynamics with optimal resuscitation and judicious vasopressor support, respiratory care designed to minimize iatrogenic injury, and early renal support is key. Preoperative and postoperative nutritional support and physical rehabilitation should remain a focus.

failure, arrhythmias leading to sudden death, hypertension, left ventricular hypertrophy, and allograft vasculopathy in heart transplantation. Neurologic complications include stroke, posterior reversible encephalopathy syndrome, infections, neuromuscular disease, seizure disorders, and neoplastic disease. Acute kidney injury occurs from immunosuppression with calcineurin inhibitors or as a result of graft failure after kidney transplantation. Gastrointestinal complications include infections, malignancy, mucosal ulceration, perforation, biliary tract disease, pancreatitis, and diverticular disease. Immunosuppression can predispose to infections and malignancy.

CRITICAL CARE CLINICS

SERIES OF RELATED INTEREST

Emergency Medicine Clinics
Available at: https://www.emed.theclinics.com/

THE CLINICS ARE AVAILABLE ONLINE!
Access your subscription at:
www.theclinics.com

Section I: Heart & Lung

Preface

Thoracic Transplantation

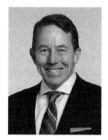

Kenneth R. McCurry, MD
Editor

Millions of people around the world suffer from chronic respiratory or chronic heart failure that could potentially benefit from lung or heart transplantation, respectively. While epidemiologically still small, the number of patients receiving thoracic transplants has grown immensely over the last 50 years. Through June 2016, more than 60,000 adult lung, 3900 adult heart-lung, and 135,000 adult heart transplants have been reported to the International Society for Heart and Lung Transplantation worldwide. In the United States alone, in 2016, more than 2300 adult lung transplants and more than 2700 adult heart transplants were performed. As a result, in this issue of *Critical Care Clinics*, we have focused on the pretransplant and posttransplant critical care of patients undergoing thoracic transplantation. While ventricular assist devices are commonly utilized to bridge patients to heart transplantation, as well as for destination therapy, we have not discussed this therapy in this issue as this was the focus of a recent issue of *Critical Care Clinics*.

In one of the articles, I provide some historical context to how we arrived at our current day approach to thoracic transplantation and outline some of the problems that are the focus of subsequent articles. As in many other areas of medicine, and surgery in particular, the pioneering physicians recognized need and demonstrated vision and (perhaps most importantly) extreme persistence in the face of failure to make these therapies the mainstream treatment options they are today. Of course, none of these therapies would be possible without the courage of those initial patients who put their lives in the hands of others for the hope of a longer and better life.

Dr Mattar, Dr Chatterjee, and Dr Loor (Texas Heart Institute at Baylor St. Luke's) highlight the rapidly evolving field of bridging to lung transplantation. While historically thought to be a poor option with poor outcomes, bridging to lung transplantation with an extracorporeal circuit has recently been increasingly utilized to support patients to lung transplantation. They provide an overview of published outcomes and very specific recommendations on selection of patients, type of extracorporeal circuit and management, and decision-making guidelines.

Dr Geube, Dr Anandamurthy, and Dr Yared (Cleveland Clinic) discuss the complex challenge of managing the lung transplant recipient in the perioperative period. They discuss the new grading system for perioperative allograft dysfunction (primary graft dysfunction), define modifiable and unmodifiable risk factors, and provide a pragmatic and comprehensive management strategy that has applicability to other forms of acute lung injury.

Dr Kaczorowski and Dr Rabin (University of Maryland) provide an up-to-date review of the issues involved and management strategies utilized in the perioperative phase following heart transplantation. They also describe the evolving field of mechanical circulatory support and options for medically refractory cardiac graft failure.

Dr Puttarajappa, Dr Bernado, and Dr Kellum (University of Pittsburgh) reflect on the common complication of renal insufficiency following thoracic transplantation. While outlining organ-specific differences, they describe the epidemiology, risk factors, pathogenesis, implications, and management and make very specific recommendations on ways to avoid further renal injury.

Dr Husain and Dr Alsaeed (University of Toronto) provide a comprehensive overview of infections seen in thoracic transplant recipients. Importantly, they provide information on the changing epidemiology of infections in this population and describe the sometimes atypical presentation that clinicians should be aware of.

I am extremely grateful to the authors for their contributions. Collectively, we hope that this issue is helpful and provides useful information to assist with patient care.

Kenneth R. McCurry, MD
Department of Thoracic and Cardiovascular Surgery
Heart and Vascular Institute and
Lerner Research Institute
Cleveland Clinic
9500 Euclid Avenue, J4-1
Cleveland, OH 44195, USA

E-mail address:
mccurrk@ccf.org

Brief Overview of Lung, Heart, and Heart-Lung Transplantation

Kenneth R. McCurry, MD

KEYWORDS

- Lung transplantation • Heart transplantation • End-stage lung disease
- End-stage heart disease

KEY POINTS

- Lung transplantation and heart transplantation are valuable options for patients with lung or cardiac failure.
- Heart-lung transplantation is a valuable treatment option for patients with lung and heart failure but has been declining in frequency.
- Lung transplant and heart transplant candidates are becoming increasingly more ill and complex, making posttransplant management more difficult.
- Outcomes following lung transplantation and heart transplantation are improving.

INTRODUCTION

Lung, heart-lung, and heart transplantation have evolved over the past several decades to become a common treatment option for patients with advanced pulmonary and cardiac disease. According to the most recent report of the International Society for Heart and Lung Transplantation (ISHLT), through June 2016, more than 60,000 adult lung, 3900 adult heart-lung, and 135,000 adult heart transplants have been reported to the ISHLT Registry worldwide.[1,2] In 2016, 140 centers reported lung transplant activity and 285 centers reported heart transplant activity to the ISHLT Registry, combining for more than 8000 thoracic transplants.[1,2] Based on this volume, critical care physicians are increasingly likely to be involved in the care of these patients. As such, the following articles in this issue outline the common issues critical care physicians face when managing these patients and present management and therapeutic strategies. Where appropriate, such as in discussion of renal complications and infectious complications, a single article is devoted to both lung transplant recipients and

Disclosure Statement: No disclosures.
Department of Cardiothoracic Surgery, Heart and Vascular Institute, Cleveland Clinic, 9500 Euclid Avenue, J4-1, Cleveland, OH 44195, USA
E-mail address: mccurrk@ccf.org

Crit Care Clin 35 (2019) 1–9
https://doi.org/10.1016/j.ccc.2018.08.005
0749-0704/19/© 2018 Elsevier Inc. All rights reserved.

criticalcare.theclinics.com

heart transplant recipients. Where management strategies diverge significantly, such as in bridging to transplant and perioperative fluid and inotropic management, separate articles are devoted to each organ. This article provides an overview discussing historical aspects and current trends in transplantation of each organ while outlining common areas of management.

HISTORICAL ASPECTS OF DEVELOPMENT OF CARDIOTHORACIC TRANSPLANTATION AND CURRENT TRENDS
Lung and Heart-Lung Transplantation

Decades of experimental work by many investigators preceded the first clinical attempts at lung and heart-lung transplantation. The main hurdles encountered were related to problems with bronchial anastomotic healing, the high immunogenicity of the lung (and the resultant need for high-level immunosuppression), and the risk of pulmonary infection. The first human lung transplant (a single lung) was performed by Dr James Hardy and colleagues[3] at the University of Mississippi in June 1963. Although the surgical procedure was initially successful, the patient survived only 18 days, succumbing to renal failure and infection. In August 1968, Dr Denton Cooley performed the first human heart-lung transplant on a 2-month-old infant, with death occurring 14 hours after the transplant.[4] Over the next 15 or so years, approximately 38 to 40 lung or heart-lung transplants were performed, with only 9 patients living more than 2 weeks and only 1 patient discharged from the hospital.[5] There were no long-term survivors, as the vast majority of patients died from the sequalae of disruption of the bronchial anastomosis during the first few weeks following the transplant. As a result, there was limited interest in pursuing clinical lung transplantation during the decade of the 1970s.

In the late 1970s to early 1980s, the Toronto Lung Transplant program embarked on further animal experimental investigation to better understand the cause of bronchial disruption and develop strategies and surgical techniques to allow successful clinical transplantation. Identifying bronchial ischemia in concert with diminished healing associated with the high doses of steroids (used for immunosuppression) as the primary cause of bronchial disruption allowed development of alternative strategies. The addition of cyclosporine, then newly introduced, to the immunosuppressive regimen with lowering of steroids as well as development of a technique to wrap the bronchial anastomosis with an omental pedicle, allowed successful bronchial healing.[6,7] These strategies along with more conservative selection of recipients (in contrast to the very ill patients in the early era) led to clinical success.

The first successful heart-lung transplant with long-term survival was performed by Dr Bruce Reitz and team[8] at Stanford University in March 1981 on a patient with primary pulmonary hypertension (PPH). The Toronto Group chose idiopathic pulmonary fibrosis (IPF) as the disease for which they would first offer single lung transplantation in the new era and, in November 1983, successfully performed a right single lung transplant on a patient with IPF.[9] The patient survived 7 years. These successes led to further innovations and expansion of the therapy. Single lung transplantation was offered to patients with emphysema and subsequently to patients with PPH. Techniques were also developed to perform double lung transplantation. Initially patients requiring double lung transplantation (such as patients with suppurative lung disease, including cystic fibrosis [CF]) were treated with heart-lung transplantation with their (normal) heart transplanted into a patient in need of heart transplantation (the domino procedure). With development of en bloc double lung transplantation (using a tracheal anastomosis) and later bilateral sequential lung transplantation (with mainstem bronchial anastomoses), patients requiring double lung transplantation could be effectively treated with good outcomes. Bilateral sequential lung transplantation (with or without the intraoperative use of mechanical circulatory support) remains the dominant technique for double lung transplantation today.

The use of heart-lung transplantation for suppurative lung disease and other indications led to a dramatic rise in these procedures in the 1980s. With more restrictive indications for heart-lung transplantation (generally reserved for those patients who cannot be treated with heart-only or lung-only transplantation due to severe pulmonary hypertension [primary or secondary] with right ventricular failure, or anatomic issues), the frequency of this procedure has declined. At its maximum, worldwide yearly volume of heart-lung transplants reached 225 in 1989 and has steadily declined to 38 reported in 2015.[1] **Fig. 1** shows the worldwide annual volume of adult and pediatric heart-lung transplants reported to the ISHLT.

Lung transplant volume also grew rapidly in the 1980s and has seen continued growth since then. Over the 2 decades spanning 1995 to 2015, worldwide yearly lung transplant volume increased from approximately 1300 to more than 4000[1] (**Fig. 2**). Although the worldwide yearly volume of lung transplants has remained at approximately 4000 for the past 3 years, in 2016, US lung transplant volume alone reached more than 2300, an all-time high.[10] The likely reasons for growth over the past 2 decades are many and include greater use of brain-dead donor lungs through utilization of organs previously considered "marginal" and the use of donation after cardiac death (DCD) donors. In the United States, in 2016, the transplant rate increased to its highest rate at 191.9 transplants per 100 waitlist years, while waitlist mortality declined slightly to 15.1 deaths per 100 waitlist years. Waitlist mortalities continue worldwide as well due to the limited availability of acceptable donor lungs for transplantation. It is hoped that greater use of lungs from DCD donors[11,12] as well as greater application of ex vivo lung perfusion technology for evaluation and

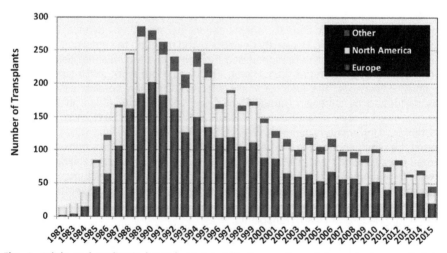

Fig. 1. Adult and pediatric heart-lung transplants: number of transplants reported by location and year. This figure includes only the heart-lung transplants that are reported to the ISHLT Transplant Registry. As such, this should not be construed as evidence that the number of heart-lung transplants worldwide has declined in recent years. (*From* Lund LH, Khush KK, Cherikh WS, et al. The Registry of the International Society for Heart and Lung Transplantation: thirty-fourth adult heart transplantation report—2017; focus theme: allograft ischemic time. J Heart Lung Transplant 2017;36(10):1037–46; with permission.)

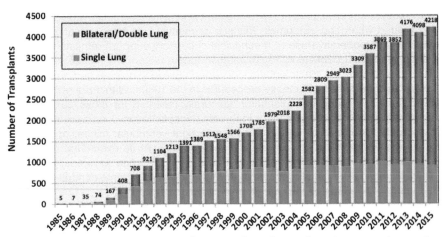

Fig. 2. Adult and pediatric lung transplants: number of transplants by year and procedure type. This figure includes only the lung transplants that are reported to the ISHLT Transplant Registry. As such, this should not be construed as representing changes in the number of lung transplants performed worldwide. (*Data from* Refs.[1,28,30,31])

reconditioning of initially unsuitable lungs for transplant[13,14] will allow continued growth and application of this therapy.

Heart Transplantation

Although Carrel and Guthrie,[15] in 1905, demonstrated the ability of the heart to tolerate and function after transplantation, attempts at preclinical and clinical orthotopic heart transplantation had to await development of cardiopulmonary bypass technology in the 1950s. Following this, many groups worked to develop and refine operative techniques to allow orthotopic cardiac transplantation. In a significant advance, Lower and Shumway[16,17] at Stanford University developed and reported the atrial cuff technique of surgical implantation and demonstrated the ability of a transplanted heart to support recipient dogs for more than 1 year. Following more work at Stanford as well as other universities, the first surgically successful human cardiac allotransplant was performed by Christian Barnard[18] in Cape Town, South Africa, in December 1967, followed closely by another successful cardiac transplant by Norman Shumway at Stanford University in January 1968.[19] Subsequently, several cardiac surgeons around the world engaged in cardiac transplantation with numerous transplants performed between 1967 and 1971. Much as with lung and heart-lung transplantation, however, outcomes with these early transplants were poor, with most patients succumbing to infection or rejection within months following transplantation. These outcomes were portrayed very publicly in a 1971 *Life Magazine* cover with the title "The Tragic Record of Heart Transplants."[20]

With many teams abandoning heart transplantation, Norman Shumway and Richard Lower persisted, and with others developed techniques for endomyocardial biopsy and its interpretation, strategies to treat acute rejection, and refined recipient selection. This significantly improved outcomes following cardiac transplantation and ushered in the era of cardiac transplantation. Cardiac transplantation volume began to grow in the early 1980s increasing rapidly through the latter half of the decade to a worldwide peak of nearly 5000 pediatric and adult heart transplants in 1993.[2] Following a decline to nearly 4000 per year in 2004, volume has steadily risen to an all-time high of 5074 heart transplants in 2015 (including 4388 adult heart transplants)[2] (**Fig. 3**). In 2016, in the US alone, 3209 pediatric and adult heart transplants (2764 adult) were performed.[21] This modest increase in volume over the past 2 decades falls far short of the need, however. Indeed, in the United States, the number of patients actively awaiting heart transplantation has continued to grow and, from 2005 to 2016, heart transplant rates declined from 129 per 100 waitlist years to 93.1 per 100 waitlist years.[21] The ongoing imbalance between supply of donor hearts and demand has continued to push the boundaries of marginal donor hearts, including the use of extracorporeal machine perfusion,[22] utilization of hearts from DCD donors,[23] and utilization of hearts from donors infected with hepatitis C (with posttransplant treatment with direct-acting antiviral agents).[24] The unmet need has also continued to drive the development of mechanical circulatory support (MCS) devices for destination therapy that began in the 1950s.[25] MCS devices are used both for destination therapy and as bridge to transplant and will be the subject of a future edition of *Critical Care Clinics*.

RECIPIENT SELECTION AND OUTCOMES
Lung and Heart-Lung Transplantation

The most common diagnosis for which lung transplantation was performed worldwide from 1995 to 2016 was chronic obstructive pulmonary disease (COPD) (36%) followed by interstitial lung disease (with various forms of pulmonary fibrosis) (30%), bronchiectasis (most commonly CF) (18%), various forms of pulmonary arterial hypertension (PAH) (4%) and various other lung diseases such as sarcoidosis and chronic rejection.[1] In the United States, COPD was the most common diagnosis of lung transplant recipients until following implementation of the lung allocation score (LAS) in 2005. The LAS prioritizes patients awaiting lung transplantation by net-transplant benefit based on predicted 1-year survival without lung transplantation and predicted 1-year post-transplant survival (weighted 2:1).[26] Implementation of the LAS system resulted in a shift in patients receiving transplants as well as a decline in waitlist mortality.[10] In 2016, 57% of US lung transplants were performed in patients with pulmonary fibrosis followed by COPD (27%) and CF (12%).[10]

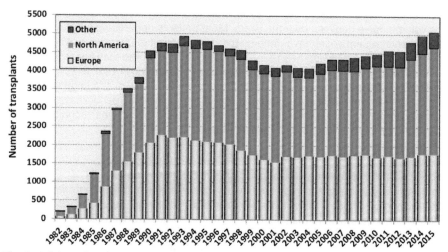

Fig. 3. Adult and pediatric heart transplants: number of transplants by year and location. This figure includes only the heart transplants that are reported to the ISHLT Transplant Registry. As such, the presented data may not mirror the changes in the number of heart transplants performed worldwide. (*Data from* Refs.[1,28,30,31])

Following the success of lung transplantation in the 1980s to 1990s, patient selection has evolved and broadened. In the United States and worldwide, patients who once would have been considered unacceptable candidates for lung transplantation are now being placed on the waitlist. Patients listed for lung transplant are increasingly more ill, have more comorbidities, and are older. In the United States, in 2016, 29.5% of lung transplants were performed in recipients 65 years or older, continuing an upward trend. Additionally, the number of patients being bridged to transplant with extracorporeal membrane oxygenation (ECMO) (either alone or with mechanical ventilation) increased from 2.3% of transplants in 2011 to 5.8% in 2016.[10] These factors, in conjunction with more comorbidities, significantly increase the complexity of posttransplant care.

Survival following lung transplantation has steadily improved over the past 3 decades, despite recent trends toward sicker recipients, and have largely been attributed to better surgical and perioperative care, changes in immunosuppression, and other factors. Worldwide, patients receiving lung transplants from 1990 to 1998 had a median survival of 4.2 years compared with 6.1 years for those transplanted from 1999 to 2008.[1] In the United States, for recipients transplanted from 2009 to 2011, posttransplant survival was 93.3% at 3 months, 85.0% at 1 year, 68.2% at 3 years, and 55% at 5 years.[10] One-year and 3-year survival rates continued a trend toward improvement, whereas 5-year survival rates remained flat (perhaps due to the increasing age of recipients or due to our inability to affect the most common cause of late death: chronic rejection). Posttransplant survival long-term is significantly associated with recipient diagnosis, with patients with CF having the best survival and patients with pulmonary fibrosis the worst.[1,10] Recipients at the extremes of age as well as those who are the most ill (as represented by higher LAS score) have lower survival than other groups.[1,10] In the first 3 years following transplantation, infection is the most common cause of death. After 3 years from transplantation, chronic lung allograft dysfunction (CLAD) is the most common cause of death and is the largest barrier to long-term success.[1,10] CLAD develops in 50% of lung recipients within 5 years and 76% of recipients within 10 years of transplant and is responsible for 50% of deaths in the first 10 years following transplant.[1,27]

As previously discussed, the indications for heart-lung transplantation, and hence the volume, have declined over the years. Most patients undergoing heart-lung transplantation in recent years have done so for various forms of pulmonary hypertension. The early survival following heart-lung transplantation is worse than lung transplantation, with a median survival of 3.3 years for those transplanted in 1982 to 2015. The risk of death is greatest early following heart-lung transplant (likely due to surgical risk and perioperative complications), whereas those who survive this period have a greater chance of long-term survival than lung transplant recipients (1-year conditional median survival of 10.3 vs approximately 8.1 years).[1]

Heart Transplantation

Ischemic cardiomyopathy (ICM) and nonischemic cardiomyopathy (NICM) are the predominant diagnoses for the vast majority of recipients of heart transplants worldwide.[2] The proportion of heart transplants performed for NICM has been increasing worldwide and represents more than 50% of recipients.[2,28] In the United States, the proportion of heart transplant candidates with ICM declined from 41.4% in 2005 to 32% in 2016, whereas the proportion of candidates with NICM rose from 45.5% to 58.1% over the same period.[21]

As with lung transplantation, heart transplant recipients are increasingly older and more complex. Worldwide, the median age of heart transplant recipients has increased to 55 with an increasing proportion of patients older than 60 and even older than 70.[2] In the United States, the proportion of heart recipients older than 65 years increased from 9.7% in 2005 to 17.4% in 2016.[21] The proportion of transplant recipients bridged with MCS has also increased significantly since 2007, with slightly more than 50% of recipients bridged worldwide.[2] The growing proportion of combined organ transplants (heart-kidney and heart-liver) has also increased recipient complexity and risk and now represents 4% of all heart transplants worldwide.[2]

Survival following heart transplantation is better than that following lung transplantation and has continued to improve. Worldwide, median survival for those recipients transplanted from 1982 to 1991 was 8.6 years, from 1992 to 2001 it was 10.5 years, and from 2002 to 2008 median survival was 12.2 years.[2] In the United States, for recipients transplanted from 2009 to 2011, posttransplant survival was 90.1% at 1 year, 83.5% at 3 years, and 78.3% at 5 years.[21] As with lung transplantation, long-term survival is lower in recipients older than 65.[2,21] In recent years (2005-June 2015), posttransplant survival is not negatively impacted by pretransplant use of ventricular assist devices but is negatively affected by pretransplant use of ECMO.[2]

IMMUNOSUPPRESSION

The goal of immunosuppression is to protect the graft from immune-mediated injury without causing short-term or long-term toxicities. In practice, that is impossible to achieve (short of achieving tolerance), and managing immunosuppression reduces to trying to achieve a balance between those 2 undesirable outcomes. Modern immunosuppressive regimens involve the use of a calcineurin inhibitor (tacrolimus or cyclosporine), an antimetabolite (most commonly mycophenolic acid), and steroids for the "maintenance phase."[29] Typically, these drugs are started at higher levels in the immediate perioperative period and weaned over time based on the patient's course, results of graft biopsies, and adverse effects. Adverse effects and complications of these drugs are common and include renal dysfunction, hypertension, glucose intolerance, infection, and malignancy. Indeed, infection is the most common cause of death in both lung and heart transplant recipients in the first few years following transplantation. Infection and renal dysfunction are discussed in subsequent articles in this issue. In some programs, recipients are routinely treated with induction therapy around the time of transplantation, which involves administration of either polyclonal (anti-thymocyte globulin) or monoclonal (interleukin-2 receptor antagonists or alemtuzumab) antibodies that either deplete graft reactive immune cells or reversibly inhibit receptors on those cells. In other programs, induction therapy is used as a strategy to avoid early (first few days to a week) exposure to calcineurin inhibitors in those patients who have suffered renal injury or who are at high risk of renal dysfunction.[29]

Lungs are more immunogenic than hearts and generally require more immunosuppression. Worldwide, more than 70% of lung transplant recipients receive some form of induction therapy around the time of transplantation compared with slightly more than 50% of heart transplant recipients.[1,2] Tacrolimus has superseded cyclosporine as the most commonly used calcineurin inhibitor and is used in 93% of lung and heart recipients worldwide.[1,2,21]

SUMMARY

Lung transplantation and heart transplantation have evolved over the past several decades to become common therapies for patients with advanced lung or heart failure. Heart-lung transplantation, although still a viable therapy, has diminished in frequency due to the ability to manage most patients with lung-only or heart-only therapy.

Lung transplant and heart transplant candidates are increasingly older and more ill, and have a greater incidence of requiring mechanical support while awaiting transplantation. All of these factors, coupled with the pervasive complications of immunosuppression, make the intensive care unit management of these patients increasing complex and difficult. Strategies to manage these issues will be discussed in subsequent articles in this issue.

REFERENCES

1. Chambers DC, Yusen RD, Cherikh WS, et al. The Registry of the International Society for Heart and Lung Transplantation: thirty-fourth adult lung and heart-lung transplantation report—2017; focus theme: allograft ischemic time. J Heart Lung Transplant 2017;36(10):1047–59.
2. Lund LH, Khush KK, Cherikh WS, et al. The Registry of the International Society for Heart and Lung Transplantation: thirty-fourth adult heart transplantation report—2017; focus theme: allograft ischemic time. J Heart Lung Transplant 2017;36(10):1037–46.
3. Hardy JD, Webb JR, Dalton ML, et al. Lung homotransplantation in man. JAMA 1963;186:1865–74.
4. Cooley DA, Bloodwell RD, Hallman GL, et al. Organ transplantation for advanced cardiopulmonary disease. Ann Thorac Surg 1969;8:30–46.
5. Venuta F, Van Raemdonck D. History of lung transplantation. J Thorac Dis 2017; 9(12):5458–71.
6. Saunders NR, Egan TM, Chamberlain D, et al. Cyclosporine and bronchial healing in canine lung transplantation. J Thorac Cardiovasc Surg 1984;88:993–9.
7. Morgan E, Lima O, Goldberg M, et al. Successful revascularization of totally ischemic bronchial autografts in dogs using omental pedicle flaps. J Thorac Cardiovasc Surg 1982;84:204–10.
8. Reitz BA, Pennock JL, Shumway NE. Simplified operative method for heart and lung transplantation. J Surg Res 1981;31:1–5.
9. Toronto Lung Transplant Group. Unilateral lung transplantation for pulmonary fibrosis. N Engl J Med 1986;314:1140–5.
10. Valapour M, Lehr CJ, Skeans MA, et al. OPTN/SRTR 2016 annual data report: lung. Am J Transplant 2018;18(Suppl 1):363–433.
11. Cypel M, Levvey B, Van Raemdonck D, et al. International Society for Heart and Lung Transplantation donation after circulatory death registry report. J Heart Lung Transplant 2015;34:1278–82.
12. Valenza F, Citerio G, Palleschi A, et al. Successful transplantation of lungs from an uncontrolled donor after circulatory death preserved in situ by alveolar recruitment maneuvers and assessed by ex vivo lung perfusion. Am J Transplant 2016;16:1312–8.
13. Steen S, Liao Q, Wierup PN, et al. Transplantation of lungs from non-heart-beating donors after functional assessment ex vivo. Ann Thorac Surg 2003;76:244–52.
14. Cypel M, Keshavjee S. Extending the donor pool: rehabilitation of poor organs. Thorac Surg Clin 2015;25:27–33.
15. Carrel A, Guthrie C. The transplantation of veins and organs. Am J Med 1905;10: 1105.
16. Lower RR, Shumway NE. Studies on orthotopic transplantation of the canine heart. Surg Forum 1960;11:18–20.
17. Lower RR, Stofer RC, Shumway NE. Homovital transplantation of the heart. J Thorac Cardiovasc Surg 1961;41:196–204.

18. Barnard CN. The operation. A human cardiac transplant: an interim report of a successful operation performed at Groote Schuur Hospital, Capetown. S Afr Med J 1967;41:1271–4.
19. Shumway NE, Dong E, Stinson EB. Surgical aspects of cardiac transplantation in man. Bull NY Acad Med 1969;45:387–93.
20. Thompson T. The tragic record of heart transplants. The year they changed hearts. Life Magazine; 1971. p. 56–70.
21. Colvin M, Smith JM, Hadley N, et al. OPTN/SRTR 2016 annual data report: heart. Am J Transplant 2018;18(Suppl 1):291–362.
22. Macdonald PS, Chew HC, Connellan M, et al. Extracorporeal heart perfusion before heart transplantation: the heart in a box. Curr Opin Organ Transplant 2016;21(3):366–442.
23. Page A, Messer S, Large SR. Heart transplantation from donation after circulatory determined death. Ann Cardiothorac Surg 2018;7(1):75–81.
24. Moayadi Y, Gulamhusein AF, Ross HJ, et al. Accepting hepatitis C virus-infected donor hearts for transplantation: multistep consent, unrealized opportunity, and the Stanford experience. Clin Transplant 2018;32(7):e13308.
25. Enciso JS. Mechanical circulatory support: current status and future directions. Prog Cardiovasc Dis 2016;58:444–54.
26. Egan TM, Murray S, Bustami RT, et al. Development of the new lung allocation system in the United States. Am J Transplant 2006;6:1212–27.
27. Yusen RD, Christie JD, Edwards LB, et al. The Registry of the International Society for Heart and Lung Transplantation: thirtieth adult lung and heart-lung transplant report—2013; focus theme: age. J Heart Lung Transplant 2013;32(10): 965–78.
28. Lund LH, Edwards LB, Dipchand AI, et al. The Registry of the International Society for Heart and Lung Transplantation: thirty-third adult heart transplantation report—2016; focus theme: primary diagnostic indications for transplant. J Heart Lung Transplant 2016;35:1158–69.
29. Benvenuto LJ, Anderson MR, Arcasoy SM. New frontiers in immunosuppression. J Thorac Dis 2018;10(5):3141–55.
30. Rossano JW, Cherikh WS, Chambers DC, et al. The Registry of the International Society for Heart and Lung Transplantation: thirty-fourth adult heart transplantation report—2017; focus theme: allograft ischemic time. J Heart Lung Transplant 2017;36(10):1060–9.
31. Goldfarb SB, Levvey BJ, Cherikh WS, et al. The Registry of the International Society for Heart and Lung Transplantation: thirty-fourth adult heart transplantation report—2017; focus theme: allograft ischemic time. J Heart Lung Transplant 2017;36(10):1070–9.

Bridging to Lung Transplantation

Aladdein Mattar, MD[a], Subhasis Chatterjee, MD[b], Gabriel Loor, MD[c],*

KEYWORDS

- End-stage lung disease • ECMO • Lung transplant • Bridging

KEY POINTS

- Extracorporeal membrane oxygenation is a valuable option for bridging critically ill patients to lung transplantation.
- ECMO bridging is generally associated with a greater perioperative risk and poorer long-term survival.
- ECMO bridging should be performed selectively for patients who are likely to survive to transplant and who are likely to survive after transplant with a good quality of life.
- Family and multidisciplinary team discussions are critical to the care of patients requiring ECMO.

INTRODUCTION

End-stage lung disease (ESLD) is a terminal disease with poor prognosis and limited treatment options. Affecting more than 25 million Americans, ESLD is the third leading cause of death in the United States and is responsible for more than 150,000 deaths annually. Since the first successful long-term lung transplantation by Cooper and colleagues[1] (Toronto) in 1983, lung transplantation has become the standard of care for selected patients with ESLD of various nonmalignant causes. More than 30,000 lung transplants have been performed worldwide. About 2000 lung transplants are

Disclosure Statement: Dr G. Loor receives funding support for the development of an extracorporeal life support in lung transplant database from Maquet and grant support for involvement in ex vivo lung perfusion trials from Transmedics.
[a] Michael E. DeBakey Department of Surgery, Division of Cardiothoracic Transplantation and Circulatory Support, Baylor College of Medicine, One Baylor Plaza, 11C33, Houston, TX 77030, USA; [b] Thoracic Surgical ICU, ECMO Program, Michael E. DeBakey Department of Surgery, Division of Cardiothoracic Transplantation and Circulatory Support, Baylor College of Medicine, CHI Baylor St. Lukes, Neurosensory Center, Mailstop BCM 390, Suite NC100T, 6501 Fannin Street, Houston, TX 77030, USA; [c] Michael E. DeBakey Department of Surgery, Division of Cardiothoracic Transplantation and Circulatory Support, Texas Heart Institute, Baylor St Luke's Medical Center, Baylor College of Medicine, 6770 Bertner Avenue, Suite C-355K, Houston, TX 77030, USA
* Corresponding author.
E-mail address: Gabriel.loor@bcm.edu

Crit Care Clin 35 (2019) 11–25
https://doi.org/10.1016/j.ccc.2018.08.006
0749-0704/19/© 2018 Elsevier Inc. All rights reserved.

performed annually in the United States; lung transplants are increasing with the highest rate to date in 2016, at 191.9 per 100 waitlist years.[2] Although most lung transplants are performed in patients with slowly progressive pulmonary disease, an increasing number requires bridging strategies due to severe acute or chronic disease.

SUMMARY/DISCUSSION
Lung Transplant: Historical

The first human lung transplant was performed on June 11, 1963, at the University of Mississippi by Hardy and colleagues. Between 1963 and 1978, 38 lung or heart and lung transplants were performed, with only 2 patients surviving beyond 2 months and none leaving the hospital. Interest in lung transplantation waned until the development of cyclosporine helped usher in a new era in transplantation. On November 7, 1983, Cooper and the University of Toronto group performed the first successful single lung transplant with survival beyond a year in a patient with pulmonary fibrosis. Many centers worldwide followed the path of the Toronto group and reported similar good outcomes in patients with pulmonary fibrosis.[1,3] Since then, more than 30,000 lung transplants have been performed worldwide.

The implementation of the lung allocation scoring (LAS) system in the United States in 2005 decreased the overall time spent on the waiting list for patients with the most urgent need for a transplant. Although implementing the LAS helped prioritize patients by urgency, many candidates died of their lung disease before a suitable organ was available. Furthermore, the number of candidates dying on the waitlist was highest in 2014 to 2015 with a mortality rate of 16.5 per 100 compared with 8.6 deaths per 100 in 2004 to 2005. This increase was likely due to the increasingly sick candidate pool.[2] Current waitlist mortality varies depending on the disease process but can range from 20% to 40% within 1 to 2 years on the list.[4]

As patients' clinical conditions deteriorate, they often require mechanical ventilation. In most cases, these patients face a near certain death without a transplant. While waiting for one, they become deconditioned and prone to develop respiratory infections and other complications.

Extracorporeal Membrane Oxygenation

Extracorporeal membrane oxygenation (ECMO) is a modality used to bridge patients to lung transplantation by providing oxygenation and removal of carbon dioxide (CO_2) with an external circuit. ECMO reduces the requirement for ventilation and can stabilize and improve end-organ perfusion. Because the early results were poor, ECMO use was limited, and many centers considered pretransplant ECMO a contraindication for lung transplantation.[5,6] However, recent advancements in the development of polymethylpentene oxygenators and newer portable, more durable circuits have increased the use of ECMO as a bridge to transplant (BTT) in select patients.[7,8]

Webb and Howard described the first use of a mechanical pump-oxygenator to support heart-lung transplantation in 1957.[9,10] In 1977, Vieth and colleagues[11] reported the first successful case of veno-arterial (VA) ECMO as a BTT in posttraumatic respiratory failure. The patient was successfully weaned from ECMO after the transplant. However, he died 10 days posttransplant of a combination of sepsis, bronchial leak, and organ size mismatch. In 1982, ECMO was used as a bridge to lung transplantation in a patient with severe paraquat poisoning. The patient was successfully weaned from VA ECMO after transplant, but ECMO was reinstituted because the paraquat poisoning recurred. The patient remained on ECMO for an additional

19 days until a second lung transplant was performed. This report was the first on the use of ECMO as a bridge to redo lung transplant. However, the patient died 93 days after the initial transplant of complications of a tracheal-innominate artery fistula.[12]

Because of the initial poor outcomes of lung transplants bridged from ECMO in the 1970s and 1980s, this practice was largely abandoned. The pretransplant use of ECMO was assumed to be associated with an unacceptably high risk for postoperative complications including infections and dehiscence. Furthermore, the results of a large multicenter, prospective, randomized trial in1979 showed no survival benefit from ECMO compared with mechanical ventilation in a non–lung transplant cohort of patients with acute respiratory failure; these findings reduced enthusiasm for this intervention.[13]

ECMO as a BTT in a patient with primary graft dysfunction was described by Jurmann and his group in 1991.[14] ECMO use gradually increased over the following 2 decades. During this period, significant improvements were made in ECMO-related technologies. This was highlighted in 2009 during the worldwide H1N1 influenza pandemic when ECMO was used successfully in a large number of patients with respiratory failure across North America, Europe, and Australia.[15] At the same time, the Conventional Ventilation or ECMO for Severe Adult Respiratory Failure (CESAR) trial in the United Kingdom demonstrated a significant survival benefit in patients with severe acute respiratory distress syndrome who were treated with ECMO as compared with those treated with conventional medical management.[16]

Impact of the Lung Allocation Score System on Bridging Strategies

The lung allocation score (LAS) is used to prioritize waiting list candidates based on a combination of waitlist urgency and posttransplant survival. Before May 2005, organ allocation was determined by length of time on the waiting list and not by medical necessity or posttransplant outcome. This approach provided an incentive for earlier listing of candidates because total time on the list led to higher prioritization. On May 4, 2005, the system for allocation of deceased donor lungs for transplant in the United States changed from allocation based on waiting time to allocation based on the LAS. The 2005 implementation of the LAS caused a significant shift for patients in need of lung transplantation. Previously, patients on ECMO may have waited for a long time before an organ became available, and the outcome always carried the risk of complications such as muscular deconditioning, thromboembolism, bleeding, and malnutrition. These factors contributed to the poor outcomes for patients on ECMO before and after lung transplantation. However, the LAS system allocates a higher urgency for patients on ECMO, which increases the chance of successfully identifying a donor organ.

Recipient Condition at Time of Transplant

The process of placing a patient on the lung transplant list begins when the lung disease approaches a critical stage. Many factors are considered including short-term prognosis, the functional status, expected clinical course, social support, quality of life, blood type, and the potential risks and benefits of transplantation. In 2015, the median wait time was 3.4 months. Despite the highest recorded transplant rate of 157 per 100 waitlist years, waitlist mortality continued a decade-long increase to a high of 16.5 deaths per 100 waitlist years.

Mason and colleagues[17] analyzed the United Network for Organ Sharing (UNOS) data from 1987 to 2008 and found that preoperative ECMO was used in only 51 patients (0.3%) in the United States. However, more recently the OPTN/SRTR (Organ Procurement and Transplantation Network/Scientific Registry of Transplant

Recipients) report from 2015 showed a substantial increase in the use of ECMO support from 2010 to 2015 (**Table 1**).[18]

Goals of Extracorporeal Membrane Oxygenation

Carefully selecting patients for bridging to lung transplant with ECMO is critical. Patient selection, cannulation approach, type of support, and appropriate adherence to inclusion and exclusion criteria are important principles when deciding on bridging strategies. The use of ECMO as a BTT for decompensating transplant candidates places patients at risk of ECMO-related complications such as bleeding and stroke. Because donor lungs are scarce, consideration should be given not just to the risk of a patient dying without transplantation but also to the achievement of good quality of life and long-term survival.

The primary goal of ECMO as a BTT is optimizing gas exchange and end-organ perfusion. Other goals include freedom from positive-pressure ventilation, mobilization, improvement of nutritional status, and psychosocial support for the patient. The threshold should be low for using tracheostomies and nasoenteric feeding tubes to facilitate weaning from the ventilator and ensuring appropriate nutritional support. Realistic expectations and care goals should be discussed with the patient and family. Optimal ECMO management includes lung-protective mechanical ventilation (4–6 mL/kg of predicted body weight, avoidance of elevated airway pressures, and positive end-expiratory pressure). Ideally, neuromuscular blockade and continuous deep sedation should be reduced or avoided for ECMO patients.

Decision to Initiate Extracorporeal Membrane Oxygenation

Indications

The main indication for ECMO as a bridge to lung transplantation is rapid pulmonary deterioration in a potential candidate with refractory hypercapnia and/or hypoxia despite optimal medical management. ECMO is also used in pretransplant patients with severe pulmonary hypertension and hemodynamic collapse. The decision to place patients on ECMO is made by a multidisciplinary team comprising lung transplant surgeons, surgical ECMO specialists, critical care intensivists, and transplant

Table 1
Recipient condition at the time of transplant

	2010		2015	
Medical condition				
Hospitalized in ICU	150	8.4%	276	13.0%
Hospitalized not in ICU	148	8.3%	242	11.8%
Not hospitalized	1487	83.3%	1530	74.5%
Hospitalization unknown	0	0.0%	16	0.8%
Vent/ECMO at transplant				
Vent + ECMO	22	1.2%	63	3.1%
Vent only	130	7.3%	64	3.1%
ECMO only	7	0.4%	33	1.6%
Neither	1626	91.1%	1895	92.2%

Abbreviation: ICU, intensive care unit.

From Valapour M, Skeans MA, Smith JM, et al. Optn/srtr 2015 annual data report: lung. Am J Transplant 2017;17(Suppl 1):413; with permission.

pulmonologists. In some cases, additional consultation from nephrologists, infectious disease specialists, and cardiologists is required. Ideally, the patient should be on the transplant list or should have nearly completed evaluation. If the patient is ineligible for lung transplant with an irreversible pulmonary process, then palliative care with end-of-life discussions may be more appropriate than ECMO. ECMO is valuable for patients with acute exacerbation requiring ventilation if it improves their ability to rehabilitate before transplant.

Absolute contraindications

Contraindications for the use of ECMO as a bridge to lung transplantation are as follows:

1. Ineligibility for lung transplant
2. Refractory bacteremia or septic shock
3. Irreversible multiorgan damage (other than lungs)
4. Severe arterial occlusive disease
5. Contraindications to systemic anticoagulation
6. Uncontrolled metastatic disease or other terminal illness that is not otherwise treatable with lung transplant
7. Acute intracerebral hemorrhage or stroke

Relative contraindications

Unfavorable prognostic factors include older age (>65 years due to impaired physiologic reserve), frailty, acute kidney injury requiring renal replacement therapy, high vasopressor requirements, a long preceding duration of mechanical ventilation (more than 7 days), obesity (body mass index >30), and allosensitization with prolonged anticipated waitlist time.[19] In essence, if a patient is a poor candidate for lung transplantation to begin with, then adding ECMO significantly escalates the risk of perioperative mortality. Success is judged by the ability to obtain a transplant, the immediate postoperative survival, and the 5- to 10-year survival. Patients with significant deterioration that will be made worse with ECMO are unlikely to make it to transplant. Patients who are already high-risk surgical candidates and who require ECMO are unlikely to survive the transplant. Most patients who require ECMO as a bridge will have a significantly impaired long-term survival compared with those who do not require ECMO; therefore, it is preferable that they not have additional risk factors that will also compromise the long-term results. The experience of the transplant center is important to consider. High-volume centers have shown better results with bridging and can likely buffer a negative outcome more so than a lower volume center. High-volume centers may have more resources to accommodate the ECMO expenditures. Nonetheless, each case is important and requires a multidisciplinary review, patient and family involvement, full disclosure, and, at times, consultation with a neighboring high-volume facility.

Technical Consideration: Venovenous Versus Venoarterial

ECMO involves taking deoxygenated blood from the patient through an outflow cannula, pumping it through a membrane oxygenator, and then returning it to the patient through an inflow cannula (**Fig. 1**). Typical ECMO configurations are venovenous (VV) and venoarterial (VA), which provide respiratory and combined respiratory and circulatory support, respectively. In VV ECMO, blood is withdrawn and returned to the central venous system after passing through a pump and oxygenator system, thus delivering oxygenated blood to the right atrium. This can be achieved with either a dual-site or a single-site configuration. In VA ECMO, blood is withdrawn from a central

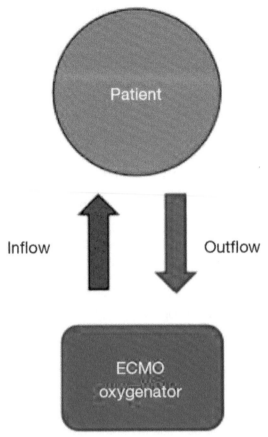

Fig. 1. ECMO cannulation: deoxygenated blood leaves the patient through an outflow cannula and is pumped through a membrane oxygenator before returning to the patient through an inflow cannula.

vein and returned to a large-caliber peripheral or central artery, providing both hemodynamic and respiratory support. The critical distinction is the status of the right ventricle and heart and if cardiac support is necessary.

Venovenous extracorporeal membrane oxygenation support

VV ECMO is the most common bridging modality for patients with advanced lung disease who are on maximum ventilator support. The goal is to prevent hemodynamic instability, irreversible end-organ damage, refractory acidosis, and pulmonary hypertension, all of which can develop from refractory hypoxemia and hypercapnia. Therefore, the early use of ECMO is warranted, before these conditions become apparent while trying to reduce the risk of complications.

The most common, easiest, and reliable method for achieving VV support involves cannulation of the femoral vein for venous outflow (deoxygenated blood) from the patient to the oxygenator and cannulation of an upper vein (subclavian or internal jugular) for the inflow (oxygenated blood) to the patient.

Technique: The patient's neck and groin are fully prepped and draped. The vein is accessed with a large-bore introducer needle under ultrasound guidance. Using the

Seldinger technique, the surgeon advances a long guide wire into the respective vein. Before advancement of the cannula, 100 to 200 units/kg of heparin are administered. Transesophageal echo (TEE) is used to document placement of the wire at the level of the right atrium. The femoral cannula is typically a long 22 to 26 French cannula with multiple side holes that is usually advanced to the level of the inferior vena cava (IVC) and the right atrium junction. Importantly, the wire must not be looped; TEE can be used to help confirm the previously specified positions. The upper vein cannula is smaller and shorter (14–16 French cannula) and is advanced to the level of the innominate vein or superior vena cava (SVC). TEE is used to document these positions. The cannulas are secured in place with multiple nonabsorbable sutures. Fluoroscopy or chest radiograph is used to confirm the position of the cannulas. They must be separated from each other to prevent recirculation. The contralateral femoral vein can be used if needed, but the risk of recirculation is greater. The cannulas are clamped, de-aired carefully, and then connected to the ECMO circuit. The flow is usually set to 3 to 4 L/min of ECMO support. Peripheral arterial blood gas is assessed from the radial line. Additional oxygen through the airway may be required depending on the contribution of the patient's native lung.

In case of recirculation, oxygenation will be compromised, and the cannulas should be adjusted accordingly. If there is concern about pulmonary hypertension, a pulmonary vasodilator such as prostacyclin or nitric oxide should be initiated. Alternatively, a right-sided TandemHeart (LivaNova, London, United Kingdom) with an oxygenator may be used. The oxygenator on the ECMO circuit oxygenates the blood while the sweep feature removes CO_2. Typical Pao_2 levels just beyond the circuit are in the 400 to 450 mm Hg range, whereas values in the periphery will range from 80 to 150 mm Hg. A radial arterial line is mandatory for assessing the peripheral blood gases. The goal after ECMO initiation is lung protective ventilation if the patient is intubated.

The advantages of this cannulation technique are as follows:

1. The procedure can be performed at the bedside, if needed, or in the operating room.
2. It is relatively straightforward for most cardiothoracic or general surgeons because they are familiar with the percutaneous wire technique.
3. This approach is particularly useful when placing cannulas emergently at an outside facility.[20]
4. Oxygenation tends to be excellent and highly predictable.

The disadvantage of using this cannulation strategy:

1. Femoral or IVC complications can be lethal.
2. In an emergency, TEE may not be available, increasing the risk of vascular complications.
3. Care must be taken to ensure the smooth passage of the femoral venous cannula because it can kink at the level of the subcutaneous tissue.
4. This approach makes the patient immobile.

The incisions are often small and can be closed with a deep single purse-string suture (nonabsorbable) through the muscle, followed by an external pressure hold for 30 minutes. Alternatively, a femoral cutdown allows exposure to the vein if it is not identified percutaneously.

The 3-stage Avalon venous cannula (MAQUET Cardiovascular, LLC, Wayne, NJ) provides inflow and outflow in one cannula. The outflow drainage to the ECMO circuit is from the tip of the cannula located in the IVC and fenestrations in the midcannula at the SVC–right atrial junction. The inflow is from an opening between these 2 points directed at the tricuspid valve (**Fig. 2**). This strategy allows ambulation and is a popular technique for postoperative support or for patients presenting with acute respiratory failure. The Avalon cannula is also inserted via the Seldinger technique but does require fluoroscopy and TEE guidance to ensure that the drainage ports are in the SVC and IVC, respectively, and that the outflow is directed toward the tricuspid valve.[21]

The advantages of this approach are patient mobility (for reconditioning/rehabilitation), increased patient comfort, and the potential decrease in the risk of infectious complications because of the absence of groin cannulation.[22] The disadvantage is that peripheral oxygenation is not always predictable and depends highly on the degree of pulmonary vascular resistance. Also, vascular complications such as IVC or right ventricular perforation can be catastrophic.[21] It is best to have a practitioner with experience performing this technique under fluoroscopy. In situations where emergency bifemoral VV ECMO is placed at the bedside, once the patient has stabilized over 48 to 72 hours, a single lumen internal jugular cannula can be placed in the cardiac catheterization laboratory in a more elective manner.

Venoarterial extracorporeal membrane oxygenation support
VA ECMO provides both respiratory and hemodynamic support, which is required for BTT patients with increased pulmonary vascular resistance and/or cardiac

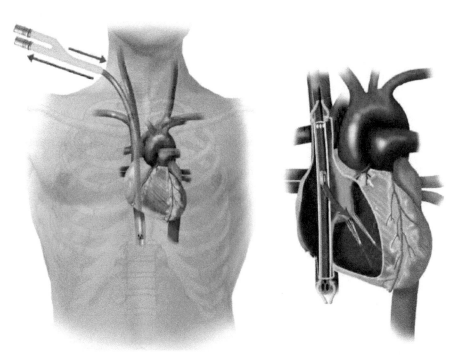

Fig. 2. Avalon cannula for VV ECMO. The Avalon cannula removes blood through a proximal and distal port in the SVC and the IVC. Oxygenated blood returns to the body through the middle inflow port oriented toward the tricuspid valve. (*From* Hirose H, Yamane K, Marhefka G, et al. Right ventricular rupture and tamponade caused by malposition of the avalon cannula for venovenous extracorporeal membrane oxygenation. J Cardiothorac Surg 2012;7:36; with permission.)

dysfunction.[23] VA ECMO can be accomplished through a variety of configurations. VA ECMO support uses an artery to deliver oxygenated blood (inflow) to the body, bypassing the pulmonary circulation, whereas a vein is used to deliver deoxygenated blood (outflow) to the ECMO oxygenator. In a recently described mobile ECMO model, a shorter percutaneous venous outflow cannula (22–24 French) is placed in the internal jugular or subclavian vein to achieve the so-called "sport model." The arterial cannula is placed directly into the axillary artery or the innominate artery usually with a tube graft.[24]

Technique: The patient's chest and neck are prepped and draped. A 6-cm subclavicular incision is made. After proximal and distal control of the axillary artery is achieved, heparin (5000 units) is administered. Next, the vessel is clamped and an 8-mm polyester graft is sewn to the axillary artery and tunneled through the subcutaneous tissue via a small counter incision. A 1/4 by 3/8-inch adaptor is secured with a heavy banding tie that is connected to the ECMO tubing. The incision is closed with absorbable sutures. The internal jugular vein cannula is advanced as described earlier. The advantage of this technique is that it allows for patient mobility. However, the disadvantage is the risk of limb hyperperfusion, which has been reported in up to 25% of cases; this complication can be reduced by starting with a lower ECMO flow setting.[25]

Alternative strategies

In patients with end-stage pulmonary hypertension and severe right heart failure, VV ECMO will not effectively deliver oxygenated blood to the body because of cardiogenic shock and/or obstruction of flow through the pulmonary vasculature. The pumpless lung assist device involves a connection between the pulmonary artery and the left atrium to bypass the lungs and provide oxygenation and right ventricular unloading.[26,27] An atrial septostomy using a balloon in cases of severe right ventricular dysfunction on VV ECMO support also allows oxygenated blood to pass into the systemic circulation.[28] Central VA ECMO typically requires a median sternotomy. A purse-string suture is placed directly on the aorta and right atrium with pledgeted sutures. After a small stab incision is made in the aorta, an arterial cannula (20–22 French) is inserted and secured to the ECMO circuit. Likewise, a venous cannula (32–34 French) is inserted through the right atrium and secured. These cannulas are often externalized through counter incisions in the upper abdomen to allow for sternal closure. Central ECMO is used in cases in which the axillary artery is too small (ie, <6–8 mm) or is insufficient to provide oxygenated blood to the periphery. The advantages of central ECMO are excellent oxygenation, lower risk of stroke, and no risk of limb complication. The disadvantages are its invasiveness and lack of patient mobility, which can be optimized by externalizing the cannulas. A small right lateral thoracotomy can also be used to limit invasiveness, although it can be technically more challenging to perform.

Outcomes

The use of ECMO and mechanical ventilator support as bridges to lung transplant has been evaluated in several trials. In a recent analysis of outcomes in the UNOS database of bridge-to-lung transplant patients in the United States, the 1-year survival rate improved from 25% in 2000 to 2002 to 74% in 2009 to 2011.[29] This improvement was likely due to a combination of technical improvements in ECMO circuit design, better medical management, avoidance of complications, and improved patient selection.[30] The study by Hayanga and colleagues[31] examined predictors for mortality and showed that patients older than 35 years (hazard ratio, 4.69; 95% confidence interval, 1.33–16.46; $P = .02$) and those with cystic fibrosis (hazard ratio, 5.38; 95% confidence interval, 1.39–20.87; $P = .03$) had worse outcomes (**Table 2**). The risk of dialysis-dependent renal failure was higher in patients who were bridged to lung transplant with ECMO. In addition, the survival rate in patients who were bridged with ECMO was worse than in those who were not bridged, but the gap in 1-year survival narrowed by the 2009 to 2011 era (74% vs 86%). Given that old age is associated with an increased risk of perioperative mortality in the same study, older patients should be cautiously considered, although patients as old as 70 years have been bridged successfully with ECMO. Improved survival outcomes depend more on patient selection, optimizing the bridge strategy, and careful weighing of competing risk factors than on having a strict age cutoff. In general, any patient older than 65 years should have very few or no additional risk factors to be considered for ECMO BTT.

Center volumes in transplantation may also be an important factor in determining outcomes for bridging. In a UNOS review, Hayanga and colleagues[32] showed an adjusted hazard ratio for mortality of 2.74 for patients who were bridged to lung transplantation with ECMO in a low-volume center (ie, 1–5 transplants/year) versus a high-volume center (ie, >15 transplants/year). This is an important consideration and suggests that transporting a patient from a low-volume center to a higher-volume center may be wise, from both a risk and quality standpoint.

In 2012, a study by Lang and colleagues[33] conducted in Vienna, Austria showed a 90% success rate in bridging patients to transplant but a 24% rate of in-hospital mortality after transplant; the median bridging time was 5.5 days (range, 1–63 days). Patients who were bridged and survived the initial 3-month period after transplant had a 5-year survival rate that was equivalent to that of patients who were not bridged (63% vs 72%, $P = .33$). This again emphasizes the importance of selecting patients who are most likely to tolerate perioperative ECMO. It also underscores the significance of optimizing patients on ECMO and knowing when the patient's condition is deteriorating and the patient may no longer be a good candidate. In a review of 26 cases of BTT, Weig and colleagues[34] showed a success rate that was lower than that reported in the Vienna study (50% vs 90%). The median time on ECMO was 33 days (range, 17–55 days). No notable differences were observed between patients who survived to transplant and those who did not. In addition, Weig and colleagues[34] studied several potential risk factors and found that patients who did not survive lung transplant after bridging had higher bilirubin levels, pulmonary artery pressures, and sequential organ failure assessment (SOFA) scores than did the surviving patients. A bilirubin level greater than 3 mg/dL and a SOFA score greater than 9 predicted a uniformly fatal outcome. Again, these are high-risk features that need to be carefully considered before committing to transplant and even before initiating ECMO.

Table 2		
Predictors for mortality with ECMO bridging		
Variables	HR (95% CI)	P Value
Age ≥35 y	4.69 (1.34–16.46)	.02
Cystic fibrosis	5.38 (1.39–20.9)	.03
Other lung diagnoses	2.49 (1.21–5.15)	.01

Abbreviations: CI, confidence interval; HR, hazard ratio.

From Hayanga AJ, Aboagye J, Esper S, et al. Extracorporeal membrane oxygenation as a bridge to lung transplantation in the united states: an evolving strategy in the management of rapidly advancing pulmonary disease. J Thorac Cardiovasc Surg 2015;149:291–6.

In a study by Crotti and colleagues,[35] the successful bridging rate was 68%. Time on ECMO was an independent factor in predicting survival after transplantation; patients who underwent transplantation after fewer than 14 days on ECMO had a 100% 1-year survival rate, and patients who were on ECMO for more than 14 days had a 50% 1-year survival rate. Mean SOFA scores from the initiation of ECMO to the end of ECMO went from 5.6 to 6.7 in the early group and from 5.2 to 9.7 in the late group. The patients on noninvasive ventilation before transplantation had a 20% mortality rate while on the waitlist and a 60% 1-year survival rate after transplantation, whereas patients requiring intubation before transplantation had a 40% mortality rate while on the waitlist and a 47% 1-year survival rate after transplantation.

Shafii and colleagues[17] showed a successful bridging to lung transplantation rate of 74%. They reported that patients who were bridged had a significantly longer hospital stay, greater coagulopathy, and higher rates of dialysis and tracheostomy. Nevertheless, they found no difference in 3-year survival rates between patients who were bridged with ECMO and those who were not. Several important complications resulted in death in ECMO patients awaiting transplantation, including renal failure (21%), sepsis (16%), diffuse intravascular coagulopathy (10%), anoxic brain injury (5%), and multisystem organ failure (5%). Patient morbidities after transplantation were also significant and included open chest management (50%), continuation of ECMO (21%), and reoperation for bleeding (29%). In 2013, 11 centers in France combined data from 36 patients who were bridged with ECMO into a registry report. Their cumulative success with bridging was 83%; however, only 56% of patients were discharged from the hospital.[36] Furthermore, only 47% of patients who were bridged were alive at 17-month follow-up. Cystic fibrosis patients had the best survival, with a 56% survival rate at 3 years from the initiation of ECMO. Toyoda and colleagues[37] reported a 77% success rate in 31 patients who were bridged with ECMO. The median duration of ECMO was 91 hours. They noted significantly higher rates of primary graft dysfunction 3 (PGD3) in patients requiring ECMO support (54% vs 6%) and a longer median hospital stay (46 vs 27 days) in the bridged group than in the nonbridged group. However, no significant difference was observed in the 2-year survival rate after transplantation, regardless of preoperative ECMO status (74% for both groups).

Collaud and colleagues[19] performed a literature review and pooled analyses to assess the role of ECMO bridging in retransplantation. They found that the 1-year overall survival rate was 48%. The intertransplant interval was a significant factor affecting survival in this group. For the subgroup of patients with an intertransplant interval of greater than 2 years and who were bridged on awake ECMO (ambulatory, communicating, low-vent requirements), the 1-year survival rate was 67%.

In another study performed at Zurich University Hospital in Switzerland, the successful bridging rate was 86%. Intensive care unit and ventilation times were significantly longer in BTT patients than in controls who were not bridged.[38] The rates of PGD3 and mortality at 2 years were also higher for bridged patients. For a subgroup of patients bridged with awake ECMO, all were alive at a median follow-up time of 10.8 months. Similarly, Lang and colleagues[33] showed that patients bridged with awake ECMO had a 2-year survival rate of 60% compared with a 2-year survival rate of 29% for patients bridged with ventilation, sedation +/− ECMO. Thus, evidence indicates that awake ECMO is a good prognostic indicator for patients who can tolerate it. It underscores the importance of identifying patients who are good candidates for awake ECMO and placing them on ECMO for BTT. This approach may require placing some patients on ECMO earlier rather than waiting too long.

Biscotti and colleagues[39] reported their 9-year experience at New York-Presbyterian/Columbia University Medical Center with a 55% success rate for

Table 3
Summary of recent studies reviewing 1-year survival outcomes of ECMO bridging conditional on receiving a lung transplant after ECMO

Single Center Studies	Number of Patients	1-y Survival
Lang et al,[33] 2012	34	63%
Shafii et al,[17] 2012	19	79%
Weig et al,[34] 2013	26	54%
Crotti et al,[35] 2013	22	79%
Lafarge et al,[36] 2013	36	60%
Inci et al,[38] 2015	26	68%
Biscotti et al,[39] 2017	40	92%

bridging with ECMO to transplant. Using univariate analysis, they identified several factors that predicted the likelihood of whether a patient will survive to transplantation. A higher percentage of inotrope or vasopressor use was noted in the nonsurvival group. In addition, a higher simplified acute physiology II score and a lower rate of ambulation were found in the group that was not successfully bridged. Consistent with the French experience described earlier, patients with cystic fibrosis had the most favorable prognosis for surviving to transplantation. Also, the need for renal replacement therapy was higher in the group of patients who did not receive a transplant. Cystic fibrosis patients had the best rate of survival after transplantation, whereas patients with interstitial lung disease had the worst rate of survival after transplantation off of ECMO (**Table 3**).

Box 1 summarizes the traits of patients on ECMO that can help predict whether an outcome will be successful after transplantation.[40] This summary is based on the

Box 1
Factors that affect posttransplant survival in patients on ECMO support

Favorable factors
  Age less than 50 years
  Normal or marginally elevated total bilirubin
  Normal or mildly elevated pulmonary artery pressures
  Less than 14-day duration on ECMO
  Low SOFA score (<6)
  Noninvasive ventilation
  Ability to participate in physical therapy (ie, "awake ECMO")

Unfavorable factors
  Age greater than 60 years
  Total bilirubin greater than 3
  Severe pulmonary hypertension
  Prolonged ECMO (>14 days)
  Prolonged mechanical ventilation
  Prolonged immobility on ECMO
  SOFA score greater than 9
  Major bleeding, infectious complications, or end-organ perfusion
  Complications on ECMO
  Retransplant with a retransplant interval less than 1 year

Abbreviations: ECMO, extracorporeal membrane oxygenation; SOFA, sequential organ failure assessment.
  Adapted from Loor G, Simpson L, Parulekar A. Bridging to lung transplantation with extracorporeal circulatory support: when or when not? J Thorac Dis 2017;9:3352–61; with permission.

above-referenced data and the authors' own institutional experience but should not be used in isolation to decide who should undergo bridging to transplantation, given that this is an evolving field.

SUMMARY

Two fundamental questions are important when deciding to place a patient on ECMO:

I. Is this patient a potential candidate for a lung transplant?
II. Is the prognosis reasonable for surviving to transplant and having quality of life and survival after transplant?

For the first question, ECMO support should be considered in any patient who is remotely close to being considered a transplant candidate and who has refractory hypoxemia or hypercapnia. At the minimum, this allows a bridge to decision. For the second question, several considerations have been described earlier and in **Box 1** that help guide multidisciplinary discussions and decisions. There is not a commitment to transplantation just because the patient is on ECMO. The multidisciplinary team and the patient's family should have daily discussions to weigh the patient's quality of life and the chance of survival.

REFERENCES

1. Cooper JD, Pearson FG, Patterson GA, et al. Technique of successful lung transplantation in humans. J Thorac Cardiovasc Surg 1987;93:173–81.
2. Valapour M. Optn/srtr 2016 annual data report: lung. Am J Transplant 2018;18: 363–433.
3. McGregor CG, Dark JH, Hilton CJ, et al. Early results of single lung transplantation in patients with end-stage pulmonary fibrosis. J Thorac Cardiovasc Surg 1989;98:350–4.
4. Levvey BJ, Whitford HM, Williams TJ, et al. Donation after circulatory determination of death lung transplantation for pulmonary arterial hypertension: passing the toughest test. Am J Transplant 2015;15:3208–14.
5. Cypel M, Keshavjee S. Extracorporeal life support as a bridge to lung transplantation. Clin Chest Med 2011;32:245–51.
6. Jurmann MJ, Haverich A, Demertzis S, et al. Extracorporeal membrane oxygenation as a bridge to lung transplantation. Eur J Cardiothorac Surg 1991;5:94–7 [discussion: 98].
7. Riley JB, Scott PD, Schears GJ. Update on safety equipment for extracorporeal life support (ecls) circuits. Semin Cardiothorac Vasc Anesth 2009;13:138–45.
8. Javidfar J, Bacchetta M. Bridge to lung transplantation with extracorporeal membrane oxygenation support. Curr Opin Organ Transplant 2012;17:496–502.
9. Hardy JD. The first lung transplant in man (1963) and the first heart transplant in man (1964). Transplant Proc 1999;31:25–9.
10. Painvin GA, Reece IJ, Cooley DA, et al. Cardiopulmonary allotransplantation, a collective review: experimental progress and current clinical status. Tex Heart Inst J 1983;10:371–86.
11. Vieth FJ. Lung transplantation. Transplant Proc 1977;9:203–8.
12. Saunders NR, Alpert HM, Cooper JD. Sequential bilateral lung transplantation for paraquat poisoning. A Case Report. The Toronto Lung Transplant group. J Thorac Cardiovasc Surg 1985;89(5):734–42.

13. Zapol WM, Snider MT, Hill JD, et al. Extracorporeal membrane oxygenation in severe acute respiratory failure. A randomized prospective study. JAMA 1979;242: 2193–6.

14. Jurmann MJ, Haverich A, Demertzis S, et al. Extracorporeal membrane oxygenation (ecmo): extended indications for artificial support of both heart and lungs. Int J Artif Organs 1991;14:771–4.

15. ANZIC Influenza Investigators, Webb SA, Pettilä V, Seppelt I, et al. Critical care services and 2009 h1n1 influenza in Australia and New Zealand. N Engl J Med 2009;361:1925–34.

16. Peek GJ, Mugford M, Tiruvoipati R, et al. Efficacy and economic assessment of conventional ventilatory support versus extracorporeal membrane oxygenation for severe adult respiratory failure (cesar): a multicentre randomised controlled trial. Lancet 2009;374:1351–63.

17. Mason DP, Thuita L, Nowicki ER, et al. Should lung transplantation be performed for patients on mechanical respiratory support? The US experience. J Thorac Cardiovasc Surg 2010;139:765–73.e1.

18. Valapour M, Skeans MA, Smith JM, et al. Optn/srtr 2015 annual data report: lung. Am J Transplant 2017;17(Suppl 1):357–424.

19. Collaud S, Benden C, Ganter C, et al. Extracorporeal life support as bridge to lung retransplantation: a multicenter pooled data analysis. Ann Thorac Surg 2016;102:1680–6.

20. Lee SG, Son BS, Kang PJ, et al. The feasibility of extracorporeal membrane oxygenation support for inter-hospital transport and as a bridge to lung transplantation. Ann Thorac Cardiovasc Surg 2014;20:26–31.

21. Hirose H, Yamane K, Marhefka G, et al. Right ventricular rupture and tamponade caused by malposition of the avalon cannula for venovenous extracorporeal membrane oxygenation. J Cardiothorac Surg 2012;7:36.

22. Jayaraman AL, Cormican D, Shah P, et al. Cannulation strategies in adult veno-arterial and veno-venous extracorporeal membrane oxygenation: techniques, limitations, and special considerations. Ann Card Anaesth 2017;20:S11–8.

23. Makdisi G, Wang IW. Extra corporeal membrane oxygenation (ecmo) review of a lifesaving technology. J Thorac Dis 2015;7:E166–76.

24. Biscotti M, Bacchetta M. The "sport model": extracorporeal membrane oxygenation using the subclavian artery. Ann Thorac Surg 2014;98:1487–9.

25. Chamogeorgakis T, Lima B, Shafii AE, et al. Outcomes of axillary artery side graft cannulation for extracorporeal membrane oxygenation. J Thorac Cardiovasc Surg 2013;145:1088–92.

26. Schmid C, Philipp A, Hilker M, et al. Bridge to lung transplantation through a pulmonary artery to left atrial oxygenator circuit. Ann Thorac Surg 2008;85:1202–5.

27. Strueber M, Hoeper MM, Fischer S, et al. Bridge to thoracic organ transplantation in patients with pulmonary arterial hypertension using a pumpless lung assist device. Am J Transplant 2009;9:853–7.

28. Kon ZN, Pasrija C, Shah A, et al. Venovenous extracorporeal membrane oxygenation with atrial septostomy as a bridge to lung transplantation. Ann Thorac Surg 2016;101:1166–9.

29. Hayanga AJ, Aboagye J, Esper S, et al. Extracorporeal membrane oxygenation as a bridge to lung transplantation in the United States: an evolving strategy in the management of rapidly advancing pulmonary disease. J Thorac Cardiovasc Surg 2015;149:291–6.

30. Combes A, Bacchetta M, Brodie D, et al. Extracorporeal membrane oxygenation for respiratory failure in adults. Curr Opin Crit Care 2012;18:99–104.

31. Hayanga JA, Murphy E, Girgis RE, et al. Extracorporeal membrane oxygenation as a bridge to lung transplantation in patients over age 70 years: a case report. Transplant Proc 2017;49:218–20.

32. Hayanga JW, Lira A, Aboagye JK, et al. Extracorporeal membrane oxygenation as a bridge to lung transplantation: what lessons might we learn from volume and expertise? Interact Cardiovasc Thorac Surg 2016;22:406–10.

33. Lang G, Taghavi S, Aigner C, et al. Primary lung transplantation after bridge with extracorporeal membrane oxygenation: a plea for a shift in our paradigms for indications. Transplantation 2012;93:729–36.

34. Weig T, Irlbeck M, Frey L, et al. Parameters associated with short- and midterm survival in bridging to lung transplantation with extracorporeal membrane oxygenation. Clin Transplant 2013;27:E563–70.

35. Crotti S, Iotti GA, Lissoni A, et al. Organ allocation waiting time during extracorporeal bridge to lung transplant affects outcomes. Chest 2013;144:1018–25.

36. Lafarge M, Mordant P, Thabut G, et al. Experience of extracorporeal membrane oxygenation as a bridge to lung transplantation in France. J Heart Lung Transplant 2013;32:905–13.

37. Toyoda Y, Bhama JK, Shigemura N, et al. Efficacy of extracorporeal membrane oxygenation as a bridge to lung transplantation. J Thorac Cardiovasc Surg 2013;145:1065–70 [discussion: 1070–1].

38. Inci I, Klinzing S, Schneiter D, et al. Outcome of extracorporeal membrane oxygenation as a bridge to lung transplantation: an institutional experience and literature review. Transplantation 2015;99:1667–71.

39. Biscotti M, Gannon WD, Agerstrand C, et al. Awake extracorporeal membrane oxygenation as bridge to lung transplantation: a 9-year experience. Ann Thorac Surg 2017;104:412–9.

40. Loor G, Simpson L, Parulekar A. Bridging to lung transplantation with extracorporeal circulatory support: when or when not? J Thorac Dis 2017;9:3352–61.

Perioperative Management of the Lung Graft Following Lung Transplantation

Mariya Geube, MD[a],*, Balaram Anandamurthy, MD[a],
Jean-Pierre Yared, MD[b]

KEYWORDS

- Lung graft • Lung transplantation • Perioperative intervention

KEY POINTS

- According to the revised definition for primary graft dysfunction, the inhaled epoprostenol and elective extracorporeal support are not part of the definition.
- Late graft dysfunction at 48- and 72-hour time points is associated with higher mortality than PGD 3 in the first 24 hours, which is usually transient and has less impact on the clinical outcome.
- Lung protective ventilation strategies supported by ARDS net data, along with permissive hypercarbia and low inspired oxygen fraction are recommended after graft implantation.
- CPB has been associated with worse early postoperative outcomes, such as graft dysfunction, bleeding and transfusion requirements, and increased duration of mechanical ventilation. Cases emergently "converted" to CPB had worse outcomes than "planned" CPB cases.
- Preclinical data suggest that nitric oxide can mitigate the inflammatory process associated with ischemia-reperfusion injury, however, these findings were not reproduced in clinical trials. Currently, inhaled pulmonary vasodilators are used as a rescu therapy, but not recommended as preemptive strategy.

INTRODUCTION

Perioperative management of patients undergoing lung transplantation is one of the most complex in cardiothoracic surgery. Certain perioperative interventions, such as mechanical ventilation, fluid management and blood transfusions, use of extracorporeal mechanical support, and pain management, may have significant impact on the lung graft function and clinical outcome. This article provides a review of perioperative interventions that have been shown to impact the perioperative course after lung transplantation.

Conflict of Interest: Nothing to disclose.
[a] Department of Cardiothoracic Anesthesiology, Cleveland Clinic Lerner College of Medicine, Case Western Reserve University, Cleveland Clinic, 9500 Euclid Avenue, J4-331, Cleveland, OH 44195, USA; [b] Department of Cardiothoracic Anesthesiology, Cleveland Clinic, 9500 Euclid Avenue, J4-331, Cleveland, OH 44195, USA
* Corresponding author.
E-mail address: geubem@ccf.org

Crit Care Clin 35 (2019) 27–43
https://doi.org/10.1016/j.ccc.2018.08.007
0749-0704/19/© 2018 Elsevier Inc. All rights reserved.

PRIMARY GRAFT DYSFUNCTION
Definition and Grading

Primary graft dysfunction (PGD) is a form of acute lung injury that develops in the initial 72 hours after lung transplantation.[1] It presents with acute hypoxemia, decreased lung compliance, and radiographic features of diffuse pulmonary infiltrates, similarly to acute respiratory distress syndrome (ARDS).[2] It remains the most important cause of early postoperative morbidity and mortality after lung transplant surgery.[3] PGD is categorized in three grades of severity, recently updated by the International Society of Heart and Lung Transplantation consensus definitions (**Table 1**).[4] The administration of inhaled pulmonary vasodilators no longer affects the grading of PGD (previously defined as grade 3). The diagnosis of PGD requires exclusion of other conditions masquerading as pulmonary edema. These are cardiogenic pulmonary edema, pneumonia, pulmonary venous flow obstruction, ARDS, pulmonary aspiration, and hyperacute rejection.[5] The radiologic findings spare the native lung in cases of single-lung transplantation, which helps to distinguish this syndrome from other clinical entities, such as left ventricular failure or ARDS.

Clinical Outcomes of Primary Graft Dysfunction

Grade 3 PGD occurs in 15% to 20% of patients and is associated with prolonged mechanical ventilation, increase the intensive care unit (ICU) length of stay, and 30-day mortality up to 50%.[6–9] In addition, late graft dysfunction at 48- and 72-hour time points is associated with higher mortality than PGD 3 in the first 24 hours, which is usually transient and has less impact on the clinical outcome.[10]

Severe form of PGD determines not only the short-term outcome after lung transplantation, but is also linked to the development of chronic allograft dysfunction, known as bronchiolitis obliterans syndrome.[11,12]

Pathogenesis and Risk Factors

PGD is a manifestation of ischemia-reperfusion injury, and the end result of series of insults, which starts in the donor after brain death, escalates during organ procurement and preservation, and peaks after reperfusion of the transplanted lungs.[13]

Table 1
PGD grading system, according to the 2016 International Society of Heart and Lung Transplantation Consensus Definition

Grade	Oxygenation	Radiographic Infiltrates
0	• Any Pao_2/Fio_2 • Extubated patient with or without supplemental oxygen	Absent
1	• Pao_2/Fio_2 >300 or • Sao_2/Fio_2 >315 • Extubated patient on supplemental oxygen with Fio_2 <30%	Present bilateral SLT, absent in the native lung
2	• Pao_2/Fio_2 200–300 or • Sao_2/Fio_2 235–315	Present bilateral SLT, absent in the native lung
3	• Pao_2/Fio_2 <200 or • Sao_2/Fio_2 <235 • Requirement for ECLS (for hypoxemia) • Mechanical ventilation with Fio_2 >50% for 48 h	Present bilateral SLT, absent in the native lung

PGD is graded by the worst Pao_2/Fio_2 ratio in the first 72 hours after allograft reperfusion.
Abbreviations: ECLS, extracorporeal life support; Pao_2/Fio_2, partial arterial oxygen pressure to fraction of inspired oxygen ratio; Sao_2, arterial oxygen saturation; SLT, single-lung transplant.

Brain death causes significant pathophysiologic changes in all organs, such as systemic inflammatory response and sympathetic storm with massive discharge of catecholamines in the circulation.[14,15] Recently, it has been postulated that the innate immunity has an important role in progression of the ischemia-reperfusion injury in a biphasic pattern.[16] The early phase is modulated by the donor lung macrophages and lymphocytes, whereas at a later stage, there is an influx of recipient T cells and neutrophils, which augment and perpetuate the inflammatory cascade in the allograft.[17] Ischemic reperfusion injury of the lung allograft is defined as a sterile inflammation of the transplanted organ with restoration of the perfusion after a period of absence of blood flow. The outburst of reactive oxygen species created as a result of interrupted and then restored blood flow to the lungs causes leukocyte adhesion, production and release of proinflammatory mediators, and disruption of the integrity of the epithelial-endothelial unit.[18]

Multiple groups have studied potential risk factors for PGD.[8,19–25] A summary of the risk factors consistently found to be associated with PGD is listed in **Table 2**.

Clinical Management of Primary Graft Dysfunction

Therapy for PGD is largely supportive and extrapolated from the ARDS literature. The main goal of ventilatory support is to minimize the volutrauma and barotrauma, and to avoid oxygen toxicity. The escalation of care for refractory hypoxemia consists of adjustment of the positive end-expiratory pressure to best respiratory system compliance, inverse ratio ventilation, initiation of inhaled pulmonary vasodilator, and extracorporeal life support.[26] Compliance with postoperative respiratory and hemodynamic protocols may prove effective in reducing the severity of PGD.[27] Therapeutic interventions, such as lung protective mechanical ventilation, restrictive fluid administration and transfusion management, avoiding cardiopulmonary bypass (CPB) during surgery, and reducing the cold ischemia time, are widely accepted to decrease the incidence of PGD, and enhance early recovery of the lung transplant recipients. As a last resort, retransplantation is considered on an individual basis, but is associated with poor survival.[28,29]

Table 2
Donor, recipient and procedure risk factors for grade-3 PGD, consistently reported in studies, based on the most recent report of International Society of Heart and Lung Transplantation

Risk Factor Category	Risk Factors for Grade-3 PGD
Donor related	• Donor age • Smoking history (dose-dependent effect) • Pulmonary aspiration • Chest trauma • Undersized donor relative to recipient
Recipient related	• Body mass index >30 • Pulmonary arterial hypertension • Idiopathic pulmonary fibrosis • Sarcoidosis
Procedural and perioperative factors	• Prolonged ischemic time • Use of cardiopulmonary bypass • Increased fraction of inspiratory oxygen • Large-volume blood transfusion

Data from Diamond J, Arcasoy S, Kennedy C, et al. Report of the International Society of Heart and Lung Transplantation working group on primary graft dysfunction, part II: epidemiology, risk factors and outcomes – a 2016 consensus group statement of the International Society for Heart and Lung Transplantation. J Heart Lung Transplant 2017;36(10):1104–13.

VENTILATORY STRATEGIES OF THE TRANSPLANTED LUNGS

The goals of mechanical ventilation after lung transplantation are to promote graft function, maintain adequate gas exchange, prevent ventilator-induced lung injury, and liberate the patient from ventilator in the shortest possible time. Immediately following implantation, the transplanted lung is suctioned of blood and secretions, and the integrity and patency of the airway anastomosis is examined with flexible bronchoscopy. After reperfusion of the ipsilateral pulmonary artery and surgical hemostasis, the lung is inflated manually to achieve maximal recruitment with slow insufflation and lung expansion. Although the role of lung protective mechanical ventilation in ARDS is well established,[30] there is a lack of strong evidence regarding ventilation mode selection and targets of gas exchange in the lung transplant population. Lung protective ventilation strategies supported by ARDS net data (tidal volume of 6 mL/kg/ideal body weight and plateau pressure <30 cm H_2O) along with permissive hypercarbia to pH greater than 7.25 are recommended.[31] Use of high tidal volume and low positive end-expiratory pressure has been detrimental to the graft function in animal experiments.[32]

Several studies have demonstrated a link between increased fraction of inspired oxygen ratio at reperfusion and a higher risk of severe PGD.[8] Therefore, the use of lowest fraction of inspired oxygen ratio to a target PaO_2 60 to 80 mm Hg (arterial oxygen saturation >91%) is recommended (**Fig. 1**).

A recent survey addressing the mechanical ventilation practice after lung transplantation has shown that most centers used the recipient's ideal body weight to select the tidal volume of the allografts, as opposed to the donor's characteristics.[33] Studies of donor/recipient lung size mismatch show that recipients of undersized allografts had higher incidence of PGD, supporting the use of donor's height when available.[34,35]

Lung allografts have disrupted nerve supply as a consequence of harvesting from the donor. Weak cough, poor respiratory mechanics caused by deconditioning, and

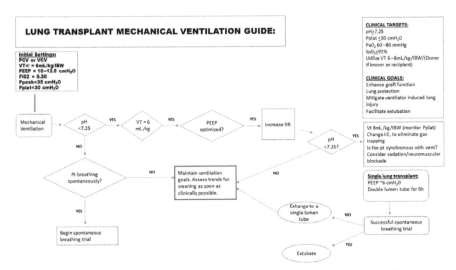

Fig. 1. Mechanical ventilation protocol after lung transplantation with bilateral and single allografts. FIO_2, fraction of inspired oxygen; I:E, inspiratory to expiratory time; IBW, ideal body weight; PCV, pressure controlled ventilation; PEEP, positive end-expiratory pressure; Ppeak, peak airway pressure; Pplat, plateau airway pressure; RR, respiratory rate; SpO_2, arterial oxygen saturation; VCV, volume-controlled ventilation; VT, tidal volume.

inadequate pain control lead to inability to clear the airway secretions. In the first several days after transplantation, the amount of secretions is increased because of sloughing of the bronchial mucosa and accumulation of necrotic debris. Thus, bronchoscopic guided bronchopulmonary toilet is of great importance to expedite tracheal extubation.

Single-Lung Transplantation: Role of Split-Lung Ventilation and the Importance of Treating the Native Lung

Single-lung transplantation (most common in chronic obstructive pulmonary disease) may present a challenge in regards to postimplantation mechanical ventilation.[36] The compliance of the native emphysematous lung is abnormally high as compared with the allograft, which tends to be stiff, because of atelectasis and ischemia-reperfusion injury. This creates a risk for dynamic hyperinflation of the native lung, described in 30% of unilateral transplantation,[37] and compression atelectasis of the transplanted lung. The uneven distribution of the tidal volume leads to ventilation/perfusion (V/Q) mismatch, respiratory failure, and hemodynamic instability from decreased preload. Early transition to spontaneous breathing and extubation is of paramount importance. Split-lung ventilation may be indicated, in case of significant difference in the mechanical properties of the two lungs (**Fig. 2**). The split-lung ventilation requires deep sedation and even muscle paralysis, because the two lungs are ventilated dyssynchronous and with different settings, thus it is poorly tolerated in lightly sedated patients. Administration of bronchodilators, mucolytics, and bronchopulmonary toilet to the native lung in the postoperative period is of utmost importance.

HEMODYNAMIC MANAGEMENT IN THE PERIOPERATIVE PERIOD
Heart-Lung Interaction Before and After Lung Transplantation

Patients with end-stage lung disease often present with secondary pulmonary arterial hypertension and various degree of right ventricular (RV) dysfunction. Induction of anesthesia poses a great risk of cardiopulmonary collapse, because of transition from spontaneous to positive pressure ventilation, anesthetic drug-related

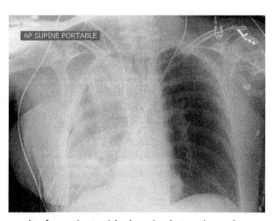

Fig. 2. Chest radiograph of a patient with chronic obstructive pulmonary disease, who underwent right lung transplantation and presented with hyperinflation of the native lung and significant opacification of the allograft (*right*), requiring split-lung ventilation. The radiograph is performed 10 hours after surgery. Note the presence of three right chest tubes, left double-lumen endotracheal tube, and pulmonary artery catheter in the main pulmonary artery.

vasodilation, and myocardial depression. Application of positive pressure ventilation decreases the preload and increases the afterload to the right ventricle, which along with the period of apnea may precipitate RV failure on induction.

The ability of a patient to tolerate bilateral sequential lung transplantation without the use of CPB is determined by the results from the preoperative pulmonary function tests and ventilation-perfusion scan. The lung with lower perfusion is transplanted first. After the pulmonary artery is clamped the entire cardiac output is diverted to the contralateral pulmonary artery, which reduces the intrapulmonary shunt; however, it significantly increases the pulmonary artery pressure. In the presence of preexisting RV dysfunction, this may precipitate severe hemodynamic instability. Preemptive institution of inotropes and inhaled pulmonary vasodilator may avoid the need for mechanical circulatory support. Surgical manipulation deep into the hilum and the left atrium can trigger arrhythmias or cause decrease in the preload, with resultant hypotension, requiring temporary vasopressor support. The release of the pulmonary artery clamp is followed by severe hypotension secondary to the pneumoplegia, metabolic acidosis, air embolism, and release of lung metabolites from the ischemic lung causing systemic vasoplegia.[38] Preemptive administration of colloid solution, vasopressor boluses, calcium, and sodium bicarbonate around the time of clamp release may attenuate these effects.

In patients with chronic pulmonary hypertension, the lung graft reperfusion is followed by a dramatic decrease in pulmonary vascular resistance. Several studies have reported an improvement of the RV function and degree of tricuspid insufficiency post lung implantation.[39,40] Typically, the left ventricular systolic function is preserved before and after lung transplantation. Increased velocities of the mitral inflow are common, indicative of increased flow to the left ventricle.[41]

The Role of Cardiopulmonary Bypass

The use of CPB varies significantly among the centers (9%–71%),[8] more often being used in bilateral lung transplantation in patients with severe pulmonary hypertension and compromised RV function. CPB is also indicated when a concomitant cardiac procedure (coronary artery bypass, valve surgery, or repair of intracardiac shunt) is anticipated. In some cases, unplanned institution of CPB is urged by the inability to tolerate one-lung ventilation (because of refractory hypoxemia or respiratory acidosis), or inability to tolerate pulmonary artery clamping (RV failure). Although CPB ensures hemodynamic stability and controlled perfusion of the lung grafts, it has been associated with worse early postoperative outcomes in several studies.[42,43] These include increased incidence of graft dysfunction, bleeding and transfusion requirements, and increased duration of mechanical ventilation. Lung transplant cases emergently "converted" to CPB had worse outcomes than "planned" CPB cases. Furthermore, in some reports, "planned" CPB cases had similar early outcomes with cases performed "off CPB."[44,45] The causal relationship of CPB with the graft dysfunction is difficult to establish, because of lack of prospective trials, different practice patterns of planned versus emergent CPB, and selection bias caused by the prevalence of pulmonary artery hypertension in the CPB cases.

Cardiopulmonary Bypass Versus Extracorporeal Membrane Oxygenation as a Means of Intraoperative Circulatory Support

The use of extracorporeal membrane oxygenation (ECMO) in the intraoperative period has been pioneered and expanded in the past decade. There are certain advantages of performing the lung transplant surgery with ECMO as an alternative to CPB. These include reduction of heparin requirements and priming volume, reduced blood contact surface in the absence of blood reservoir and cardiotomy suction, reduced inflammatory response and coagulopathy, and decreased transfusion requirements.[46] Several studies reported more favorable early postoperative outcomes with the use of ECMO compared with CPB during lung transplantation. These include lower rate of perioperative blood transfusions, shorter period of mechanical ventilation and ICU stay, and lower reoperation rate.[47–49] ECMO can be continued in the early postoperative period allowing for controlled perfusion of the lung allografts and avoiding ventilator-associated lung injury during the immediate postimplantation period.[50] The short- and mid-term mortality rate was found to be similar with the two techniques.[51] A common feature of all studies is their single-center retrospective design, and historical comparison of cohorts of preceding use of CPB, followed by change of practice to ECMO.

The Use of Inhaled Pulmonary Vasodilators in Lung Transplantation

Inhaled pulmonary vasodilators have been studied in experimental and clinical trials in lung transplantation for their potential beneficial effect on the ischemia-reperfusion injury, independent of their effect on the pulmonary arterial tone.[52–54] Preservation and reperfusion of the lung allograft significantly reduce the levels of intrinsic nitric oxide. Preclinical data suggest that nitric oxide can mitigate the inflammatory processes associated with ischemia-reperfusion injury, inhibit neutrophil and platelet adhesion to the pulmonary endothelium, decrease oxidative stress, and prevent endothelial dysfunction.[55–57] These findings, although promising, were not reproduced in clinical trials.[58–60] There is significant variation of the dosing regimen and timing of the therapy in these studies, which may explain the inconsistency in the results. Development of the PGD is a complex process that involves several stages of the lung transplant process, so its course may not be altered by an agent, started at the time of reperfusion. Thus, the rationale for prophylactic use of nitric oxide to prevent PGD remains unproven and is not recommended.[30,61] Currently, inhalational pulmonary vasodilators are used for the following indications: (1) in patients with moderate pulmonary arterial hypertension to facilitate intraoperative management during pulmonary artery clamping; (2) hemodynamic instability caused by RV dysfunction, to avoid the need for CPB; (3) in hypoxemia during one-lung ventilation; and (4) refractory hypoxemia in severe form of PGD.[62] The improved oxygenation is caused by the regional vasodilation of the ventilated lung units with significant improvement of the ventilation perfusion ratio. Nitric oxide and epoprostenol showed similar efficacy in hemodynamic and respiratory endpoints.[63]

PERIOPERATIVE FLUID ADMINISTRATION AND CARDIAC OUTPUT MANAGEMENT

Lung allografts are at high risk for developing postoperative pulmonary edema and fluid replacement should be considered with caution. There are several mechanisms explaining the increased predisposition to lung edema. The ischemia-reperfusion injury results in distortion of the endothelial integrity and extravasation of fluid. A decrease in alveolar fluid clearance from disruption of the lymphatic drainage during the lung procurement further aggravates this process.[64,65] In addition, administration of fluid and blood products augment the lung injury by increasing the hydrostatic forces in the pulmonary circulation. Augmentation of cardiac output with inotropic medications may also contribute by increasing the amount of flow through the lung allografts. Thus, it is advisable to maintain adequate, but not high cardiac output state after lung reperfusion.

Few studies focus on the relationship between perioperative fluid management and subsequent development of PGD. Several exploratory reports suggest that elevated cardiac filling pressures and administration of colloid solutions are associated with hypoxemia and prolonged mechanical ventilation.[66,67] In a large retrospective study, Geube and colleagues[68] showed that the total amount of intra-operative fluids and red blood cell concentrates were associated with grade 3 PGD. Each additional liter of fluid intraoperatively increased the odds for grade 3 PGD by 22%. The association of blood transfusion with PGD was confirmed in other reports.[8,25]

POSTOPERATIVE CONSIDERATIONS UNIQUE TO PATIENTS WITH LUNG TRANSPLANTATION

Diaphragmatic Paralysis

The incidence of phrenic nerve injury after lung transplantation occurs in 5% to 9% and it is higher in bilateral lung transplantation.[69,70] It results from stretching or direct surgical injury, and presents clinically with paradoxic breathing pattern, on transition from full mechanical ventilator support to spontaneous breathing. Phrenic nerve injury should be suspected in case of early extubation failure in the absence of graft dysfunction or infection. It often results in prolonged mechanical ventilation, need for tracheostomy, and prolonged hospital stay.[71] The diagnosis is usually suspected clinically and confirmed by fluoroscopic examination of the diaphragm, and supine and sitting spirometry.

Impact of Perioperative Correction of Metabolic Alkalosis in Patients with Chronic Respiratory Acidosis, on Post-transplant Weaning from Mechanical Ventilation

Patients with chronic obstructive pulmonary disease and cystic fibrosis often present for lung transplantation with chronic respiratory acidosis and compensatory metabolic alkalosis, with elevated serum bicarbonate levels. After reperfusion of the lung allograft, it is common for some degree of metabolic acidosis to occur because of cardiovascular instability, ischemia-reperfusion injury, and use of CPB. As a consequence, the serum bicarbonate level decreases and is often left uncorrected, as long as it is in "normal" range. Maintenance of a normal pH is achieved by increasing minute ventilation and decreasing $Paco_2$ from its chronically elevated levels to a lower "normal" value. Because arterial CO_2 rapidly equilibrates with the cerebrospinal fluid, whereas bicarbonate ions require many hours to diffuse across the blood-brain barrier, the cerebrospinal fluid pH remains elevated for a substantial duration after surgery before an equilibrium is achieved. The central respiratory drive remains depressed as long as cerebrospinal fluid pH remains substantially higher than the arterial pH, leading to failure to wean from mechanical ventilation. Transition to spontaneous mode of ventilation in this situation risks increased pulmonary vascular resistance and RV failure, because of central hypoventilation. Thus, in patients who present with compensated chronic respiratory acidosis, it is advisable to maintain serum bicarbonate level and $Paco_2$ close to baseline intraoperatively.

Lung Size/Chest Wall Mismatch

Donor-recipient matching is directed by the predicted total lung capacity based on height, age, and gender.[28] Oversized grafts may lead to compression of cardiac chambers and inability to close the chest. Postoperatively, large allografts cause dyspnea because of flattening and impaired motion of the diaphragm, with resultant atelectasis. In significant donor-recipient size mismatch, volume reduction surgery, such as wedge lung resection, may be considered.[72]

Pulmonary Thromboembolism

During lung procurement process, the bronchial arterial supply is disrupted, making the lung parenchyma totally dependent on pulmonary artery blood flow. An acute thromboembolic event may cause catastrophic ischemia to the lung graft, resulting in pulmonary infarct.[73] In case of a single-lung transplantation, the emboli lodge preferentially in the transplanted lung, because it has lower pulmonary vascular resistance and receives most of the blood flow. This may lead to acute respiratory and RV failure.

Pulmonary Venous Flow Obstruction

Pulmonary venous anastomosis involves attachment of small atrial cuff along with the ipsilateral pulmonary veins to the recipient's left atrium. Pulmonary venous flow could be compromised secondary to anastomotic stenosis, thrombosis, or torsion. Clinically, pulmonary venous flow obstruction presents with unilateral pulmonary edema. Intraoperative transesophageal echocardiography is an excellent tool to monitor the flow pattern in the pulmonary veins after lung implantation (**Fig. 3**).

In single-lung transplantation, the allograft receives higher blood flow compared with the native lung, and is expected to have higher velocities; however, normal phasic flow pattern should be present on spectral Doppler examination. Other factors that may affect the velocities in the pulmonary veins are high cardiac output and decreased compliance of the left ventricle.[74] Criteria for anastomosis revision are venous diameter less than 0.5 cm and pulmonary venous flow peak velocity greater than 1 m/s with blunted flow pattern.[75]

Postoperative Pain Control

Optimal pain regimen after lung transplantation is difficult to standardize in the presence of three different surgical approaches: (1) anterolateral thoracotomy, (2) clamshell incision, and (3) sternotomy. Thoracic epidural analgesia has been established

A　　　　　　　　　　**B**

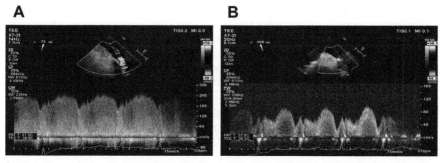

Fig. 3. Intraoperative transesophageal echocardiographic images demonstrating interrogation of the left upper pulmonary vein with spectral Doppler in a patient after bilateral lung transplantation. (*A*) Continuous-wave Doppler in addition to color flow Doppler interrogation of the left upper pulmonary vein after lung transplantation. Note the blunted flow pattern and the absence of distinguished waveforms. Because of the high velocities in the pulmonary vein, a continuous-wave Doppler was applied as opposed to pulse-wave Doppler. Peak velocity greater than 1.0 m/s and blunted flow pattern are pathognomonic for pulmonary venous flow obstruction. (*B*) Pulse-wave Doppler interrogation of the left upper pulmonary vein after release of the obstruction. Note the restoration of the normal phasic flow pattern along with normal velocity on spectral Doppler. Color flow Doppler demonstrates laminar flow in the left upper pulmonary vein.

as the gold standard for postoperative pain management following thoracotomy or clamshell approach,[76] and has proven efficacious and well tolerated after lung transplantation.[77] Preoperative placement of an epidural catheter has disadvantages, such as a possibility of surgery cancellation, time constraint at the beginning of surgery, unplanned use of CPB and associated coagulopathy, and prolonged need for mechanical ventilation postoperatively. Epidural catheter may be considered before tracheal extubation; however, performing the procedure in an intubated and sedated patient carries additional risks.

There are two new regional techniques gaining popularity after thoracotomy for nontransplant surgery, which have been anecdotally used in patients after lung transplantation. Serratus anterior plane block[78,79] and erector spinae plane block[80] are chest wall blocks performed under ultrasound guidance, delivered as single shot or catheter-based continuous analgesia. These techniques are performed any time after surgery in awake or sedated patients, independent of their coagulation status. The feasibility of the chest wall blocks after lung transplantation is to be determined. The use of multimodal analgesia regimen is advisable, combining regional techniques with nonopioid agents and early transition to oral medications.

Postoperative Delirium

Incidence of postoperative delirium after lung transplantation is 29% to 40%. Obesity (body mass index, >30), use of benzodiazepines, CPB, and bilateral transplantation have been associated with postoperative delirium.[81] Prophylactic measures include avoidance of benzodiazepines, daily reorientation, early rehabilitation, and use of antipsychotics. Idiopathic hyperammonemia after lung transplantation has a similar presentation and is easily mistaken for typical ICU delirium. It is uncommon but portends worse prognosis. Diagnosis is usually established by elevated serum ammonia level postoperatively. It may be a result of infection from urea splitting organisms that need to be identified and treated.[82]

Postoperative Gastroparesis and Gastroesophageal Reflux

Gastrointestinal complications occur frequently after lung transplantation, with gastroesophageal reflux disorder and gastroparesis being the most common. They are common in end-stage lung disease[83] and are exacerbated by vagus nerve injury and immunosuppression after surgery. Gastroesophageal reflux disease presents with a variety of clinical symptoms in these patients, such as early satiety, delayed gastric emptying, nausea, anorexia, and vomiting.[84] In most cases, spontaneous recovery is observed with supportive treatment, including prokinetics and total parenteral nutrition. A small number of patients require surgical treatment with fundoplication, which has been shown to have protective effect against development of bronchiolitis obliterans syndrome.[85]

PERIOPERATIVE CONSIDERATIONS IN PATIENTS WITH DIFFERENT UNDERLYING DISEASE PRESENTING FOR LUNG TRANSPLANTATION

There are unique perioperative challenges pertinent to different causes of end-stage lung disease, requiring specific clinical management. The indications for lung transplantation are grouped into several categories depending on the underlying lung pathology: obstructive (chronic obstructive pulmonary disease), suppurative (cystic fibrosis), interstitial (idiopathic pulmonary fibrosis), and vascular (primary pulmonary arterial hypertension) (**Table 3**).

Table 3
Unique challenges in the perioperative management for different underlying lung disease processes and proposed treatment strategies

Lung Disease	Perioperative Considerations	Management Strategies
Chronic obstructive lung disease	• Risk of pneumothorax • Dynamic hyperinflation • Unequal distribution of the alveolar ventilation in single-lung transplantation • Lower risk for PGD • Significant $Etco_2/Paco_2$ gradient caused by increased dead space	• Allow for long expiration time (I:E 1:2.5 or 1:3.0) • Low extrinsic PEEP • Ensure muscle paralysis • Administer bronchodilators before induction • Consider split-lung ventilation in severe cases • Continue to treat the native lung
Idiopathic pulmonary fibrosis	• Often pulmonary hypertension • Poor tolerance to one-lung ventilation	• Apply prolonged inspiratory time (I:E 1:1) • Lungs have low recruitment potential, applying high PEEP does not provide benefit, but does increase the airway pressures • Continue to treat the native lung (lung protective ventilation)
Cystic fibrosis	• Chronic respiratory acidosis • Recurrent infections with multidrug resistant organisms • Thick bronchial secretions • Risk for bleeding during surgical dissection • Previous thoracic procedures • Malnutrition • Diabetes mellitus • Chronic liver disease	• Intubation with large endotracheal tube for tracheobronchial toilet, which increases the tolerance to one-lung ventilation • Diluted betadine irrigation of the tracheobronchial tree • Perioperative antibiotic coverage according to the recipient antibiograms • Plan for early nutrition
Primary pulmonary arterial hypertension	• Severe pulmonary arterial hypertension and RV dysfunction • At high risk for cardiopulmonary collapse during induction in general anesthesia and positive pressure ventilation • High risk for PGD and prolonged intubation after lung transplantation • Presence of systolic heart failure is an indication for heart-lung transplantation	• Judicious induction of anesthesia and slow transition of spontaneous breathing to positive pressure ventilation • Avoid prolonged period of apnea, which precipitates RV failure • Plan early for preinduction inotropic support and RV afterload reduction • CPB indicated in the setting of severe pulmonary arterial hypertension • Optimize modifiable factors of pulmonary vascular resistance, such as oxygenation, ventilation, and acid base balance

Abbreviations: $Etco_2$, end tidal carbon dioxide level; I:E, inspiratory to expiratory time; $Paco_2$, partial arterial carbon dioxide pressure; PEEP, positive end-expiratory pressure.
   Data from Refs.[86–88]

GAPS OF KNOWLEDGE AND FUTURE DIRECTIONS IN THE PERIOPERATIVE CARE OF THE LUNG TRANSPLANT PATIENT

Identifying the presence of modifiable perioperative risk factors for PGD may help to apply certain measures early after lung transplantation. Tidal volumes, role of postimplantation ECMO, early rehabilitation, and prophylaxis of delirium are all important aspects of perioperative care lung transplant recipients. There are only a few studies addressing the appropriate ventilatory modality after lung transplantation, and the current practice is heavily influenced by the literature accumulated in ARDS. The optimal hemoglobin level and transfusion threshold have not been established. VV ECMO has shown a growing role in the perioperative management of lung transplant patients, but its role intraoperatively is yet to be established in large prospective trials. High-volume fluid administration is likely detrimental and presents a modifiable risk factor for development of PGD; however, there are no controlled studies to evaluate the magnitude of this presumed effect. Future experience will show the applications and feasibility of the chest wall blocks for postoperative pain control after lung transplantation, which may replace the thoracic epidural analgesia, because of their simplicity, efficacy, and safety.

REFERENCES

1. Christie J, Carby M, Bag R, et al. Report of the ISHLT working group on primary graft dysfunction part II: definition. A consensus statement of the International Society for Heart and Lung Transplantation. J Heart Lung Transplant 2005;24(10): 1454–9.
2. Oto T, Levvey B, Snell G, et al. Potential refinements of the International Society for Heart and Lung Transplantation primary graft dysfunction grading system. J Heart Lung Transplant 2007;26:435.
3. Lee J, Christie J. Primary graft dysfunction. Clin Chest Med 2011;32:279–93.
4. Snell G, Yusen R, Weill D, et al. Report of the ISHLT working group on primary graft dysfunction, part I: definition and grading – a 2016 consensus group statement of the International Society of Heart and Lung Transplantation. J Heart Lung Transplant 2017;36(10):1097–103.
5. Tejwani V, Panchabhai T, Kotloff R, et al. Complications of lung transplantation, a roentgenographic perspective. CHEST 2016;149(6):1535–45.
6. Prekker M, Nath D, Walker A, et al. Validation of the proposed International Society for Heart and Lung Transplantation grading system for primary graft dysfunction after lung transplantation. J Heart Lung Transplant 2006;25(4):371–8.
7. Prekker M, Herrington C, Hertz M, et al. Early trends in PaO2/fraction of inspired oxygen ratio predict outcome in lung transplant recipients with severe primary graft dysfunction. Chest 2007;132(3):991–7.
8. Diamond J, Lee J, Kawut S, et al, Lung Transplant Outcomes Group. Clinical risk factors for primary graft dysfunction after lung transplantation. Am J Respir Crit Care Med 2013;187:527–34.
9. Arcasoy S, Fisher A, Hachem R, et al. Report of the ISHLT working group on primary graft dysfunction part V: predictors and outcomes. J Heart Lung Transplant 2005;24(10):1451–3.
10. Christie J, Bellamy S, Ware L, et al. Construct validity of the definition of primary graft dysfunction after lung transplantation. J Heart Lung Transpl 2010;29: 1231–9.

11. Daud S, Yusen R, Meyers B, et al. Impact of immediate primary lung allograft dysfunction on bronchiolitis obliterans syndrome. Am J Respir Crit Care Med 2007;175(5):507–13.

12. Huang H, Yusen R, Meyers B, et al. Late primary graft dysfunction after lung transplantation and bronchiolitis obliterans syndrome. Am J Transplant 2008; 8(11):2454–62.

13. Gelman A, Fisher A, Huang H, et al. Report of the ISHLT working group on primary graft dysfunction part III: Mechanisms. A 2016 consensus group statement of the International Society of Heart and Lung Transplantation. J Heart Lung Transpl 2017;36(10):1115–20.

14. Weissa S, Kotschb K, Francuskia M, et al. Brain death activates donor organs and is associated worse ischemia reperfusion injury after liver transplantation. Am J Transplant 2007;7:1584–93.

15. Avlonitis V, Wigfiels C, Golledge H, et al. Early hemodynamic injury during donor brain death determines severity of primary graft dysfunction after lung transplantation. Am J Transplant 2007;7:83–90.

16. Diamnod J, Wigfield C. Role of innate immunity in primary graft dysfunction after lung transplantation. Curr Opin Organ Transplant 2013;18:518–23.

17. Fiser S, Tribble C, Long S, et al. Pulmonary macrophages are involved in reperfusion injury after lung transplantation. Ann Thorac Surg 2001;71(4):1134–8.

18. Porteous M, Diamond J, Christie J. Primary graft dysfunction: lessons learned about the first 72h after lung transplantation. Curr Opin Organ Transplant 2015; 20:506–14.

19. Shah R, Diamond J, Cantu E, et al. Objective estimates improve risk stratification for primary graft dysfunction after lung transplantation. Am J Transplant 2015; 15(8):2188–96.

20. Christie J, Kotloff R, Pochettino A, et al. Clinical risk factors for primary graft failure following lung transplantation. Chest 2003;124:1232–41.

21. Perrot M, Bonser R, Dark J, et al, ISHLT Working Group on Primary Lung Graft Dysfunction. Report of the ISHLT working group on primary lung graft dysfunction part III: donor-related risk factors and markers. J Heart Lung Transpl 2005;24: 1460–7.

22. Whitson BA, Nath DS, Johnson AC, et al. Risk factors for primary graft dysfunction after lung transplantation. J Thorac Cardiovasc Surg 2006;131:73–80.

23. Kuntz C, Hadjiliadis D, Ahya V, et al. Risk factors for early primary graft dysfunction after lung transplantation: a registry study. Clin Transplant 2009;23:819–30.

24. Fang A, Stunder S, Kawut S, et al, Lung Transplant Outcome Group. Elevated pulmonary artery pressure is a risk factor for primary graft dysfunction following lung transplantation for idiopathic pulmonary fibrosis. Chest 2011;139(4):782–7.

25. Liu Y, Liu Y, Su L, et al. Recipient-related clinical risk factors for primary graft dysfunction after lung transplantation. A systemic review and meta-analysis. PLos One 2014;9(3):e92773.

26. Raemdonck D, Matthew H, Hertz M, et al. Report of the ISHLT working group on primary graft dysfunction part IV: prevention and treatment: a 2016 consensus group statement of the International Society for Heart and Lung Transplantation. J Heart Lung Transpl 2017;36(10):1121–36.

27. Currey J, Pilcher D, Davies A, et al. Implementation of a management guideline aimed at minimizing the severity of primary graft dysfunction after lung transplant. J Thorac Cardiovasc Surg 2010;139:154–61.

28. Shargall Y, Guenther G, Ahya V, et al. Report of the ISHLT working group on primary lung graft dysfunction part VI: treatment. J Heart Lung Transpl 2005;24(10): 1489–500.

29. Kawut S. Lung retransplantation. Clin Chest Med 2011;32:367–77.

30. Fan E, Brodie D, Slutsky A. Acute respiratory distress syndrome. Advances in diagnosis and treatment. JAMA 2018;319(7):698–710.

31. Barnes L, Reed R, Parekh K, et al. Mechanical ventilation for the lung transplant recipient. Curr Pulmonol Rep 2015;4(2):88–96.

32. De Perrot M, Imai Y, Volgyesi G, et al. Effect of ventilator, induced lung injury on the development of reperfusion injury in a rat lung transplant Model. J Thorac Cardiovasc Surg 2002;124:1137–44.

33. Beer A, Reed R, Bolukbas, et al. Mechanical ventilation after lung transplantation. An international survey of practices and preferences. Ann Am Thorac Soc 2014; 11:546–53.

34. Eberlein M, Reed R, Bolukbas S, et al. Lung size mismatch and primary graft dysfunction after bilateral lung transplantation. J Heart Lung Transpl 2015;34: 233–40.

35. Dezube R, Arnaoutakis G, Reed R, et al. The effect of lung-size mismatch on mechanical ventilation tidal volumes after bilateral lung transplantation. Interact Cardiovas Thorac Surg 2013;16:275–81.

36. Christie J, Edwards L, Kucheryavaya A, et al. The registry of the International Society of Heart and Lung Transplantation: twenty-seventh official adult lung and heart-lung transplant report—2010. J Heart Lung Transpl 2010;29(10):1104–18.

37. Fuehner T, Kuehn C, Welte T, et al. ICU care before and after lung transplantation. Chest 2016;150(2):442–50.

38. Castillo M. Anesthetic management for lung transplantation. Curr Opin Anesthesiol 2011;24:32–6.

39. Kato T, Armstrong H, Schulze C, et al. Left and right ventricular functional dynamics determined by echocardiograms before and after lung transplantation. Am J Cardiol 2015;116(4):652–9.

40. Gorter T, Verschuuren E, van Veldhuisen D, et al. Right ventricular recovery after bilateral lung transplantation for pulmonary arterial hypertension. Interact Cardiovasc Thorac Surg 2017;24:890–7.

41. Kusunose K, Tsutsui R, Bhatt K, et al. Prognostic value of RV function before and after lung transplantation. JACC Cardiovasc Imaging 2014;7(11):1084–94.

42. Nagendran M, Maruthappu M, Sugand K. Should double lung transplant be performed with or without cardiopulmonary bypass? Interactive Cardiovasc Thorac Surg 2012;12:799–805.

43. Wang Y, Kurichi J, Blumenthal N, et al. Multiple variables affecting blood usage in lung transplantation. J Heart Lung Transpl 2006;25:533–8.

44. Sabashnikov M, Garcia-Saez D, Zych B, et al. The role of cardiopulmonary bypass in lung transplantation. Clin Transplant 2015;30:202–9.

45. Burdett C, Butt T, Lordan J, et al. Comparison of single lung transplant with and without the use of cardiopulmonary bypass. Interactive Cardiovasc Thorac Surg 2012;15:432–6.

46. Nazarnia S, Subramaniam K. Pro: veno-arterial extracorporeal membrane oxygenation (ECMO) should be used routinely for bilateral lung transplantation. J Cardiothorac Vasc Anesth 2017;31:1505–8.

47. Machuca T, Collaud S, Mercier O, et al. Outcomes of intraoperative extracorporeal membrane oxygenation versus cardiopulmonary bypass for lung transplantation. J Thorac Cardiovasc Surg 2015;149:1152–7.

48. Biscotti M, Yang J, Sonett J, et al. Comparison of extracorporeal membrane oxygenation versus cardiopulmonary bypass for lung transplantation. J Thorac Cardiovasc Surg 2014;148:2410–6.
49. Hoechter D, von Dossow V, Winter H, et al. The Munich Lung Transplant Group: intraoperative extracorporeal circulation in lung transplantation. Thorac Cardiovasc Surg 2015;63:706–14.
50. Ius F, Kuehn C, Tudorache I, et al. Lung transplantation on cardiopulmonary support: venoarterial extracorporeal membrane oxygenation outperformed cardiopulmonary bypass. J Thorac Cardiovasc Surg 2012;144:1510–6.
51. Bermudez C, Shiose A, Esper S, et al. Outcomes of intraoperative venoarterial extracorporeal membrane oxygenation versus cardiopulmonary bypass during lung transplantation. Ann Thorac Surg 2014;98:1936–43.
52. Ardehali A, Laks H, Levine M, et al. A prospective trial of inhaled nitric oxide in clinical lung transplantation. Transplantation 2001;72:112–5.
53. Moreno I, Vicente A, Leon M, et al. Effects of inhaled nitric oxide on primary graft dysfunction in lung transplantation. Transplant Proc 2009;41:2210–2.
54. Yerebaken C, Ugurlucan M, Bayraktar S, et al. Effects of inhaled nitric oxide following lung transplantation. J Card Surg 2009;24:269–74.
55. Kurose I, Wolf R, Grisham M, et al. Modulation of ischemia/reperfusion-induced microvascular dysfunction by nitric oxide. Circ Res 1994;74:376–82.
56. Bhabra M, Hopkinson D, Shaw T, et al. Low-dose nitric oxide inhalation during the initial reperfusion enhances rat lung graft function. Ann Thorac Surg 1997;63: 339–44.
57. Moreno I, Mir A, Vicente R, et al. Analysis of interleukin-6 and interleukin-8 in lung transplantation: correlation with nitric oxide administration. Transplant Proc 2008; 40:3082.
58. Meade M, Granton J, Matte-Martyn A, et al, the Toronto Lung Transplant Program. A randomized trial of inhaled nitric oxide to prevent ischemia-reperfusion injury after lung transplantation. Am J Respir Crit Care Med 2003;167:1483–9.
59. Botha P, Jeyakanthan M, Rao J, et al. Inhaled nitric oxide for modulation of ischemia-reperfusion injury in lung transplantation. J Heart Lung Transpl 2007; 26:1199.
60. Perrin G, Roch A, Michelet P, et al. Inhaled nitric oxide does not prevent pulmonary edema after lung transplantation measured by lung water content: a randomized clinical study. Chest 2006;129:1024–30.
61. Tavare A, Tsakok T. Does prophylactic inhaled nitric oxide reduce morbidity and mortality after lung transplantation? Interactive Cardiovasc Thorac Surg 2011;13: 516–20.
62. Pasero D, Martin E, Davi A, et al. The effect of inhaled nitric oxide after lung transplantation. Minerva Anesthesiol 2010;76:353–61.
63. Khan T, Schnickel G, Ross D, et al. A prospective, randomized, crossover pilot study of inhaled nitric oxide versus inhaled prostacyclin in heart transplant and lung transplant recipients. J Thorac Cardiovasc Surg 2009;138:1417–24.
64. Ware L, Golden J, Finkbeiner W, et al. Alveolar epithelial fluid transport capacity in reperfusion lung injury after lung transplantation. Am J Respir Crit Care Med 1999;159:980–8.
65. Sugita M, Ferraro P, Dagenais A, et al. Alveolar liquid clearance and sodium channel expression are decreased in transplanted canine lungs. Am J Respir Crit Care Med 2003;167:1440–50.

66. Pilcher D, Scheinkestel C, Snell G, et al. High central venous pressure is associated with prolonged mechanical ventilation and increased mortality after lung transplantation. J Thorac Cardiovasc Surg 2005;129:912–8.

67. McLlroy D, Pilcher D, Snell G. Does anesthetic management affect early outcomes after lung transplant? An exploratory analysis. Br J Anaesth 2009;102:506–14.

68. Geube M, Perz-Protto S, McGrath T, et al. Increased intraoperative fluid administration is associated with severe primary graft dysfunction after lung transplantation. Anesth Analg 2016;122:1081–8.

69. Sano Y, Oto T, Toyooka S, et al. Phrenic nerve paralysis following lung transplantation. Kyobu Geka 2007;60:993–7.

70. Ferdinande P, Bruyninckx F, van Raemdonck D, et al. Phrenic nerve dysfunction after heart-lung and lung transplantation. J Heart Lung Transpl 2004;23(1):105.

71. Maziak D, Maurer J, Kesten S. Diapgragmatic paralysis: a complication of lung transplantation. Ann Thorac Surg 1996;61(1):170.

72. Shigemura N, Orhan Y, Bhama J, et al. Delayed chest closure after lung transplantation: techniques, outcomes, and strategies. J Heart Lung Transpl 2014;33:741–8.

73. Potestio C, Jordan D, Kachulis B. Acute postoperative management after lung transplantation. Best Pract Res Clin Anesthesiol 2017;31:273–84.

74. Gonzalez-Fernandez C, Gonzalez-Castro A, Rodriguez-Borregan J, et al. Pulmonary venous obstruction after lung transplantation. Diagnostic advantages of transesophageal echocardiography. Clin Transplant 2009;23:975–80.

75. Schulman L, Anandarangam T, Leibowitz D, et al. Four-year prospective study of pulmonary venous thrombosis after lung transplantation. J AM Soc Echocardiogr 2001;14:806.

76. Feltracco S, Barbieri S, Milevoj M, et al. Thoracic epidural analgesia in lung transplantation. Transplant Proc 2010;42:1265–9.

77. Cason M, Naik A, Grimm J, et al. The efficacy and safety of epidural based analgesia in a case series of patients undergoing lung transplantation. J Cardiothorac Vasc Anesth 2014;29(1):126–32.

78. Blanco R, Parras T, McDonnell J, et al. Serratus plane block: a novel ultrasound-guided thoracic wall nerve block. Anaesthesia 2013;68:1107–13.

79. Bossolasco M, Bernardi E, Fenoglio L. Continuous serratus plane block in a patient with multiple rib fractures. J Clin Anesth 2017;38:85–6.

80. Forero M, Adhikary S, Lopez H, et al. The errector spinae plane block. A novel analgesic technique in thoracic neuropathic pain. Reg Anesth Pain Med 2016;41:1–7.

81. Anderson B, Chelsey C, Theodore M, et al. Incidence, risk factors, and clinical implications of post-operative delirium in lung transplant recipients. J Heart Lung Transpl 2018;37(6):755–62.

82. Chen C, Bain K, Iuppa J, et al. Hyperammonemia syndrome after lung transplantation: a single center experience. Transplantation 2016;100(3):678–84.

83. D'Ovidio F, Singer LG, Hadjiliadis D, et al. Prevalence of gastroesophageal reflux in end-stage lung disease candidates for lung transplant. Ann Thorac Surg 2005;80(4):1254–60.

84. Leal S, Sacanell J, Riera J, et al. Early postoperative management of lung transplantation. Minerva Anestesiol 2014;80:1234–45.

85. Biswas R, Elnahas S, Serrone R, et al. Early fundoplication is associated with slower decline in lung function after lung transplantation in patients with gastroesophageal reflux disease. J Thorac Cardiovasc Surg 2018;155(6):2762–71.e1.

86. Nicoara A, Anderson-Dam J. Anesthesia for lung transplantation. Anesthesiol Clin 2017;35:473–89.
87. Lee J, Hadjiliadis D, Aahya V, et al. Risk factors for early vs late primary graft dysfunction. Am J Respir Crit Care Med 2008;177:A396.
88. Morrell M, Pilewski J. Lung transplantation for cystic fibrosis. Clin Chest Med 2016;37:127–38.

Perioperative Management of the Cardiac Transplant Recipient

Joseph Rabin, MD[a], David J. Kaczorowski, MD[b],*

KEYWORDS

- Heart transplant • Perioperative management • Primary graft dysfunction
- Extracorporeal membrane oxygenation • Ventricular assist device
- Mechanical circulatory support

KEY POINTS

- Achieving desired outcomes after cardiac transplantation requires meticulous attention to optimizing hemodynamics through careful titration of inotropes and vasopressors as well as management of the patient's volume status.
- The right ventricular function of the transplanted heart must be carefully monitored and managed, particularly in the setting of recipient pulmonary hypertension.
- Arrhythmias, bleeding and coagulopathy, renal dysfunction, and vasoplegia may be encountered and special considerations are necessary in this setting of cardiac transplantation.
- Primary graft dysfunction is a problematic complication that may occur after cardiac transplantation, and mechanical circulatory support or other measures may be required for successful management of the patient in this scenario.

INTRODUCTION

Immediately following completion of a heart transplant, the patient is transferred to the cardiac surgery intensive care unit (CSICU) for continuous monitoring and recovery from the operation. Although many of the initial postoperative considerations apply universally to all patients who have undergone cardiac surgery, some potential complications and necessary interventions are unique to cardiac transplant patients. Hemodynamic lability in the early postoperative period is common after cardiac surgery and is often multifactorial. A patient's preload, afterload, and contractility need

[a] R Adams Cowley Shock Trauma Center, University of Maryland School of Medicine, 22 South Greene Street, Baltimore, MD 21201, USA; [b] Division of Cardiac Surgery, Department of Surgery, University of Maryland School of Medicine, 110 South Paca Street, 7th Floor, Baltimore, MD 21201, USA
* Corresponding author.
E-mail address: Dkaczorowski@som.umaryland.edu

Crit Care Clin 35 (2019) 45–60
https://doi.org/10.1016/j.ccc.2018.08.008
0749-0704/19/© 2018 Elsevier Inc. All rights reserved.

criticalcare.theclinics.com

to be optimized to achieve ideal cardiac performance and cardiac output. Achieving ideal cardiac performance will often require fluid resuscitation to optimize the preload, inotropes to support the contractility and function of a labile myocardium, and finally, vasopressors to raise afterload and support the mean arterial pressure (MAP) in the setting of vasodilatation. In addition to these considerations, primary graft dysfunction (PGD) can be a catastrophic complication after cardiac transplantation, and mechanical circulatory support may be required to support the patient. This review highlights some of the perioperative management strategies that can be used to help manage the cardiac transplant patient population.

HEMODYNAMIC MONITORING

Patients arrive to the CSICU from the operating room intubated and with multiple modalities for continuous hemodynamic monitoring based on the guidelines published by the International Society for Heart and Lung Transplant (ISHLT).[1] Such monitoring devices include an arterial line for continuous blood pressure monitoring and a Swan Ganz pulmonary artery (PA) catheter to monitor PA pressures, central venous pressure (CVP), and cardiac output. As with other cardiac surgery patients, chest tubes are placed to drain residual blood and monitor for postoperative hemorrhage. Other noninvasive monitors include a continuous electrocardiographic monitoring of heart rate and rhythm, oxygen saturation, end tidal carbon dioxide (CO_2), and urine output with a Foley catheter. Such real-time data enable the critical care physician to accurately assess a patient's hemodynamic and physiologic condition and provide the capability to quickly detect physiologic derangements at the earliest possible time.

It is common for newly transplanted hearts to require vasoactive support[2] in the early postoperative period, and the ISHLT guidelines suggest using inotropic support (**Table 1**) over the first few days to support the newly implanted heart and slowly wean the support over the following few days as the patient recovers.[1] There are various causes of early hemodynamic compromise, including bleeding, primary and secondary graft dysfunction, arrhythmia, vasoplegia, pulmonary hypertension, and a systemic inflammatory response or SIRS. There are also 3 critical variables that impact a patient's hemodynamic status and include the volume status or preload, the resistance or afterload, and the contractility or efficiency of the heart.[3] Later in a patient's recovery, other complications can adversely impact the hemodynamics, including respiratory failure, renal failure, fluid overload, and infection.

COAGULOPATHY, BLEEDING, AND PRODUCT ADMINISTRATION

Bleeding can have a deleterious impact on all the variables that contribute to cardiac function and simultaneously result in a decreased preload, increased afterload, and compromised contractility. Bleeding is often identified from high chest tube output and may be the result of a coagulopathy due to prolonged cardiopulmonary bypass, preoperative anticoagulation and antiplatelet medication, hypothermia, incomplete heparin reversal, or from a surgical source.[4] Management often involves the transfusion of blood and blood products to replace the blood loss, to correct coagulopathies and acidosis, and for careful assessment for the potential of development of tamponade. This diagnosis should always be considered especially when confronted with low cardiac output.[5] Many institutions have bleeding management guidelines that outline the routine for transfusion of blood and products by the intensive care unit team while simultaneously discussing the potential for mediastinal reexploration with the surgical team. At the authors' institution, more than 300 mL of bleeding within the first hour requires immediate intervention that includes platelet transfusion

Table 1
Vasoactive medications commonly used to support the cardiac transplant recipient

	Mechanism	Primary Effects	Limitations
Inotropic agents			
Epinephrine	β-Agonist with α effects at higher doses	Improves CO via ↑ contractility and HR α-Agonist at higher dose also ↑ BP	Tachycardia and arrhythmias Associated with metabolic acidosis
Isoproterenol	β-Agonist	Improves CO via ↑ contractility and HR Also reduces PVR helping RV function	Arrhythmias and tachycardia Associated with ↑ O_2 demand
Milrinone	Phosphodiesterase III inhibitor	Improves CO via ↓ afterload (SVR & PVR) from ↑ cAMP and small ↑ contractility	Hypotension
Dobutamine	Pure β-agonist	Improves CO via ↑ contractility and HR	Tachycardia (> epi) and arrhythmias
Vasopressor agents			
Norepinephrine	α-Agonist with β effects	Increases BP and SVR	↑ SVR may compromise visceral perfusion
Vasopressin	Acts on vasomotor V_1 and renal V_2 receptors	Increase BP in patients with vasoplegia	↑ Intestinal vasoconstriction may compromise visceral perfusion/ischemic bowel
Dopamine	β- and α-agonist at higher doses	↑ Contractility, HR, SVR, and BP	Tachycardia and arrhythmias
Phenylephrine	Pure α-agonist	Increases SVR and BP	Has no cardiac support and ↑ SVR may compromise visceral perfusion

Abbreviations: BP, blood pressure; cAMP, cyclic adenosine monophosphate; CO, cardiac output; HR, heart rate; PVR, pulmonary vascular resistance; SVR, systemic vascular resistance.

followed by fresh frozen plasma and blood if bleeding continues at a high rate. Transfusion goals are for international normalized ratio less than 1.8, platelets greater than 100, and hemoglobin greater than 8.0, while actively optimizing the patient's temperature, controlling agitation, and correcting acidosis. To mitigate the potential of developing postoperative tamponade in patients who are coagulopathic, these patients may intentionally be left with an open chest, packed, taken to the CSICU, and brought back for delayed closure once the coagulopathy has been corrected.[6]

Patients with low cardiac output and postoperative bleeding that is persistent or recently corrected must be ruled out for cardiac tamponade. Tamponade, especially in the early postoperative period, may have a nonspecific presentation and should be suspected in situations involving decompensating hemodynamics and low cardiac output requiring increasing vasopressor support.[7] Although a transthoracic echocardiogram (TTE) may demonstrate the presence of an effusion and resulting tamponade, it may not be able to identify posterior or isolated collections. Therefore, even with a negative TTE, tamponade remains a clinical diagnosis that warrants a low threshold for mediastinal reexploration in the appropriate clinical setting or at least further evaluation with a transesophageal echocardiogram.[8]

Fluid administration or fluid resuscitation is often necessary in the early postoperative period.[4,9] Nevertheless, it is important to identify the underlying cause of such fluid requirements because continued fluid requirements are often an indication of other critical conditions for which alternative treatment strategies may be indicated, such as hemorrhage, cardiac dysfunction, pneumothorax, or tamponade. Excessive volume administration after ideal filling pressures have been achieved may ultimately be counterproductive, as described by the Starling curve, and result in right ventricular (RV) distension and iatrogenic RV failure, further complicating the hemodynamics.[10]

VASOPLEGIA

Vasoplegia is a condition of hypotension secondary to severe vasodilation that often leads to inadequate end-organ perfusion or shock requiring significant vasopressor support. Despite the severe hypotension, the cardiac output is characteristically normal or hyperdynamic. The cause of this shock state is uncertain but thought to be associated with an inflammatory response to the operation and/or cardiopulmonary bypass support that leads to loss of vascular tone and exceptionally low systemic vascular resistance, ultimately resulting in high vasopressor requirements.[5,11,12] Risk factors for development of post–heart transplant vasoplegia have been reported to include higher body surface area and body mass index, history of thyroid disease, prior cardiac surgery and mechanical support, and longer cardiopulmonary bypass time and ischemic time.[11] Treatment involves titrating infusions of vasopressors (see **Table 1**) to improve vascular tone and restore an adequate perfusion pressure often targeting a minimal MAP of 65 to 70 mm Hg. Catecholamines are an essential class of such medications that act on α-1 adrenergic receptors to stimulate vascular smooth muscle contraction and subsequent vessel constriction. Vasoactive medications include norepinephrine, phenylephrine, epinephrine, and dopamine. Although there is no clear evidence that one is any better than another, dopamine has been associated with the development of arrhythmias and is rarely a first-line agent.[12–14] Phenylephrine lacks any β or inotropic affect and was shown to be associated with a significant decrease in internal mammary artery graft flow when compared with norepinephrine after coronary artery bypass surgery.[15] In this context and without other evidence that demonstrates improved outcomes, phenylephrine is not routinely used at the authors' institution in this setting. Rather, norepinephrine is the first-line catecholamine that is infused,[5] whereas epinephrine is primarily used for directed inotropic support. Although norepinephrine has been shown not to cause hyperlactatemia after cardiac surgery, it also has been shown to be associated with a reduced mortality in patients with septic shock, making it a first-line agent in that setting.[13,14]

Other options for treating vasoplegia include vasopressin and methylene blue. Vasopressin is a noncatecholamine that binds to other receptors, including the arginine vasopressin receptor, oxytocin receptor, and purinergic receptor.[14,16] Administration of this agent has been shown to reduce the need for catecholamine infusions and may also help in the context of vasopressin deficiency after cardiopulmonary bypass.[13,14,16] Although there is inadequate evidence to conclusively determine whether vasopressin should or should not be used as a first-line agent for vasoplegia, a recent study does appear to suggest that there may be some outcomes benefit when used early.[16] However, vasopressin must be used with care because high doses have been associated with mesenteric ischemia.[5,12] Finally, methylene blue has been shown to reduce the vasopressor requirements in patients with vasoplegia and also shown to reverse this condition in a heart transplant patient. These observations suggests that methylene blue may also be considered as an additional agent that can be administered early in the management of vasoplegia, whereas its exact indication and timing remain ambiguous based on the current, limited existing data.[12–14,17,18]

INOTROPIC AND CHRONOTROPIC SUPPORT

Myocardial function after heart transplantation is often labile, and the ISHLT guidelines recommend administration of continuous inotropic support (see **Table 1**) during the perioperative and early postoperative period.[1] Low cardiac output and myocardial dysfunction are frequently encountered after cardiac surgery in general and are associated with multiple causes, including reperfusion injury, inadequate myocardial protection, inflammatory response, and pulmonary hypertension.[9] These conditions also apply to the heart transplant patient with increased concern for reperfusion injury and inadequate myocardial protection in conjunction with duration of ischemic time.[2,19] Also, donor brain death before procurement of the allograft may impair its function and increase its susceptibility to later insult.[1,19] An additional cause for post-transplant myocardial dysfunction may also be related to the depletion of catecholamines from transplanted human hearts, which is thought to be secondary to its denervation.[20]

In cases of severe left ventricular (LV) dysfunction requiring significant inotropic support, other causes requiring emergent treatment need to also be considered, such as cardiac tamponade and acute rejection. Otherwise, LV dysfunction is frequently managed with infusions of isoproterenol, dobutamine, milrinone, or epinephrine. Isoproterenol has inotropic, chronotropic, and vasodilatory affects, making it an excellent choice especially in patients requiring heart rate support. Milrinone provides inotropic support in addition to afterload reduction and is often used in patients with pulmonary hypertension. Finally, dobutamine, a pure β-agonist and epinephrine providing β and α support, can also be used.[1,2] This inotropic support is often continued for at least 3 to 5 days after transplant and slowly weaned off as the heart recovers.

RIGHT VENTRICULAR FAILURE AND PULMONARY HYPERTENSION

Acute right heart failure is a frequent complication after heart transplant. It may result from the development or worsening of pulmonary hypertension or actual RV failure associated with ischemia, arrhythmias, or PGD.[3,19] Severe RV failure may be a manifestation of PGD.[21] Alternatively, RV dysfunction may also be a physiologic response of a normal right ventricle after it has been implanted into a patient with significant chronic pulmonary hypertension.[22]

Management strategies to treat RV dysfunction and pulmonary hypertension focus on optimizing myocardial perfusion, preload, and contractility while reducing the pulmonary vascular resistance and its resulting RV afterload. Preload optimization is challenging, because excessive preload leads to RV dilation, dysfunction, and failure. Patients are routinely treated with inotropic support to enhance contractility with agents such as epinephrine and isoproterenol, which can also improve chronotropic function. Milrinone is another inotropic agent that also helps reduce afterload and pulmonary hypertension, although its administration may be limited by hypotension and vasopressor requirements. Other medications that have been shown to contribute to pulmonary vasodilation and effectively reduce pulmonary vascular resistance include inhaled nitric oxide and inhaled prostacyclin or epoprostenol (Flolan), which often have a minimal effect on the systemic arterial pressures.[21–23] Inhaled prostacyclin was shown to be easier to administer, to have no risk of met-hemoglobinemia, and to be cheaper than inhaled nitric oxide, making this a potentially preferable option.[23]

Because hypoxia and hypercarbia lead to increased pulmonary vascular resistance, optimal oxygenation and correction of hypoxia and hypercarbia are essential to successful management of pulmonary hypertension and RV dysfunction. Arterial blood gas and end tidal CO_2 monitoring can help direct ventilator changes to insure the patient is not acidotic with optimal oxygenation and ventilation.[4] Finally, in patients with continued RV failure refractory to medical management, early consideration for other mechanical support with a ventricular assist device (VAD) or extracorporeal membrane oxygenation (ECMO) is advised and is discussed in more detail later.[21]

ARRHYTHMIA

Arrhythmias are frequently encountered following cardiac surgery and especially heart transplantation.[4] Ventricular tachycardia (VT) or fibrillation (VF) is the most concerning but least common early posttransplant arrhythmia. Although patients are initially treated with cardioversion for sustained VT or VF, they will often require further workup, including an angiogram to assess the coronary anatomy and an endomyocardial biopsy to rule out rejection.[1,24] Nonsustained VT is more frequent in the early postoperative period and is frequently managed with electrolyte optimization and antiarrhythmic medication. Late-onset VT may be associated with a vasculopathy or severe ventricular dysfunction requiring placement of a defibrillator,[24] whereas other late conduction abnormalities may be due to coronary artery disease.[25]

Bradycardia and supraventricular tachyarrhythmias are more common after heart transplant and likely associated with denervation, ischemic time with related secondary sinus node damage, rejection, electrolyte abnormalities, and myocardial irritability from inflammation or inotropic support.[24,25] Bradycardia and sinus node dysfunction are frequently encountered in the early period after a transplant. Sinus node injury has been shown to be reduced when a bicaval technique, rather a biatrial technique, is used for the transplant. The bicaval technique is associated with lower postoperative pacing requirements and fewer tachyarrhythmias.[26,27] Still, the implantation procedure involves denervation of the allograft. As a result, the newly transplanted heart lacks parasympathetic vagal inputs, leading to an expected heart rate of about 100, whereas heart rates less than 90 are often considered a relative bradycardia. Such relative bradycardia should be treated by temporary atrial pacing between 90 and 110 beats per minute and by starting isoproterenol or theophylline until the return of the appropriate heart rate.[1,3,24]

Atrial fibrillation and atrial flutter are common tachyarrhythmias encountered after heart transplant and other cardiac surgery. Treatment generally involves optimizing electrolytes, particularly potassium and magnesium. Amiodarone may be considered a first-line antiarrhythmic,[1,9,24] although amiodarone must be administered with care especially if cyclosporine is part of the immune suppression regimen, due to its associated drug interactions that increase levels of immune suppression.[24,28] Other agents to consider include sotalol and procainamide. Beta-blockers are commonly used after routine cardiac surgery. However, their use may be limited in the early postoperative period after heart transplant because bradycardia should be avoided and many patients are already being administered inotropic support. Calcium channel blockers also require very judicious consideration because they are associated with negative inotropic affects, which should be avoided after a heart transplant.[1] Calcium channels may also have drug interactions with immunosuppressive medications, leading to tacrolimus and cyclosporine toxicity.[24,28] Atrial fibrillation that occurs beyond 2 weeks after transplant also increases the concern for rejection and LV dysfunction and should be evaluated accordingly.[1,3]

VENTILATOR SUPPORT

Patients typically arrive in the CSICU intubated and on mechanical ventilation. Once the patient is hemodynamically stable with a closed chest, the ventilator should be weaned and the patient extubated as soon as possible. Mechanical ventilation can contribute to increased intrathoracic pressures and subsequent pulmonary hypertension. However, inadequate ventilation can lead to hypercarbia, respiratory acidosis, and increased pulmonary vascular resistance, which can also negatively impact cardiac function. When the patient achieves hemodynamic stability and the ventilator can be weaned, the patient is started on pressure support trials, and diuresis can be considered to remove excess volume.[3,4] Earlier extubation reduces the risk of developing ventilator-associated morbidities, such as ventilator-associated pneumonia and deconditioning.

RENAL AND VOLUME STATUS

Renal function and volume status often serve as indicators of cardiac function, and there appears to be an increased risk of kidney injury once the CVPs are too high for optimal Starling curve cardiac performance. Such elevated right-sided cardiac pressures create an elevated renal venous pressure, which reduces renal perfusion and leads to acute kidney injury (AKI).[1] This relationship emphasizes the careful balance that is necessary in achieving an ideal volume status. Hypovolemia results in poor cardiac performance and AKI due to hypoperfusion, whereas excessive volume loading can lead to both RV dysfunction and AKI secondary to venous congestion. Fluid overload also increases the risk of edema and impaired oxygenation leading to the development of respiratory failure and/or abdominal compartment syndrome.[10]

Strategies to optimize renal function and volume status include maintaining adequate renal perfusion pressure by maintaining an MAP of at least 65 to 70 mm Hg. A combination of fluid, with a goal CVP goal of 5 to 12 mm Hg, to optimize cardiac performance in conjunction with inotropes and vasopressors is frequently used.[1,4,9] In cases of hypervolemia and elevated filling pressures, diuresis and/or renal replacement therapy is initiated to remove volume, reduce right-sided venous congestion, and improve both cardiac and renal function.[1] Finally, careful immune suppression management is essential to prevent AKI due to its nephrotoxic potential. Close monitoring of renal function and levels of immune suppression in conjunction with pharmacy and the multidisciplinary care team is essential for the overall care of the heart transplant patient.

MANAGEMENT OF PRIMARY GRAFT DYSFUNCTION
Definition and Pathogenesis of Primary Graft Dysfunction

A donor cardiac allograft may be subjected to several potential insults around the time of transplant, which may have an adverse impact on its function after transplant. Such potential insults include myocardial injury after donor brain death, ischemia/reperfusion, immunologic injury, and others as well. The disparate potential causes for cardiac allograft dysfunction have made it difficult to define and quantify the incidence of PGD in the past. In 2013, a consensus conference was convened at the annual meeting of the ISHLT. Based on the best available evidence, survey data, and expert opinion, a consensus statement was issued that classified cardiac allograft dysfunction into either PGD or secondary graft dysfunction.[19] In contrast to PGD, secondary graft dysfunction was defined as graft dysfunction whereby a clear discernible cause could be identified. Potential causes of graft dysfunction include problems such as hyperacute rejection, severe recipient pulmonary hypertension, or surgical complications, including uncontrolled bleeding or anastomotic problems. PGD was subclassified into PGD-LV, which includes LV and biventricular dysfunction, and PGD-RV, which includes RV dysfunction in isolation. Furthermore, a severity scale for PGD-LV was defined, with grades including mild, moderate, and severe.

Although the mechanisms that result in PGD are incompletely understood, several factors thought to participate in its pathogenesis have been identified. Brain death has been shown to have adverse effects on myocardial function. Furthermore, the insult to the graft that occurs as a result of both cold and warm ischemia and subsequent reperfusion is clearly a critical component. The inflammatory milieu in the recipient may also be important in the development of PGD. As such, several clinical risk factors for PGD have been identified and have been clearly outlined in the ISHLT consensus statement.[19] These risk factors include factors specific to the donor, recipient risk factors, and procedural risk factors (**Table 2**).

Management

Cardiac allograft dysfunction can be a devastating complication after cardiac transplantation. Potential causes of secondary graft dysfunction, including anastomotic kinking or narrowing, should be sought and eliminated. The initial management of mild or moderate PGD is medical. Inotropic support, ventilator settings, and acid/base status should be optimized. Inhaled nitric oxide or prostaglandins along with a phosphodiesterase inhibitor should be considered, particularly in the setting of RV dysfunction, and are recommended by the ISHLT consensus statement in this setting.[19] If PGD is severe or medical therapy is ineffective, then mechanical support must be considered. Mechanical support may also be useful in cases of secondary graft dysfunction until the underlying cause is sought and corrected.

Mechanical Circulatory Support for Management of Cardiac Allograft Dysfunction

A variety of different mechanical support strategies have been used to support patients with cardiac allograft dysfunction. These strategies range from the use of an intra-aortic balloon pump (IABP) to extracorporeal membrane oxygenation or VADs (**Table 3**). The appropriate mechanical support modality depends on the clinical scenario as well as the degree of graft dysfunction.

Intra-Aortic Balloon Pump

An IABP provides counterpulsation, which may both unload the left ventricle and provide improved coronary perfusion during diastole. An IABP is an attractive first-line

Table 2		
Risk factors for primary graft dysfunction		
Donor Characteristics	**Recipient Characteristics**	**Operative Factors**
Age	Age	Ischemic time
Female donor	Preoperative temporary mechanical	Size mismatch
Cause of death	support	High-volume transfusion
Cardiac dysfunction	LVAD	Emergency transplant
Inotrope requirement	Preoperative mechanical ventilation	Redo heart transplant
Prolonged cardiac arrest	Elevated PVR	Prolonged cardiopulmonary
Trauma	Amiodarone use	bypass
	Recipient CVP >10 mm Hg	Noncardiac organ donation
	Recipient inotrope use	

Data from Refs.[19,54–56]

Table 3
Mechanical circulatory support options for allograft graft dysfunction

Modality	Advantages	Disadvantages
IABP	Easy insertion Image guidance is not mandatory Anticoagulation is not mandatory	Partial hemodynamic support No ability to provide gas exchange Limited data for use in the setting of allograft dysfunction
ECMO	Full hemodynamic support Provides gas exchange May be placed centrally or peripherally	Anticoagulation is generally required May not provide optimal LV unloading Aortic root thrombus or LV thrombus may form if pulsatility is absent
Temporary VAD	May be used in LV, RV, or BiV configurations May provide superior ventricular unloading Percutaneous options are available	Gas exchange may not be possible Percutaneous modalities generally require image guidance Device cost may be higher

Abbreviation: BiV, biventricular.

mode of mechanical support because it is generally fast and easy to insert and requires only small-bore arterial access. It can be inserted either in the operating room or at the bedside. Imaging modalities, such as fluoroscopy or transesophageal echocardiography, may be useful to guide insertion and positioning, but are not mandatory for successful placement. An additional advantage is that anticoagulation is also not mandatory for an IABP, which may be important in the early perioperative period. Although these features are attractive, an IABP may provide only partial hemodynamic support. Furthermore, its ability to support the right ventricle is less clear. Last, an IABP provides no mechanism for oxygenation or carbon dioxide removal, which may be an important consideration if the recipient has significant pulmonary edema.

Traditionally, because of their beneficial effects on coronary perfusion as well as LV unloading, IABPs have been most commonly used in the setting of ischemic coronary disease, including acute myocardial infarction with or without cardiogenic shock and high-risk percutaneous coronary intervention.[29] Despite the potential physiologic benefits of IABPs, there has been substantial controversy over their true clinical benefit.[29–31] Interestingly, single-center retrospective studies have demonstrated benefit in supporting patients with decompensated congestive heart failure with improvement in hemodynamic parameters after IABP insertion.[32,33] Accordingly, other reports have demonstrated that IABPs can be used successfully as a bridge to heart transplantation.[34,35] Although IABPs are used to support patients with allograft dysfunction after heart transplant,[36] there are few data points to guide their use in this setting. Because an IABP can provide only partial hemodynamic support and does not assist with gas exchange, use of an IABP should be reserved for patients with mild degrees of graft dysfunction and without significant pulmonary edema.

Extracorporeal Membrane Oxygenation

In distinction to an IABP, ECMO can provide full hemodynamic support as well as both oxygenation and carbon dioxide removal. For these reasons, ECMO is applicable in the setting of isolated RV or LV failure, biventricular failure, pulmonary failure, or any combination of these. ECMO can be established either centrally or peripherally, and a variety of different cannulation strategies can be used depending on the clinical scenario. Central cannulation can be easily performed in the operating room and generally provides excellent ECMO flows with little risk of limb ischemia. Peripheral cannulation can be performed either in the operating room or at the bedside. A peripheral strategy may expedite definitive chest closure but may carry a more significant risk of limb complications. With either central or peripheral cannulation, anticoagulation is required, which can be problematic in the setting of coagulopathy and bleeding. Anticoagulation is particularly important if the ventricle is so severely impaired that there is little or no ejection of blood during systole. Under these conditions, stagnation of blood in the aortic root and ventricle can result in thrombus formation, which is undesirable and may result in catastrophic complications. Last, although ECMO generally provides excellent flow of oxygenated blood to the organs, it may not unload the left ventricle.[37]

Marasco and colleagues[38] reported on a retrospective cohort of 239 heart transplants at a single center between 2000 and 2009. Of these, 54 patients experienced some degree of PGD, and 39 patients required support with ECMO. The investigators found that 87% of patients were able to be successfully weaned from ECMO, and 74.3% survived to discharge. Survival of the patients who required ECMO was significantly worse compared with patients who did not require ECMO. However, when early deaths in the ECMO group were excluded, long-term survival was similar in both groups, suggesting that if the patient survives the early perioperative period, good long-term survival can be achieved. Of note, there were no significant differences observed in survival of patients who were cannulated centrally versus those who were peripherally cannulated. Complications, including reoperation for bleeding, renal failure, pneumonia, and sepsis, were common in both groups but did not significantly differ based on the cannulation strategy.[38]

In another retrospective single-center study, D'Alessandro and coinvestigators[39] reported outcomes of 54 patients supported with ECMO for PGD after cardiac transplantation. Overall, 50% of these patients survived to discharge. Central cannulation was performed in 26 patients, and 28 patients underwent peripheral cannulation. Survival and complication rates were similar between the groups, except that the peripheral cannulation group had a higher rate of vascular complications. Importantly, although the overall survival of patients with PGD was worse than those who did not suffer PGD, the long-term conditional survival was similar for those salvaged with ECMO compared with the patients who did not have PGD.[39]

Ventricular Assist Devices

By providing both hemodynamic support and gas exchange, ECMO can serve as a very useful means for supporting patients with PGD after cardiac transplantation. However, because of the requirement for anticoagulation and lack of LV unloading associated with ECMO, it may not be ideal for supporting all patients with PGD. Rather, temporary VAD may be preferable in the early perioperative period when coagulopathy is often present and ventricular recovery is desired. Temporary VADs may be used in isolated RV, isolated LV, or biventricular configurations. Generally, temporary left ventricular assist devices (LVADs) do not provide gas exchange, but an oxygenator can be added to the circuit of some devices.

A variety of different temporary VADs are available for clinical use. One commonly used device is the Thoratec CentriMag (Abbott, Abbott Park, IL, USA). This device contains a magnetically levitated impeller and can deliver nearly 10 L of flow per minute (**Fig. 1**A, B). A variety of different cannulation strategies can be used, and it can be used as either a right or left isolated VAD or in a biVAD configuration. A recent review of the literature and meta-analysis found that the CentriMag could be effectively used in a

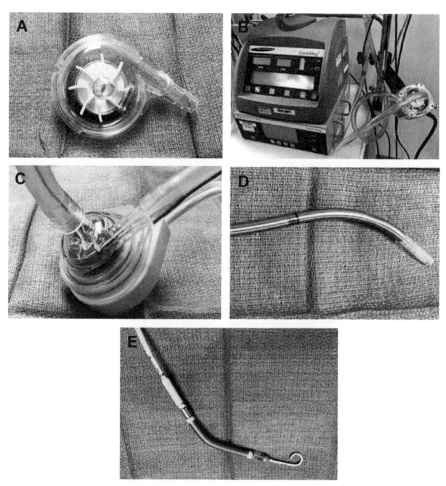

Fig. 1. Temporary left ventricular assist devices. (*A*) CentriMag blood pump featuring a magnetically levitated impeller. (*B*) CentriMag console. (*C*) TandemHeart pump. (*D*) Tandem-Heart transseptal cannula. (*E*) Impella left ventricular assist device.

broad variety of clinical settings.[40] The CentriMag was used in 38 patients with PGD after cardiac transplantation in one study with a 50% 30-day survival.[41] One-year survival in this cohort was only 32% however.[41] Bhama and colleagues[42] reported 60% survival to hospital discharge in heart transplant recipients with either PGD or graft failure due to acute rejection when support with the CentriMag was used.

Another example of a temporary LVAD is the TandemHeart (Tandem Life, Pittsburgh, PA, USA). This system features a transseptal cannula that can be percutaneously placed from the femoral vein into the left atrium with return to the arterial system, thereby providing hemodynamic support with LV decompression (**Fig. 1**C, D). Placement of the transseptal cannula requires image guidance. The TandemHeart has been used as a bridge to recovery in the setting of early acute cellular rejection[43] as well as a bridge to transplantation,[44] but there are few data points on its use in the setting of PGD. Of note, a system featuring a dual lumen cannula that can be percutaneously placed via the right internal jugular vein for isolated RV support is also available. This system has been used for RV support in a variety of different clinical settings, including early RV failure after heart transplant.[45]

The Impella (Abiomed, Danvers, MA, USA) is a small axial flow device that is placed via the femoral or axillary artery, either percutaneously or surgically, and crosses the aortic valve into the left ventricle (**Fig. 1**E). The Impella 5.0 can produce 5 L per minute of flow but generally requires surgical insertion, whereas the Impella CP can be inserted percutaneously but produces lower peak flows. Another version, the Impella RP, is designed to be used as a right ventricular assist device (RVAD). Impellas have been successfully used to support patients with severe acute cardiac allograft rejection[46,47] and early RV dysfunction after heart transplantation.[48]

In a retrospective analysis of 597 heart transplant recipients over an 8-year period, Takeda and colleagues[49] found that 7.4% of these patients developed severe PGD and required mechanical support. The investigators compared outcomes between patients with PGD that were supported with a continuous flow external VAD versus those that were supported with ECMO. Of the patients with severe PGD, hospital survival was better in the group of patients supported with ECMO (81%) compared with those supported with a VAD (59%). Although this finding did not reach statistical significance, patients supported with ECMO required a significantly shorter duration of mechanical support, had significantly less bleeding requiring reoperation, and a lower incidence of renal failure requiring dialysis.[49] Because of the retrospective nature of this study, it is impossible to draw definitive conclusions from the data. Furthermore, ECMO was disproportionately used in more recent patients.

In another study, Taghavi and coinvestigators retrospectively[50] compared the use of an isolated RVAD versus ECMO for RV failure after cardiac transplantation. Of 963 patients who underwent transplantation at their center between 1984 and 2003, 28 required mechanical circulatory support for RV failure. Of these, 15 were supported with an RVAD and 13 were supported with ECMO. The overall hospital mortality was 57%. There was a trend toward improved survival in the group of patients supported with ECMO compared with those who underwent RVAD insertion, but this did not reach statistical significance. A significantly greater proportion of patients could be successfully weaned from ECMO (77%) than from an RVAD (13%). Accordingly, more patients required retransplantation in the RVAD group (40%) compared with the ECMO group (1%). There was also greater graft survival in the ECMO group (54%) compared with the RVAD group (7%).[50] These results suggest that ECMO may be preferable for the management of severe RV failure after cardiac transplantation. However, this is a relatively small, retrospective study from a single center. Other confounding factors exist as well. For example, in this study, only the patients who underwent ECMO received nitric oxide, which may be beneficial to RV function. For these reasons, it is difficult to draw definitive conclusions regarding the benefit of an RVAD versus ECMO for RV failure after cardiac transplantation.

Multiple different mechanical support modalities may be used in isolation or combination in the management of severe allograft dysfunction after cardiac transplantation as well. Mihaljevic and colleagues[51] reported on 1417 heart transplants over nearly a 20-year period. Of these, 53 required mechanical circulatory support. Mechanical support was required within 1 week of transplant in 39. ECMO was used most commonly (43 patients), and some patients who were initiated on ECMO were later transitioned to either BiVADs or RVADs. Patients with isolated RV failure underwent RVAD insertion (6 patients), and 2 of these patients were transitioned to ECMO. BiVADs were used as the initial strategy in 4 patients. The overall 1-year survival in this cohort was 40%. The type of device used for support did not affect survival. Importantly, the investigators note that the long-term survival of patients who were successfully weaned from mechanical support was comparable to the expected long-term survival after cardiac transplantation.[51]

Retransplantation

Mechanical circulatory support may be used to a support a recipient in the setting of graft dysfunction. However, if the graft does not ultimately recover, retransplantation may be considered as an option. In the setting of early allograft dysfunction, retransplantation can be challenging for many reasons. The recipient may not be in an ideal physiologic state after the initial allograft has failed. Pulmonary edema, renal failure, hepatic failure, vasoplegia, and coagulopathy may be present and may act as barriers to achieving a successful outcome. An open sternum or resternotomy may increase the risk of wound infection. Certainly, a second major operation in a short period of time may place substantial physiologic stress on a patient.

Outcomes of cardiac retransplantation performed within 90 days of initial transplant were examined by Iribarne and colleagues[52] using data from the United Network of Organ Sharing on 26,804 adult heart transplant recipients between 1995 and 2008. Among these, only 90 patients (0.34%) underwent retransplantation. The investigators found that the median survival of patients undergoing retransplantation was only 1.6 years compared with 10.5 years for the primary heart transplant recipients. The patients who underwent retransplant also had higher rates of perioperative complications. In this study, the recipients undergoing retransplant were more likely to have preoperative renal or hepatic insufficiency, mechanical ventilation, inotropic support, and mechanical circulatory support compared with recipients of primary heart transplants. When the investigators controlled for these differences in recipient characteristics, they found that the observed differences in mortality and complications were no longer significant.[52] These results suggest that the poor preoperative condition of many of the recipients at the time of retransplantation adversely impacts upon the outcomes of early retransplantation for cardiac graft failure. A recent meta-analysis also reported that retransplantation was associated with lower overall survival compared with primary heart transplant.[53]

REFERENCES

1. Costanzo MR, Dipchand A, Starling R, et al. The International Society of Heart and Lung Transplantation Guidelines for the care of heart transplant recipients. J Heart Lung Transplant 2010;29:914–56.
2. Schumacher KR, Gajarski RJ. Postoperative care of the transplanted patient. Curr Cardiol Rev 2011;7:110–22.
3. Vega E, Schroder J, Nicoara A. Postoperative management of heart transplant patients. Best Pract Res Clin Anaesthesiology 2017;31:201–13.
4. Stephens RS, Whitman GJR. Postoperative critical care of the adult cardiac surgical patient. Part I: routine postoperative care. Crit Care Med 2015;43:1477–97.
5. Stephens RS, Whitman GJR. Postoperative critical care of the adult cardiac surgical patient. Part II: procedure-specific considerations, management of complications, and quality improvement. Crit Care Med 2015;43:1995–2014.
6. Stulak JM, Romans T, Cowger J, et al. Delayed sternal closure does not increase late infection risk in patients undergoing left ventricular assist device implantation. J Heart Lung Transplant 2013;31:1115–9.
7. Carmona P, Matea E, Casanovas I, et al. Management of cardiac tamponade after cardiac surgery. J Cardiothorac Vasc Anesth 2012;26:302–11.

8. McCanny P, Colreavy F. Echocardiographic approach to cardiac tamponade in critically ill patients. J Crit Care 2017;39:271–7.

9. St. Andre AC, DelRossi A. Hemodynamic management of patients in the first 24 hours after cardiac surgery. Crit Care Med 2005;33:2082–93.

10. Holte K, Sharrock NE, Kehlet H. Pathophysiology and clinical implications of perioperative fluid excess. Br J Anaesth 2002;89:622–32.

11. Patarroyo M, Simbaqueba C, Shrestha K, et al. Pre-operative risk factors and clinical outcomes associated with vasoplegia in recipients of orthotopic heart transplantation in the contemporary era. J Heart Lung Transplant 2012;31:282–7.

12. Fischer GW, Levin MA. Vasoplegia during cardiac surgery: current concepts and management. Semin Thorac Cardiovasc Surg 2010;22:140–4.

13. Egi M, Bellomo R, Langenberg C, et al. Selecting a vasopressor drug for vasoplegic shock after adult cardiac surgery: a systematic literature review. Ann Thorac Surg 2007;83:715–23.

14. Shaefi S, Mittel A, Klick J, et al. Vasoplegia after cardiovascular procedures-Pathophysiology and targeted therapy. J Cardiothorac Vasc Anesth 2018;32:1013–22.

15. Dinardo JA, Bert A, Schwartz MJ, et al. Effects of vasoactive drugs on flows through left internal mammary artery and saphenous vein grafts in man. J Thorac Cardiovasc Surg 1991;102:730–5.

16. Hajjar LA, Vincent JL, Galas FRBG, et al. Vasopressin versus norepinephrine in patients with vasoplegic shock after cardiac surgery. Anesthesiology 2017;126:85–93.

17. Levin RL, Degrange MA, Bruno GF, et al. Methylene blue reduces mortality and morbidity in vasoplegic patients after cardiac surgery. Ann Thorac Surg 2004;77:496–9.

18. Kofidis T, Struber M, Wilhelmi M, et al. Reversal of severe vasoplegia with single dose methylene blue after heart transplantation. J Thorac Cardiovasc Surg 2001;122:823–4.

19. Kobashigawa J, Zuckermann A, Macdonald P, et al. Report from a consensus conference on primary graft dysfunction after cardiac transplantation. J Heart Lung Transplant 2014;33:327–40.

20. Regitz V, Bossaller C, Strasser R, et al. Myocardial catecholamine content after heart transplantation. Circulation 1990;82:620–3.

21. Hadad H, Isaac D, Legare JF, et al. Canadian Cardiovascular Society Consensus Conference update on cardiac transplantation 2008: executive summary. Can J Cardiol 2009;25:197–205.

22. Simsch O, gromann T, knosalla C, et al. The intensive care management of patients following heart transplant at the Deutsches Herzzentrum Berlin. Appl Cardiopulm Pathophysiol 2011;15:230–40.

23. DeWet CJ, Affleck DG, Jacobson E, et al. Inhaled prostacyclin is safe, effective and affordable in patients with pulmonary hypertension, right heart dysfunction, and refractory hypoxemia after cardiothoracic surgery. J Thorac Cardiovasc Surg 2004;127:1058–67.

24. Thajudeen A, Stecker EC, Shehata M, et al. Arrhythmias after heart transplantation: mechanisms and management. J Am Heart Assoc 2012;1(2):e001461. Available at: https://doi-org.proxy-hs.researchport.umd.edu/10.1161/JAHA.112.001461.

25. Leonelli FM, Dunn JK, Young JB, et al. Natural History, determinants, and clinical relevance of conduction abnormalities following orthotopic heart transplantation. Am J Cardiol 1996;77:47–51.

26. El Gamel A, Yonan NA, Grant S, et al. Orthotopic cardiac tranasplantation: a comparison of standard and bicaval Wythenshawe techniques. J Thorac Cardiovasc Surg 1995;109:721–30.

27. Weiss ES, Nwakanma LU, Russell SB, et al. Outcomes in bicaval versus biatrial techniques in heart tranplantation: an analysis of the UNOS database. J Heart Lung Transplant 2008;27:178–83.

28. Page RL II, Miller GG, Lindenfeld J. Drug therapy in the heart transplant recipient. Part IV: drug-drug interactions. Circulation 2005;111:230–9.

29. van Nunen LX, Noc M, Kapur NK, et al. Usefulness of intra-aortic balloon pump counterpulsation. Am J Cardiol 2016;117:469–76.

30. Unverzagt S, Buerke M, de Waha A, et al. Intra-aortic balloon pump counterpulsation (IABP) for myocardial infarction complicated by cardiogenic shock. Cochrane Database Syst Rev 2015;(27):CD007398.

31. Ahmad Y, Sen S, Shun-Shin MJ, et al. Intra-aortic balloon pump therapy for acute myocardial infarction: a meta-analysis. JAMA Intern Med 2015;175:931–9.

32. den Uil CA, Galli G, Jewbali LS, et al. First-line support by intra-aortic balloon pump in non-ischaemic cardiogenic shock in the era of modern ventricular assist devices. Cardiology 2017;138:1–8.

33. Fried JA, Nair A, Takeda K, et al. Clinical and hemodynamic effects of intra-aortic balloon pump therapy in chronic heart failure patients with cardiogenic shock. J Heart Lung Transplant 2017;36(4):S137–8.

34. Gjesdal O, Gude E, Arora S, et al. Intra-aortic balloon counterpulsation as a bridge to heart transplantation does not impair long-term survival. Eur J Heart Fail 2009;11:709–14.

35. Estep JD, Cordero-Reyes AM, Bhimaraj A, et al. Percutaneous placement of an intra-aortic balloon pump in the left axillary/subclavian position provides safe, ambulatory long-term support as bridge to heart transplantation. JACC Heart Fail 2013;1:382–8.

36. Dronavalli VB, Rogers CA, Banner NR. Primary cardiac allograft dysfunction-validation of a clinical definition. Transplantation 2015;99:1919–25.

37. Esposito ML, Shah N, Dow S, et al. Distinct effects of left or right atrial cannulation on left ventricular hemodynamics in a swine model of acute myocardial injury. ASAIO J 2016;62:671–6.

38. Marasco SF, Vale M, Pellegrino V, et al. Extracorporeal membrane oxygenation in primary graft failure after heart transplantation. Ann Thorac Surg 2010;90:1541–6.

39. D'Alessandro C, Aubert S, Golmard JL, et al. Extra-corporeal membrane oxygenation temporary support for early graft failure after cardiac transplantation. Eur J Cardiothorac Surg 2010;37:343–9.

40. Borisenko O, Wylie G, Payne J, et al. Thoratec CentriMag for temporary treatment of refractory cardiogenic shock or severe cardiopulmonary insufficiency: a systematic literature review and meta-analysis of observational studies. ASAIO J 2014;60:487–97.

41. Thomas HL, Dronavalli VB, Parameshwar J, et al, Steering Group of the UK Cardiothoracic Transplant Audit. Incidence and outcome of Levitronix CentriMag support as rescue therapy for early cardiac allograft failure: a United Kingdom national study. Eur J Cardiothorac Surg 2011;40:1348–54.

42. Bhama JK, Kormos RL, Toyoda Y, et al. Clinical experience using the Levitronix CentriMag system for temporary right ventricular mechanical circulatory support. J Heart Lung Transplant 2009;28:971–6.

43. Velez-Martinez M, Rao K, Warner J, et al. Successful use of the TandemHeart percutaneous ventricular assist device as a bridge to recovery for acute cellular rejection in a cardiac transplant patient. Transplant Proc 2011;43:3882–4.
44. Bruckner BA, Jacob LP, Gregoric ID, et al. Clinical experience with the Tandem-Heart percutaneous ventricular assist device as a bridge to cardiac transplantation. Tex Heart Inst J 2008;35:447–50.
45. Ravichandran AK, Baran DA, Stelling K, et al. Outcomes with the tandem protek duo dual-lumen percutaneous right ventricular assist device. ASAIO J 2018; 64(4):570–2.
46. Chandola R, Cusimano R, Osten M, et al. Use of Impella 5L for acute allograft rejection postcardiac transplant. Thorac Cardiovasc Surg 2012;60:302–4.
47. Samoukovic G, Al-Atassi T, Rosu C, et al. Successful treatment of heart failure due to acute transplant rejection with the Impella LP 5.0. Ann Thorac Surg 2009;88:271–3.
48. Bennett MT, Virani SA, Bowering J, et al. The use of the Impella RD as a bridge to recovery for right ventricular dysfunction after cardiac transplantation. Innovations (Phila) 2010;5:369–71.
49. Takeda K, Li B, Garan AR, et al. Improved outcomes from extracorporeal membrane oxygenation versus ventricular assist device temporary support of primary graft dysfunction in heart transplant. J Heart Lung Transplant 2017;36:650–6.
50. Taghavi S, Zuckermann A, Ankersmit J, et al. Extracorporeal membrane oxygenation is superior to right ventricular assist device for acute right ventricular failure after heart transplantation. Ann Thorac Surg 2004;78:1644–9.
51. Mihaljevic T, Jarrett CM, Gonzalez-Stawinski G, et al. Mechanical circulatory support after heart transplantation. Eur J Cardiothorac Surg 2012;41:200–6.
52. Iribarne A, Hong KN, Easterwood R, et al. Should heart transplant recipients with early graft failure be considered for retransplantation? Ann Thorac Surg 2011;92: 520–7.
53. Rizvi SA, Luc JGY, Choi JH, et al. Outcomes and survival following heart retransplantation for cardiac allograft failure: a systematic review and meta-analysis. Ann Cardiothorac Surg 2018;7:12–8.
54. Russo MJ, Iribarne A, Hong KN, et al. Factors associated with primary graft failure after heart transplantation. Transplantation 2010;90:444–50.
55. Nicoara A, Ruffin D, Cooter M, et al. Primary graft dysfunction after heart transplantation: incidence, trends, and associated risk factors. Am J Transplant 2018;18:1461–70.
56. Segovia J, Cosío MD, Barceló JM, et al. RADIAL: a novel primary graft failure risk score in heart transplantation. J Heart Lung Transplant 2011;30:644–51.

Renal Complications Following Lung Transplantation and Heart Transplantation

Chethan M. Puttarajappa, MD, MS[a],*, Jose F. Bernardo, MD, MPH[a],
John A. Kellum, MD, MCCM[b]

KEYWORDS

- Heart transplantation • Lung transplantation • Acute kidney injury • Dialysis
- Continuous renal replacement therapy

KEY POINTS

- Renal complications are common following heart and/or lung transplantation and lead to increased morbidity and mortality.
- Perioperative heart and lung function predict the development of acute kidney injury (AKI) following transplantation.
- Protective lung ventilation and optimization of right heart function are key to reducing AKI following lung and heart transplantation.
- Renal impairment occurs early after transplantation given multiple risk factors for AKI in the peritransplant setting, and continues in the long-term from chronic calcineurin inhibitor use.
- Patients with residual renal impairment should have close nephrology follow-up for appropriate pre–end-stage renal disease care and timely referral to kidney transplantation.

INTRODUCTION

Renal complications are common following transplantation of thoracic organs and lead to increased morbidity and mortality, both short-term and long-term. Renal dysfunction is also associated with increased mortality for patients while on the on the transplant wait list. The presence of significant renal impairment, such as dialysis dependence, is a relative contraindication for heart and/or lung transplantation at most centers, and such patients are often listed for a simultaneous kidney transplantation.

Disclosures: None.
[a] Renal-Electrolyte Division, University of Pittsburgh Medical Center, 3550 Terrace Street, Pittsburgh, PA 15261, USA; [b] Department of Critical Care Medicine, Center for Critical Care Nephrology, University of Pittsburgh Medical Center, 3550 Terrace Street, Pittsburgh, PA 15261, USA
* Corresponding author. 3459 5th Avenue, Room N 755-2, Pittsburgh, PA 15213.
E-mail address: puttarajappacm@upmc.edu

Crit Care Clin 35 (2019) 61–73
https://doi.org/10.1016/j.ccc.2018.08.009
0749-0704/19/© 2018 Elsevier Inc. All rights reserved.
criticalcare.theclinics.com

Several factors contribute to the impaired renal function in these patients, including the interplay between cardiopulmonary and renal hemodynamics, complex perioperative issues, and exposure to nephrotoxic medications, most commonly calcineurin inhibitors (**Fig. 1**).

EPIDEMIOLOGY, RISK FACTORS, AND PATHOGENESIS
Heart Transplantation

Renal dysfunction in the setting of heart failure, referred to as cardiorenal syndrome (acute and chronic), is commonly a result of a combination of reduced left-ventricular cardiac output, impaired right-ventricular function with high venous pressures and edema, deleterious effects of the compensatory neurohormonal mechanisms such as the renin angiotensin aldosterone system, and escalating doses of diuretics.[1] Five percent of patients listed for heart transplantation (HT) have a glomerular filtration rate (GFR) less than 30 mL/min at listing and 2% to 3% are on dialysis.[2] Additionally, the prevalence among wait-list candidates of risk factors for kidney disease, such as diabetes and hypertension, is high with 20% to 25% having diabetes and 40% to 50% having a history of hypertension.[2]

Postoperative acute kidney injury (AKI) after HT is common and has been reported in up to 70% of HT recipients, with 20% to 40% having KDIGO (Kidney Disease: Improving Global Outcomes) stage II AKI or higher, and 5% to 6% needing renal replacement therapy (RRT).[3–5] Risk factors for postoperative AKI in the setting of HT are impaired baseline renal function, presence of diabetes mellitus, occurrence of transplant surgery–related complication (commonly right-ventricular failure), and early initiation of calcineurin inhibitor immunosuppression.[3] Preoperative right heart pressures also appear to influence the risk of AKI following HT. A recent study found that higher right atrial pressures and reduced pulmonary artery pulsatility index (PAPi) (right atrial pressure-to-pulmonary capillary wedge pressure ratio) were both strong predictors of AKI following HT.[6] These results suggest that the hemodynamic condition of the patient before HT, especially right-sided pressures, influence post-transplant AKI risk.

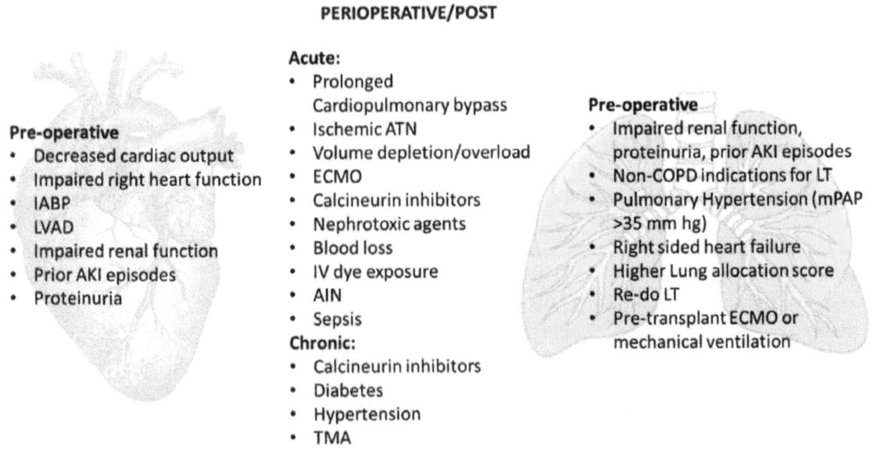

PERIOPERATIVE/POST

Acute:
- Prolonged Cardiopulmonary bypass
- Ischemic ATN
- Volume depletion/overload
- ECMO
- Calcineurin inhibitors
- Nephrotoxic agents
- Blood loss
- IV dye exposure
- AIN
- Sepsis

Chronic:
- Calcineurin inhibitors
- Diabetes
- Hypertension
- TMA

Pre-operative
- Decreased cardiac output
- Impaired right heart function
- IABP
- LVAD
- Impaired renal function
- Prior AKI episodes
- Proteinuria

Pre-operative
- Impaired renal function, proteinuria, prior AKI episodes
- Non-COPD indications for LT
- Pulmonary Hypertension (mPAP >35 mm hg)
- Right sided heart failure
- Higher Lung allocation score
- Re-do LT
- Pre-transplant ECMO or mechanical ventilation

Fig. 1. Risk factors for renal impairment following HT and/or LT. COPD, chronic obstructive pulmonary disease; IABP, intra-aortic balloon pump; IV, intravenous; LVAD, left ventricular assist device; mPAP, mean pulmonary artery pressure; TMA, thrombotic microangiopathy.

Other factors that are also likely playing a role but less well defined in HT settings are pretransplant proteinuria, previous AKI events and extent of recovery, and exposure to nephrotoxic medications and intravenous iodinated contrast. Patients with demonstrated pretransplant improvement in GFR after mechanical circulatory support have a lower risk of renal impairment after HT than those who do not demonstrate such improvements pretransplantation.[7]

Lung Transplantation

Unlike the well-studied heart-kidney interactions of cardiorenal syndrome, the contribution and underlying pathophysiology of respiratory failure causing renal dysfunction is unclear. There is some suggestion that hypoxia and hypercarbia may themselves affect renal blood flow, and water and salt handling.[8] In general, however, renal impairment in the pretransplant setting is not as common in lung transplant (LT) candidates when compared with HT. The proportion of patients with significant renal impairment (dialysis requirement) at the time of LT is less than 1%.[9] This low prevalence is partly due to the exclusion of patients with advanced renal failure as candidates for LT. Despite this low prevalence of baseline renal impairment, patients undergoing an LT procedure still experience significant renal impairment posttransplantation. AKI is very common, occurring in up to two-thirds of the patients with as much as 5% to 8% needing dialysis in the first few months after transplantation.[10,11] Risk factors for AKI after lung transplantation include higher lung allocation score at listing and at transplantation, mean pulmonary artery pressures greater than 35 mm Hg, LT for causes other than chronic obstructive pulmonary disease, re-do LT, higher baseline creatinine, use of extracorporeal membrane oxygenation (ECMO) or mechanical ventilation pretransplantation, and prolonged duration of cardiopulmonary bypass.[10–12] The implementation of lung allocation score (LAS) has led to sicker patients receiving transplantation, which is reflected in the higher incidence of dialysis requiring renal failure in the post-LAS era.[12] Similar to HT, patients with decompensated organ failure (eg, requiring mechanical ventilation) pretransplant are at increased risk for AKI posttransplant. Even outside of transplantation, mechanical ventilation is strongly associated with increased risk for AKI. Although this risk is confounded by disease severity, protective lung ventilation reduces risk for dialysis and increase dialysis-free survival in patients with acute respiratory distress syndrome.[13] Thus, maintaining lung protection, even for pretransplant patients, is prudent.

Postoperatively, primary graft dysfunction (PGD) complicates LT in up to 30% of patients, and management of these patients often involves a fluid restrictive strategy.[14,15] This often leads to both increased airway pressures on mechanical ventilation and escalating doses of diuretics, both risk factors for AKI. Additionally, the relative volume-depleted state of these patients predisposes them to increased risk of AKI from calcineurin inhibitors, iodinated contrast, and nephrotoxic medications.

Long-Term Risks After Transplantation

In addition to the acute events contributing to AKI in the postoperative setting, patients with HT and LT are at increased risk for chronic kidney disease (CKD) over the ensuing years.[9] Renal dysfunction of some form develops in approximately half of HT recipients by 5 years posttransplantation.[16] The incidence of end-stage kidney disease (ESKD), defined as need for chronic dialysis or kidney transplantation, develops in approximately 5% by year 5 and 10% to 12% 10 years posttransplantation.[9,16] Similarly, the incidence of chronic dialysis 1, 5, and 10 years after LT is 3.8%, 7.2%, and 7.9%, respectively.[9,17]

IMPACT OF RENAL FAILURE

Both AKI and CKD/ESKD have a significant impact on patient survival after HT and LT.

Heart Transplantation

Patients developing postoperative AKI requiring RRT have an increased risk of in-hospital and overall 1-year mortality. Studies have reported 1-year mortality of 28% to 38% in these patients.[3–5] Advanced CKD (estimated GFR<30 mL/min) and ESKD requiring dialysis also portend an elevated risk of mortality after transplantation.[9,16] In addition, it has been shown that patients who need chronic dialysis after HT have a mortality risk that is higher than a matched cohort of nontransplant patients on chronic dialysis.[18]

Lung Transplantation

Postoperative AKI is associated with longer duration of hospital stay, increased short-term and 1-year mortality, and elevated risk of CKD.[10,11,17] Dialysis-dependent renal failure has the highest risk of 1-year and 5-year mortality when controlled for multiple other clinical variables, with a 3 to 7 times higher risk of patient mortality compared with patients without dialysis.[12,17]

DIAGNOSIS AND MANAGEMENT

There are several key components to the management of renal complications arising after HT and LT. These vary according to the setting, and timing of renal impairment after transplantation but generally comprise the following issues (**Fig. 2**):

- Identification of at-risk patient population
- Early recognition and diagnoses of AKI
- Protective lung ventilation
- Management of heart failure (both left-sided and right-sided)
- Avoiding secondary insults
- Careful attention to volume management and fluid composition
- Appropriate utilization of dialysis therapies
- Modifications to immunosuppressive therapy
- Timely referral to kidney transplantation

Identification of At-Risk Patient Population

Before listing patients for isolated HT or LT, it is important to identify patients who may have underlying CKD of a sufficient degree that would require them to undergo a simultaneous kidney transplantation along with the HT or LT. Although there are clear guidelines established for simultaneous liver and kidney transplantation, similar guidelines for heart-kidney and lung-kidney are not available. In general, presence of reduced GFR before transplantation should prompt evaluation to assess chronicity and reversibility of renal impairment. This is particularly true before HT, where patients may have some amount of reversible renal impairment from cardiorenal physiology. As noted before, improvement in GFR with mechanical circulatory support (MCS) is a favorable risk factor.[7] In select circumstances, a kidney biopsy might provide evidence of underlying chronicity in the form of moderate to severe interstitial fibrosis and tubular atrophy, which will allow for appropriate listing for a simultaneous heart-kidney transplantation.[19] in general, there has been an increase in the numbers of simultaneous heart-kidney transplantation, whereas simultaneous lung-kidney transplantation is quite rare.[20–22]

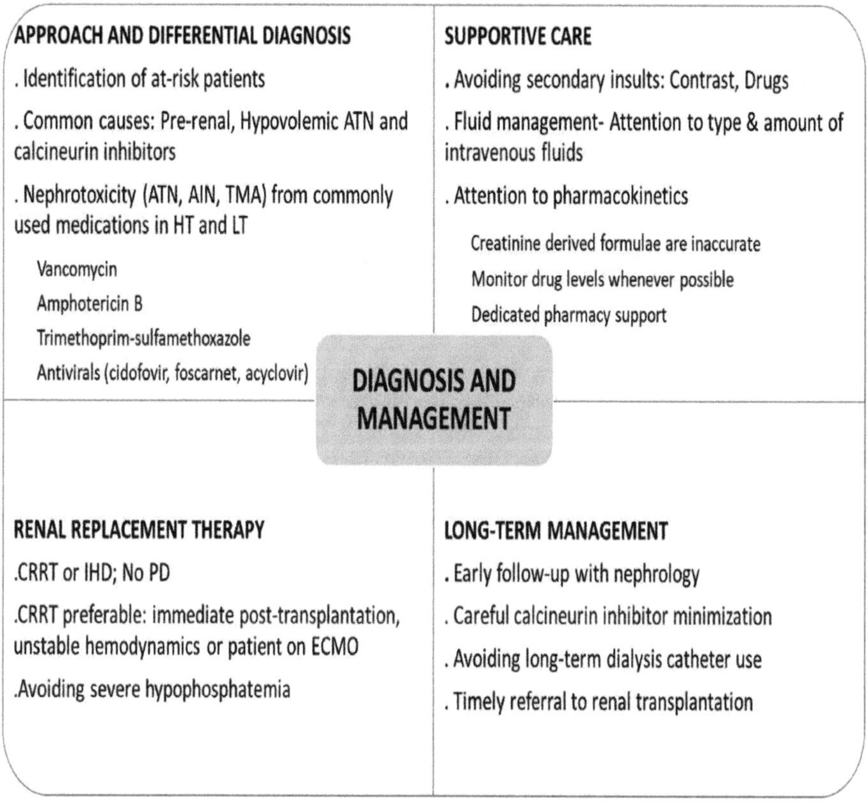

APPROACH AND DIFFERENTIAL DIAGNOSIS

. Identification of at-risk patients

. Common causes: Pre-renal, Hypovolemic ATN and calcineurin inhibitors

. Nephrotoxicity (ATN, AIN, TMA) from commonly used medications in HT and LT

   Vancomycin

   Amphotericin B

   Trimethoprim-sulfamethoxazole

   Antivirals (cidofovir, foscarnet, acyclovir)

SUPPORTIVE CARE

. Avoiding secondary insults: Contrast, Drugs

. Fluid management- Attention to type & amount of intravenous fluids

. Attention to pharmacokinetics

   Creatinine derived formulae are inaccurate

   Monitor drug levels whenever possible

   Dedicated pharmacy support

DIAGNOSIS AND MANAGEMENT

RENAL REPLACEMENT THERAPY

.CRRT or IHD; No PD

.CRRT preferable: immediate post-transplantation, unstable hemodynamics or patient on ECMO

.Avoiding severe hypophosphatemia

LONG-TERM MANAGEMENT

. Early follow-up with nephrology

. Careful calcineurin inhibitor minimization

. Avoiding long-term dialysis catheter use

. Timely referral to renal transplantation

Fig. 2. Approach to diagnosis and management of renal impairment after HT and/or LT.

Identifying patients at risk of postoperative AKI based on their pretransplant risk factors and operative course is important. In general, patients in the hospital or intensive care unit (ICU) at the time of transplantation, on mechanical ventilation or ECMO or MCS, re-do transplantation, moderate or severe pulmonary hypertension, and preexisting renal impairment are the patients at highest risk. It is important to note that many patients undergoing HT or LT have underlying poor functional and nutritional status leading to muscle wasting. Diagnosing renal impairment using creatinine alone in these patients may lead to under or delayed recognition of AKI events.

Etiology of Acute Kidney Injury in the Posttransplant Setting

Most AKI events are related to 1 or more of the following etiologies: volume depletion (absolute or reduced effective circulatory volume), acute tubular necrosis (ATN), and the renal hemodynamic effects of calcineurin inhibitors (CNIs). Other possible etiologies that should be considered in the right clinical setting are acute interstitial nephritis (AIN), obstructive uropathy, and drug-induced thrombotic microangiopathy (TMA). Routine renal ultrasounds in patients with AKI are not useful unless there is a prior history of urinary tract obstruction.[23] The diagnosis of CNI-induced TMA is often missed or delayed due to the nonspecific clinical manifestations (ie, anemia, creatinine elevation, thrombocytopenia) in the ICU setting.[24] Additionally, not all patients with TMA manifest the full clinical spectrum, which adds to the diagnostic difficulty. TMA in transplant recipients was originally described mostly with cyclosporine and often managed by switching to tacrolimus. However, several reports have subsequently described cases of TMA with both tacrolimus and mammalian target of rapamycin (mTOR) inhibitors (sirolimus and everolimus).[25] Diagnosis is aided by documenting elevation of lactate dehydrogenase and presence of microangiopathic hemolytic anemia (MAHA) with demonstration of schistocytes. ADAMTS-13 enzyme activity should be checked to rule out thrombotic thrombocytopenic purpura (TTP); ADAMTS-13 activity in TTP is usually less than 10%, whereas it is usually greater than 10% in drug-related MAHA.[26] Treatment involves supportive care and discontinuation of the offending drug. Although plasmapheresis is often performed, its use in drug-induced MAHA is controversial and not clearly proven.[25,27]

Biomarkers for Acute Kidney Injury

Several biomarkers have been investigated in AKI for prediction and risk stratification. The recently approved test for urinary tissue inhibitor of metalloproteinases-2 (TIMP-2) and insulinlike growth factor binding protein 7 (IGFBP7) has been found to improve the prediction of AKI in patients undergoing cardiac surgery, over and above the clinical variables.[28,29] The test provides an AKI risk score based on the urinary concentration of both markers multiplied together. Results of [TIMP-2]•[IGFBP7] >0.3 represent high risk for AKI, and this result can be incorporated as an automatic alert to prompt health care providers to institute AKI preventive measures, including reducing nephrotoxins and improving hemodynamics.[28]

Avoiding Secondary Insults

Timely recognition of AKI should be followed by a multipronged approach to reduce secondary nephrotoxic insults. This should be a concerted team effort and appropriate communication among all the involved health care providers. Key components of these preventive measures are as follows:

- Limiting exposure to nephrotoxins
  - Antimicrobials:
    - Most patients in the posttransplant setting who develop AKI often have infectious complications and are exposed to different classes of nephrotoxins. These include vancomycin, aminoglycoside antibiotics (gentamicin, neomycin, tobramycin) that induce tubular apoptosis and/or necrosis, amphotericin B, which causes afferent arteriole vasoconstriction and tubule-toxicity, and antivirals (acyclovir, foscarnet and cidofovir), which cause AKI through various mechanisms such as intratubular crystallization leading to crystal-induced nephropathy and direct tubular toxicity.[30,31]
    - Careful attention should be paid to vancomycin trough levels, because higher trough levels have increased risk of vancomycin nephropathy.[32] In addition, a pharmacist-driven protocolized vancomycin dosing can increase the proportion of patients who achieve the goal trough concentrations.[33] Although vancomycin dosing based on trough concentration is commonly used as a surrogate for the area under the curve/minimum inhibitory concentration (AUC/MIC) ratio, using the AUC/MIC ratio approach has been shown in small studies to reduce the number of vancomycin doses required and has the potential to further reduce supratherapeutic levels.[34]
    - Several studies have shown a significant risk of AKI with vancomycin and piperacillin-tazobactam combination.[35,36] Hence, the use of this

combination should be chosen wisely. In addition, timely de-escalation of antibiotics based on culture results and clinical status is vital.

- ■ Drug-induced AIN can often go unrecognized and should always be included in the differential diagnosis of unexplained AKI, particularly when the onset of renal impairment is subacute and developing over days. Common culprits are beta-lactam antibiotics, and trimethoprim-sulfamethoxazole used commonly as a prophylactic agent against *Pneumocystis jiroveci* infection in transplant recipients. Diagnosis is often made clinically though presence of peripheral eosinophilia, and urine eosinophils increase the likelihood of AIN diagnosis. The offending drug should be eliminated and, if severe, a short course of steroids can be given.
- ○ Iodinated contrast: The risk of contrast-mediated AKI has decreased over time, possibly due to judicious use of contrast and availability of iso-osmolar and low-osmolar iodinated contrast agents.[37,38] Still, the risk of contrast is likely not fully eliminated, and it is important to adequately volume expand before and after contrast exposure. However, it should be noted that patients often may already be in a volume-expanded state in the ICU and care should be taken to avoid further volume overloading such patients. In addition, there is no benefit of bicarbonate fluids or acetylcysteine in the prevention of contrast nephropathy.[39]
- ○ CNIs: Nephrotoxicity caused by these agents has been appropriately called the Achilles heel of transplantation. The CNIs, tacrolimus and cyclosporine, are the drugs with best efficacy for rejection prevention but they come with a substantial price of nephrotoxicity.[40] Although the exact molecular mechanisms of toxicity are not fully established, the major effects are hemodynamic (renal vasoconstriction) in the short-term, and chronic arteriolar changes and interstitial fibrosis in the long-term.[40]
  - ■ If possible, the introduction of CNIs can be delayed in the presence of AKI, but is usually not done given the risk of rejection. More often, the approach taken is to maintain target trough levels at the lower end of the desired range. Eighty-five percent to 95% of tacrolimus is within the erythrocytes, and 60% of tacrolimus in plasma is bound to albumin and other plasma proteins.[41] Several factors affect the pharmacokinetics of these drugs in the ICU setting: altered liver metabolism, drug interactions (azoles, antiseizure medications), impaired/altered gut absorption, use of ECMO, anemia, and hypoalbuminemia. Hence, daily trough measurements are crucial in the ICU setting. Additionally, whole-blood levels are preferred over plasma levels.[41]

Careful Attention to Volume Management and Fluid Composition

- Type of intravenous fluids: Due to their increased cost, lack of clear benefit and potential for toxicity of some agents (eg, starch), colloids are not recommended for fluid resuscitation in most transplant patients. Among the crystalloids, recent evidence (in acute and critically ill patients not receiving transplants) suggests that balanced crystalloids, such as lactated Ringer solution and PlasmaLyte, are associated with lower incidence of AKI and better patient outcomes.[42,43]
- Volume of intravenous fluids: Multiple observational studies have shown deleterious outcomes with volume overload in the ICU, suggesting that extra care should be taken to avoid excessive fluid administration.[44,45] Careful monitoring of urine output and fluid balance may help reduce mortality in patients with

AKI.[46] In addition, more than one-third of the LT recipients have PGD, where this issue is of even more importance.[14,15]

Appropriate Utilization of Dialysis Therapies

- Continuous renal replacement therapy (CRRT) versus intermittent hemodialysis (IHD): neither modality has been shown to be superior in general in the ICU setting and choice is often made based on hemodynamic stability and local practice patterns. CRRT will allow for easier management of volume status and is often preferred in the immediate postoperative setting. Our practice is to use CRRT rather than IHD for initial management of severe AKI in both HT and LT patients.
- Peritoneal dialysis (PD) is in general avoided in the acute settings unless the patient was already on PD, which is uncommon. Even in those situations, hemodialysis will be preferred for easier management of fluid and electrolyte problems arising in the acute setting.
- Patients on ECMO: For patients on veno-arterial or veno-venous ECMO, CRRT is better suited given the hemodynamic instability and the advantage of making rapid changes to treatment.[47] CRRT can be delivered by either using an in-line hemofilter or by integrating a standard CRRT machine to the extracorporeal circuit.[47] The CRRT machine is usually connected to the venous limb of the ECMO circuit. Because the inflow pressure into the CRRT machines will be positive (unlike the usual negative pressures), the alarm settings will need to be adjusted.[47] Blood should be ultimately returned to the patient after passing through the oxygenator to allow for air and clot trapping. Each center should develop appropriate RRT protocols for these settings.
- Management of electrolytes, macronutrients, and micronutrients:
  - Hypophosphatemia is common and affects one-third of the patients on CRRT.[48] Unlike IHD, phosphorus elimination is increased with CRRT due to the time-dependent clearance of phosphorus by CRRT. Hypophosphatemia usually develops on day 2 or 3, and when severe (ie, <1 mg/dL) can cause muscle weakness and possibly increase duration of mechanical ventilation.[49] Daily monitoring of serum phosphorus levels along with intravenous or oral supplementation is necessary to avoid severe hypophosphatemia. An alternative is to add phosphorus to CRRT solutions or use commercially available phosphate-containing CRRT solutions. Commercial solutions avoid the risk of human errors that may occur when phosphate is added by individual hospital pharmacies.[48]
  - Patients on dialysis should receive 25 to 35 kcal/kg per day of total energy intake along with at least 1.5 to 1.8 g/kg per day of protein/amino acid supplementation. Higher protein requirement occurs due to catabolic states and loss of amino acids in the CRRT effluent.[50] In addition, there is loss of water-soluble vitamins and trace elements with dialysis; these should be replaced to avoid deleterious effects.[50]
- Drug dosing considerations: A detailed guidance is beyond the scope of this article. Salient points are noted as follows.[51]
  - There are difficulties in accurately estimating GFR in AKI and in ICU settings. Formulae using creatinine might overestimate GFR in patients with low muscle mass. Additionally, all creatinine-derived formulae require a steady-state creatinine; rate of change can guide estimation but is not fully reliable
  - GFR-based dosing recommendations mostly come from studies in patients with stable CKD and may not fully apply to patients with AKI.

- The volume of distribution is often increased in the AKI setting due to volume-overload issues. Higher loading doses are often needed in these settings.
- Drug removal by hemodialysis is 25% to 50% higher when high-flux dialyzers are used compared with low-flux dialyzers.
- Drugs removed by dialysis should be given postdialysis session.
- Therapeutic drug monitoring should be used whenever possible.
- For CRRT, dosing can be based on the total estimated creatine clearance provided by CRRT and any residual renal function. The usual values are in the 25 to 40 mL/min range.

MANAGEMENT OF CHRONIC RENAL IMPAIRMENT

As a result of posttransplant renal events, a significant number of patients with HT and LT develop CKD or end-stage renal disease (ESRD). Given the central role of CNI toxicity in the development of chronic renal impairment, management strategies for such patients have revolved around the minimization or elimination of CNIs. The development of mTOR inhibitors (sirolimus and everolimus) has led to numerous attempts by many investigators to attempt minimization or elimination of CNIs in HT and LT recipients. Most of these studies have been either uncontrolled studies or contained small sample sizes with only intermediate outcomes of GFR or renal functions assessed over a short period.[52–55] Well-controlled studies looking at hard outcomes, such as dialysis or renal transplantation, in the setting of CNI minimization or avoidance are lacking. It is important to note that mTOR inhibitors are associated with increase of glomerular proteinuria, and affect wound healing. Belatacept is a non-CNI immunosuppressive agent that blocks costimulatory blockade and has been approved for use in kidney transplantation. It has been shown to preserve renal function better compared with CNIs but with an accompanied increased risk of early rejections.[56] Its use however in HT and LT have been reported in only a handful of cases.

KIDNEY TRANSPLANTATION AFTER HEART OR LUNG TRANSPLANTATION

Patients who develop dialysis-dependent renal failure after HT or LT have significantly worse survival when compared with HT or LT patients without dialysis.[16,17] They also have worse survival when compared with patients on dialysis due to native kidney failure or those with a failed kidney transplantation(KT).[57,58] KT for patients with history of either prior HT or LT is associated with a significant survival benefit compared to waiting on the KT waiting list.[57] The overall patient and graft survival for patients undergoing KT after HT or KT are however inferior to patients undergoing first KT or repeat KT.[58]

SUMMARY

Renal complications after HT or LT are common and contribute to significant mortality and morbidity. Renal impairment occurs early after transplantation given multiple risk factors for AKI in the peritransplant setting, and continues in the long-term from chronic CNI use. Efforts should be focused on preserving native renal function by avoiding secondary insults in the postoperative phase. Care of patients developing severe AKI in the posttransplant setting should be multidisciplinary and involve good coordination among transplant physicians, nephrologists, intensivists, infectious disease specialists, nutritionists, and ICU pharmacists. Patients with residual renal impairment should have close nephrology follow-up for appropriate pre-ESRD care and timely referral to kidney transplantation.

REFERENCES

1. Cruz DN, Gheorghiade M, Palazzuoli A, et al. Epidemiology and outcome of the cardio-renal syndrome. Heart Fail Rev 2011;16(6):531–42.
2. Singh TP, Almond CS, Taylor DO, et al. Decline in heart transplant wait list mortality in the United States following broader regional sharing of donor hearts. Circ Heart Fail 2012;5(2):249–58.
3. Fortrie G, Manintveld OC, Caliskan K, et al. Acute kidney injury as a complication of cardiac transplantation: incidence, risk factors, and impact on 1-year mortality and renal function. Transplantation 2016;100(8):1740–9.
4. De Santo LS, Romano G, Amarelli C, et al. Implications of acute kidney injury after heart transplantation: what a surgeon should know. Eur J Cardiothorac Surg 2011;40(6):1355–61 [discussion: 1361].
5. Gude E, Andreassen AK, Arora S, et al. Acute renal failure early after heart transplantation: risk factors and clinical consequences. Clin Transplant 2010;24(6): E207–13.
6. Guven G, Brankovic M, Constantinescu AA, et al. Preoperative right heart hemodynamics predict postoperative acute kidney injury after heart transplantation. Intensive Care Med 2018;44(5):588–97.
7. Singh M, Shullo M, Kormos RL, et al. Impact of renal function before mechanical circulatory support on posttransplant renal outcomes. Ann Thorac Surg 2011; 91(5):1348–54.
8. Kilburn KH, Dowell AR. Renal function in respiratory failure. Effects of hypoxia, hyperoxia, and hypercapnia. Arch Intern Med 1971;127(4):754–62.
9. Ojo AO, Held PJ, Port FK, et al. Chronic renal failure after transplantation of a nonrenal organ. N Engl J Med 2003;349(10):931–40.
10. Rocha PN, Rocha AT, Palmer SM, et al. Acute renal failure after lung transplantation: incidence, predictors and impact on perioperative morbidity and mortality. Am J Transplant 2005;5(6):1469–76.
11. Fidalgo P, Ahmed M, Meyer SR, et al. Incidence and outcomes of acute kidney injury following orthotopic lung transplantation: a population-based cohort study. Nephrol Dial Transplant 2014;29(9):1702–9.
12. Banga A, Mohanka M, Mullins J, et al. Characteristics and outcomes among patients with need for early dialysis after lung transplantation surgery. Clin Transplant 2017;31(11).
13. Brower RG, Matthay MA, Morris A, et al. Ventilation with lower tidal volumes as compared with traditional tidal volumes for acute lung injury and the acute respiratory distress syndrome. N Engl J Med 2000;342(18):1301–8.
14. Snell GI, Yusen RD, Weill D, et al. Report of the ISHLT Working Group on Primary Lung Graft Dysfunction, part I: definition and grading-A 2016 Consensus Group statement of the International Society for Heart and Lung Transplantation. J Heart Lung Transplant 2017;36(10):1097–103.
15. Van Raemdonck D, Hartwig MG, Hertz MI, et al. Report of the ISHLT Working Group on primary lung graft dysfunction Part IV: prevention and treatment: a 2016 Consensus Group statement of the International Society for Heart and Lung Transplantation. J Heart Lung Transplant 2017;36(10):1121–36.
16. Lund LH, Khush KK, Cherikh WS, et al. The Registry of the International Society for Heart and Lung Transplantation: thirty-fourth adult heart transplantation report-2017; focus theme: allograft ischemic time. J Heart Lung Transplant 2017;36(10):1037–46.

17. Chambers DC, Yusen RD, Cherikh WS, et al. The Registry of the International Society for Heart and Lung Transplantation: thirty-fourth adult lung and heart-lung transplantation report-2017; focus theme: allograft ischemic time. J Heart Lung Transplant 2017;36(10):1047–59.

18. Alam A, Badovinac K, Ivis F, et al. The outcome of heart transplant recipients following the development of end-stage renal disease: analysis of the Canadian Organ Replacement Register (CORR). Am J Transplant 2007;7(2):461–5.

19. Labban B, Arora N, Restaino S, et al. The role of kidney biopsy in heart transplant candidates with kidney disease. Transplantation 2010;89(7):887–93.

20. Schaffer JM, Chiu P, Singh SK, et al. Heart and combined heart-kidney transplantation in patients with concomitant renal insufficiency and end-stage heart failure. Am J Transplant 2014;14(2):384–96.

21. Ruderman I, Sevastos J, Anthony C, et al. Outcomes of simultaneous heart-kidney and lung-kidney transplantations: the Australian and New Zealand experience. Intern Med J 2015;45(12):1236–41.

22. Yerokun BA, Mulvihill MS, Osho AA, et al. Simultaneous or sequential lung-kidney transplantation confer superior survival in renal-failure patients undergoing lung transplantation: a national analysis. J Heart Lung Transplant 2017;36(4):S95.

23. Podoll A, Walther C, Finkel K. Clinical utility of gray scale renal ultrasound in acute kidney injury. BMC Nephrol 2013;14:188.

24. Boyer NL, Niven A, Edelman J. Tacrolimus-associated thrombotic microangiopathy in a lung transplant recipient. BMJ Case Rep 2013;2013 [pii:bcr2012007351].

25. Ponticelli C, Banfi G. Thrombotic microangiopathy after kidney transplantation. Transpl Int 2006;19(10):789–94.

26. Scully M, Cataland S, Coppo P, et al. Consensus on the standardization of terminology in thrombotic thrombocytopenic purpura and related thrombotic microangiopathies. J Thromb Haemost 2017;15(2):312–22.

27. Schwartz J, Padmanabhan A, Aqui N, et al. Guidelines on the use of therapeutic apheresis in clinical practice-evidence-based approach from the writing committee of the American Society for Apheresis: the Seventh Special Issue. J Clin Apher 2016;31(3):149–62.

28. Levante C, Ferrari F, Manenti C, et al. Routine adoption of TIMP2 and IGFBP7 biomarkers in cardiac surgery for early identification of acute kidney injury. Int J Artif Organs 2017;40(12):714–8.

29. Oezkur M, Magyar A, Thomas P, et al. TIMP-2*IGFBP7 (Nephrocheck(R)) measurements at intensive care unit admission after cardiac surgery are predictive for acute kidney injury within 48 hours. Kidney Blood Press Res 2017;42(3):456–67.

30. Sawyer MH, Webb DE, Balow JE, et al. Acyclovir-induced renal failure. Clinical course and histology. Am J Med 1988;84(6):1067–71.

31. Berns JS, Cohen RM, Stumacher RJ, et al. Renal aspects of therapy for human immunodeficiency virus and associated opportunistic infections. J Am Soc Nephrol 1991;1(9):1061–80.

32. Luque Y, Louis K, Jouanneau C, et al. Vancomycin-associated cast nephropathy. J Am Soc Nephrol 2017;28(6):1723–8.

33. Hirano R, Sakamoto Y, Kitazawa J, et al. Pharmacist-managed dose adjustment feedback using therapeutic drug monitoring of vancomycin was useful for patients with methicillin-resistant *Staphylococcus aureus* infections: a single institution experience. Infect Drug Resist 2016;9:243–52.

34. Stoessel AM, Hale CM, Seabury RW, et al. The impact of AUC-based monitoring on pharmacist-directed vancomycin dose adjustments in complicated methicillin-resistant *Staphylococcus aureus* infection. J Pharm Pract 2018. 897190018764564.

35. Hammond DA, Smith MN, Li C, et al. Systematic review and meta-analysis of acute kidney injury associated with concomitant vancomycin and piperacillin/tazobactam. Clin Infect Dis 2017;64(5):666–74.

36. Navalkele B, Pogue JM, Karino S, et al. Risk of acute kidney injury in patients on concomitant vancomycin and piperacillin-tazobactam compared to those on vancomycin and cefepime. Clin Infect Dis 2017;64(2):116–23.

37. Bucher AM, De Cecco CN, Schoepf UJ, et al. Is contrast medium osmolality a causal factor for contrast-induced nephropathy? Biomed Res Int 2014;2014:8.

38. Wilhelm-Leen E, Montez-Rath ME, Chertow G. Estimating the risk of radiocontrast-associated nephropathy. J Am Soc Nephrol 2017;28(2):653–9.

39. Weisbord SD, Gallagher M, Jneid H, et al. Outcomes after angiography with sodium bicarbonate and acetylcysteine. N Engl J Med 2018;378(7):603–14.

40. Naesens M, Kuypers DR, Sarwal M. Calcineurin inhibitor nephrotoxicity. Clin J Am Soc Nephrol 2009;4(2):481–508.

41. Sikma MA, van Maarseveen EM, van de Graaf EA, et al. Pharmacokinetics and toxicity of tacrolimus early after heart and lung transplantation. Am J Transplant 2015;15(9):2301–13.

42. Self WH, Semler MW, Wanderer JP, et al. Balanced crystalloids versus saline in noncritically ill adults. N Engl J Med 2018;378(9):819–28.

43. Semler MW, Self WH, Wanderer JP, et al. Balanced crystalloids versus saline in critically ill adults. N Engl J Med 2018;378(9):829–39.

44. Grams ME, Estrella MM, Coresh J, et al. Fluid balance, diuretic use, and mortality in acute kidney injury. Clin J Am Soc Nephrol 2011;6(5):966–73.

45. Teixeira C, Garzotto F, Piccinni P, et al. Fluid balance and urine volume are independent predictors of mortality in acute kidney injury. Crit Care 2013;17(1):R14.

46. Jin K, Murugan R, Sileanu FE, et al. Intensive monitoring of urine output is associated with increased detection of acute kidney injury and improved outcomes. Chest 2017;152(5):972–9.

47. Askenazi DJ, Selewski DT, Paden ML, et al. Renal replacement therapy in critically ill patients receiving extracorporeal membrane oxygenation. Clin J Am Soc Nephrol 2012;7(8):1328–36.

48. Bellomo R, Cass A, Cole L, et al. The relationship between hypophosphataemia and outcomes during low-intensity and high-intensity continuous renal replacement therapy. Crit Care resuscitation 2014;16(1):34–41.

49. Heung M, Mueller BA. Prevention of hypophosphatemia during continuous renal replacement therapy—an overlooked problem. Semin Dial 2018;31(3):213–8.

50. Honore PM, De Waele E, Jacobs R, et al. Nutritional and metabolic alterations during continuous renal replacement therapy. Blood Purif 2013;35(4):279–84.

51. Matzke GR, Aronoff GR, Atkinson AJ Jr, et al. Drug dosing consideration in patients with acute and chronic kidney disease—a clinical update from Kidney Disease: improving Global Outcomes (KDIGO). Kidney Int 2011;80(11):1122–37.

52. Demirjian S, Stephany B, Abu Romeh IS, et al. Conversion to sirolimus with calcineurin inhibitor elimination vs. dose minimization and renal outcome in heart and lung transplant recipients. Clin Transplant 2009;23(3):351–60.

53. Gullestad L, Iversen M, Mortensen SA, et al. Everolimus with reduced calcineurin inhibitor in thoracic transplant recipients with renal dysfunction: a multicenter, randomized trial. Transplantation 2010;89(7):864–72.

54. Raichlin E, Khalpey Z, Kremers W, et al. Replacement of calcineurin-inhibitors with sirolimus as primary immunosuppression in stable cardiac transplant recipients. Transplantation 2007;84(4):467–74.

55. de Pablo A, Santos F, Sole A, et al. Recommendations on the use of everolimus in lung transplantation. Transplant Rev (Orlando) 2013;27(1):9–16.
56. Vincenti F, Rostaing L, Grinyo J, et al. Belatacept and long-term outcomes in kidney transplantation. N Engl J Med 2016;374(4):333–43.
57. Cassuto JR, Reese PP, Sonnad S, et al. Wait list death and survival benefit of kidney transplantation among nonrenal transplant recipients. Am J Transplant 2010; 10(11):2502–11.
58. Lonze BE, Warren DS, Stewart ZA, et al. Kidney transplantation in previous heart or lung recipients. Am J Transplant 2009;9(3):578–85.

Infections in Heart and Lung Transplant Recipients

Mohammed Alsaeed, MD[a,b], Shahid Husain, MD, MS, FECMM, FRCP[a,*]

KEYWORDS

- Infections • Lung transplant • Heart transplant • Critical care

KEY POINTS

- Sepsis is the leading cause of admission to intensive care unit in heart/lung transplant recipients.
- Heart/lung transplant recipients with infection are less likely to present with fever and leukocytosis, but rather with organ dysfunction.
- Bloodstream infections are more common in the first 3 months posttransplant and are associated with high mortality.
- Pneumonia is the leading cause of infection in heart/lung transplant recipients especially in the first year posttransplant.
- Bacteria are the leading cause of infection in heart/lung transplant patients but always look for viral and fungal causes.

INTRODUCTION

Heart and lung transplantation has become the treatment modality of choice for end-stage cardiac and pulmonary disease. The critical care unit is the first step toward recovery and normal life afterward. According to the International Society for Heart and Lung transplantation in 2017, there were more than 60,000 lung transplants and 4000 heart-lung transplants performed worldwide that were reported to their registry.[1] With the rapidly increasing number of transplants, critical care physicians are more likely to be involved in the specialized care of these types of patients. The morbidity and mortality following heart and/or lung transplantation is largely due to infection and rejection-related complications.[2,3] Critical care physicians should be aware of the

Disclosure Statement: S. Husain has received grant funding from Merck (Canada) and Astellas (Canada) and consultancy fees from Cidara. M. Alsaeed has nothing to disclose.
[a] Division of Infectious Diseases, Multi-Organ Transplant Program, Department of Medicine, University of Toronto, University Health Network, 585 University Avenue, 11 PMB 138, Toronto, Ontario M5G 2N2, Canada; [b] Division of Infectious Diseases, Department of Medicine, Prince Sultan Military Medical City, Makkah Al Mukarramah Road, As Sulimaniyah, Riyadh 12233, Saudi Arabia
* Corresponding author.
E-mail address: shahid.husain@uhn.ca

Crit Care Clin 35 (2019) 75–93
https://doi.org/10.1016/j.ccc.2018.08.010
0749-0704/19/© 2018 Elsevier Inc. All rights reserved.

common infections that develop in this population. In this article, the authors review the epidemiology, risk factors, specific clinical syndromes, and most frequent opportunistic infections in heart and/or lung transplant recipients and provide a practical approach of empirical management.

EPIDEMIOLOGY

Since the first lung and heart transplantations performed in the 1960s, there has been significant advancement in organ preservation, surgical techniques, immunosuppression, and postoperative care that has made long-term survival a reality. Despite these advancements, posttransplant infectious complications remain a significant contributor to overall morbidity and mortality.[4]

The epidemiology of infections has changed over time, which is primarily due to widespread use of different prophylactic strategies. Classically, infections in solid organ transplant patients have been divided into 3 periods[5]:

- Early period posttransplant (first month) has been attributed mostly to nosocomial pathogens.
- Intermediate period (2 to 6 months) has been attributed mostly to opportunistic pathogens.
- Late period (more than 6 months) has been attributed mostly to community pathogens.

This approach is simple but is rigid and has its limitations. It fails to take into account several factors such as type of transplant, antimicrobial prophylaxis, induction immunosuppression, and nosocomial exposure of the patient.

RISK FACTORS

The risk factors for heart and/or lung transplant recipients continue to change overtime but are broadly classified into recipient, donor, and graft (transplanted organ) factors. These factors are listed in **Box 1**. The evaluation of these risk factors is important when a critically ill heart and/or lung transplant recipient is seen in the intensive care unit (ICU).

SPECIFIC CLINICAL SYNDROMES
Sepsis

Sepsis has been studied extensively in the past 3 decades, but despite the growing number of solid organ transplant (SOT) patients worldwide the definition of sepsis has never been validated in these patients.[6,7] Solid organ transplant patients may lack classical signs and symptoms probably due to their immunosuppressed state, which blunts the inflammatory response.

They are less likely to present with fever and leukocytosis, but rather with organ dysfunction. Another important issue is that many other noninfectious transplant-related complications can mimic the clinical presentation of sepsis such as primary graft dysfunction and rejection.[8–11]

Sepsis is the leading cause of admission to hospital and critical care unit in solid organ transplant recipients. Trzeciak and colleagues[12] looked retrospectively into 325 emergency room visits by SOT patients; 6% were lung and heart transplant patients. The leading cause of admission was infections (35%); around 12% had severe sepsis and required ICU care. In comparison with nontransplant, SOT patients are 3 times more likely to be admitted with sepsis.

Box 1
Risk factors for heart and/or lung transplant recipients

Recipient Factors

- Age
- Diabetes
- Hypogammaglobulinemia
- Renal failure
- No immunity against CMV, toxoplasmosis, EBV, VZV
- Latent infection TB, CMV, HSV, VZV, EBV, endemic mycosis
- Colonization with MDR.
- Immunosuppressive therapy
- Rejection
- Environmental exposure (gardener, animals, caves, travel)
- Native lung colonization

Donor Factors

- Bacterial or fungal allograft colonization
- Allograft latent infection (toxoplasma, CMV, other viruses, endemic mycosis, TB)

Transplantation

- Allograft injury (ischemia, preservation)
- Complexity and length of surgery
- Postsurgical care (mechanical ventilation, intravenous catheters, drains, bladder catheters, extracorporeal membrane oxygenation)
- Transfusion
- Intensive care stay

Abbreviations: CMV, cytomegalovirus; EBV, Epstein-Barr virus; HSV, herpes simplex virus; MDR, multidrug resistance; TB, tuberculosis; VZV, varicella zoster virus.

Sepsis is also a predominant cause of intensive care readmission and death. Pietrantoni and colleagues[13] looked into 210 lung transplant recipients for ICU readmission after initial 30-day posttransplant period over a 4-year period and found 46% admission due to sepsis with a mortality rate approaching 52%.

Kalil and colleagues[14] compared mortality in blood culture–proven sepsis in SOT patients and non-SOT patients. They surprisingly found that SOT patients had better survival at 28 days and 90 days in comparison to non-SOT patients. This could be explained by the fact that the transplant group was more likely to receive appropriate initial antibiotic therapy. They also found SOT recipients had 20 times more nosocomial infections than non-SOT recipients.

Inadequate empirical antibiotic therapy is associated with poor outcome in SOT patients. Hamandi and colleagues[15] looked into 312 SOT patients admitted with culture-proven sepsis. Fifty-four percent of patients received inadequate therapy with a mortality approaching 25% while a mortality of only 7% in those who received appropriate empirical antibiotic therapy.

The choice of appropriate antibiotic therapy depends on many factors, including the knowledge of colonization with multidrug-resistant organisms, recent antibiotic exposure, source of infection, local epidemiology, and any recent procedures or surgeries.[10]

Bloodstream Infections

Bloodstream infections is a well-recognized problem among heart/and or lung transplant patients. It is associated with graft loss and increased mortality. The incidence of bloodstream infections in heart transplant approaches 16%, whereas in lung transplants this goes up to 25%.[16,17]

Rodríguez and colleagues[16] looked into 309 consecutive heart transplant patients for bloodstream infections and found an incidence of 15.8% with direct mortality of 12.2% related to bloodstream infection. Over the 15-year study period they noted a decline in the incidence of bloodstream infections, which they attributed to a change in immunosuppression regimens, antimicrobial protocols, and better improvement in infection control measures. They also observed that most of the bloodstream infections occurred within the first 2 months after transplantation and around 65% were nosocomial. The most common source of infection was pulmonary. Almost half (55.3%) were gram-negative, followed closely by gram-positive (44.6%), whereas only one case of candidemia was noted.

Palmer and colleagues[17] looked into 176 consecutive lung transplant recipients for bloodstream infections and found an incidence of 25%. Risk factors associated with bacteremia are as follows: younger age, have cystic fibrosis, have undergone bilateral lung transplant, or have undergone pretransplant mechanical ventilation. In comparison to lung transplant patients without bloodstream infection, patients who had a first bloodstream infection had higher mortality. The most common source of infection was pneumonia. During the transplant period, gram-negative bacteria (46%) and candida (23%) were the most common cause of bloodstream infections, whereas after transplant discharge gram-positive organisms (38%) were more prevalent.

Husain and colleagues[18] have also looked prospectively into bacteremia among lung transplant recipients: they found that 50% of bacteremias in the first posttransplant year were pulmonary in origin. After 1 year, the proportion of bacteremias that were due to pulmonary infection declined to 26.7% and vascular catheters emerged as a leading source of bacteremia (53.3%). Mortality rate at 28 days after the onset of bacteremia was 25%. Multiple antibiotic–resistant (multidrug-resistant [MDR]) organisms were isolated in 48% of the bacteremia episodes. Patients with cystic fibrosis were more likely to have MDR (35% vs 8%). The approach to gram-negative and positive bacteremia in heart and/or lung transplant recipients is summarized in **Figs. 1** and **2**.

Vascular catheters should always be considered as a source of bloodstream infection in the ICU. Most exit site infections can be treated with antiinfective therapy without line removal. However, vascular catheters should be immediately removed in patients with septic shock, septic phlebitis, and tunnel or port pocket infections. Catheter infections with certain organisms such as *Staphylococcus aureus*, *Pseudomonas aeruginosa*, nontuberculous mycobacteria, yeast, and molds should also be removed. Treating catheter-related bloodstream infection in heart and/or lung transplant patients is similar to treating other patients according to published guidelines.[19,20]

Candida bloodstream infection in critically ill patients is usually severe and life threatening. Although uncommon in heart and lung transplant recipients, it is nevertheless associated with significant mortality and morbidity. Gadre and colleagues[21] have looked into 1053 lung transplant patients for candida bloodstream infections. Only 11 patients (1.04%) developed candidemia. Most patients were hospitalized

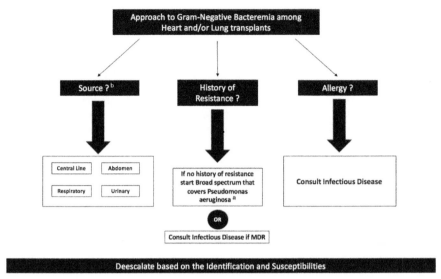

Fig. 1. The approach to gram-negative bacteremia in heart and/or lung transplant recipients. [a] Based on hospital susceptibility pattern. [b] By proper imaging and cultures.

pretransplant and exposed to high-dose steroids, antibiotics, and immunomodulators in the 3 months before transplant. Posttransplant, extra-corporeal life support was also associated with increased risk for candidemia, with the most common source being surgical site infection and the most common species being *Candida albicans*. Mortality was more than 50%.

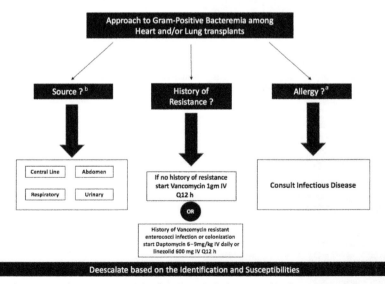

Fig. 2. The approach to gram-positive bacteremia in heart and/or lung transplant recipients. [a] If allergic to first-line drugs consult an Infectious Disease Specialist. [b] By proper imaging and culture.

Treatment for candida bloodstream infection in heart and/or lung transplant patients is similar to other patient population based on 2016 Infectious Disease Society of America guidelines. There is no randomized study for the treatment of candidemia in this heart and/or lung transplant recipients.[22] Delaying empirical treatment of candida bloodstream infection until positive blood cultures may pretend to worse outcome in this patient population.[23] However, empirical management with an echinocandin did not increase the survival in 2 randomized controlled trails in nonneutropenic candidemic individuals.[24,25] In patients with septic shock attributed to candida infection, delaying appropriate antifungal treatment and proper source control is associated with worse outcome.[26] The approaches to suspected and confirmed candidemia are summarized in **Figs. 3** and **4**.

Pneumonia

Pneumonia is the leading cause of infection in both heart and lung transplant patients. Two separate studies from Spain looked into pneumonia among heart and lung transplant patients. The first study was a multicenter retrospective study that evaluated 307 heart transplant recipients for pneumonia and found that 20% of patients developed pneumonia; 75% of episodes of pneumonia were in the first 3 months after transplant and 60% of the organisms were opportunistic.[27] The second study was a multicenter prospective study that observed 236 lung transplant patients for 180 days; 85 episodes of pneumonia were documented with an incidence of 72 episodes/100 lung transplant years; around 44% developed pneumonia in the first month; 82% were

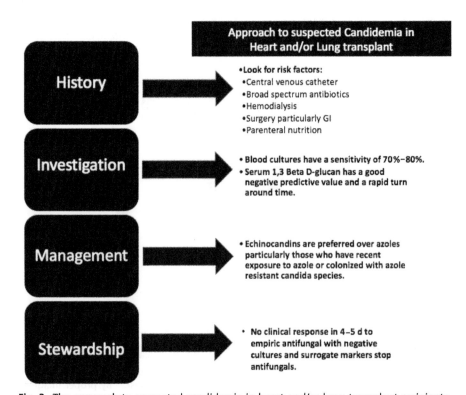

Approach to suspected Candidemia in Heart and/or Lung transplant

History
- •Look for risk factors:
- •Central venous catheter
- •Broad spectrum antibiotics
- •Hemodialysis
- •Surgery particularly GI
- •Parenteral nutrition

Investigation
- • Blood cultures have a sensitivity of 70%–80%.
- • Serum 1,3 Beta D-glucan has a good negative predictive value and a rapid turn around time.

Management
- • Echinocandins are preferred over azoles particularly those who have recent exposure to azole or colonized with azole resistant candida species.

Stewardship
- • No clinical response in 4–5 d to empiric antifungal with negative cultures and surrogate markers stop antifungals.

Fig. 3. The approach to suspected candidemia in heart and/or lung transplant recipients.

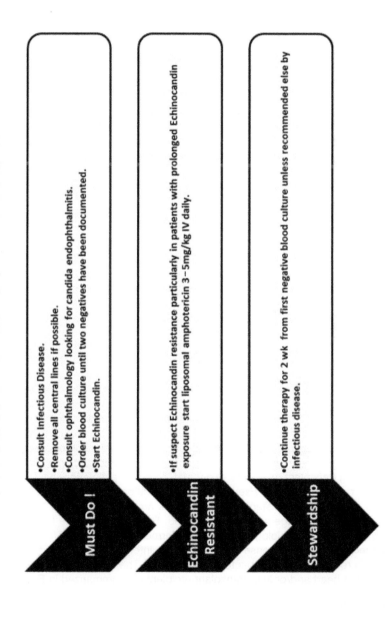

Approach to confirmed Candidemia

Must Do !
- Consult Infectious Disease.
- Remove all central lines if possible.
- Consult ophthalmology looking for candida endophthalmitis.
- Order blood culture until two negatives have been documented.
- Start Echinocandin.

Echinocandin Resistant
- If suspect Echinocandin resistance particularly in patients with prolonged Echinocandin exposure start liposomal amphotericin 3–5mg/kg IV daily.

Stewardship
- Continue therapy for 2 wk from first negative blood culture unless recommended else by infectious disease.

Fig. 4. The approach to confirmed candidemia in heart and/or lung transplant recipients.

bacterial and 72% were due to gram-negative organisms most commonly *Pseudomonas*. The study also showed reduced survival at 1 year in patients who had developed an episode of pneumonia (74%) as compared with those who did not develop pneumonia (99%).[28]

Lung transplant recipients have the greatest risk of developing pneumonia for several reasons, including continuous and direct exposure of the allograft to microbes, denervation of the allograft with subsequent impairment of cough reflex and mucociliary clearance; impaired lymphatic drainage; complications associated with anastomosis[29]; transmission of infection from donor lungs[30]; infection from native lung in single lung transplantation; and need for prolonged mechanical ventilatory support.[31]

Understanding the epidemiologic characteristics is of paramount importance in predicting the suspected cause of pneumonia; for example, local ecology of MDR organisms,[32] recent exposure to sick contacts particularly viral infections in children, history of travel to endemic areas for fungal and mycobacterial infections,[33] recent exposure to construction sites or environmental source for *Aspergillus* or *Nocardia*[34] and water sources such as *Legionella* or nontuberculous mycobacteria.[35]

Clinical presentation can differ according to the pathogen. Typical presentation with fever may be absent due to immunosuppression. Dry cough is present with cytomegalovirus (CMV) and *Pneumocystis jiroveci* pneumonias (PJP).[36,37] Hemoptysis is more frequent with *Aspergillus* pneumonia.[38] Nosocomial pneumonias usually have an acute presentation, whereas *Mycobacterium tuberculosis* has a subacute presentation.[39]

Diagnosis of pneumonia particularly in lung transplantation may be difficult, because the presence of organisms in the airway may reflect airway colonization. Moreover, other noninfectious cause, especially acute cellular rejection or primary graft dysfunction, may mimic pneumonia. **Fig. 5** summarizes the diagnostic criteria for proven pneumonia in heart and lung recipients.[40]

Respiratory viruses, CMV, and fungi should be worked up as potential cause of pneumonia.[41] Computed tomography is more sensitive than regular X-rays in detecting pulmonary complications in immunosuppressed individuals. Although being nonspecific, certain characteristics on radiograph images can favor certain causes such as bilateral interstitial infiltrates go with PJP, whereas the presence of cavitation indicates an *Aspergillus* infection.[42] Bronchoscopy and bronchoalveolar lavage are crucial tools for evaluating respiratory symptoms in heart and/or lung transplant recipients. A transbronchial biopsy provides an excellent route for excluding allograft rejection.[43] **Fig. 6** summarizes the diagnostic tests for the evaluation of pneumonia.

Empirical treatment of pneumonia depends on prior colonization or infection, especially in lung transplant recipients. In general, empirical antibiotics should cover gram-negative bacteria including *Pseudomonas*. In addition, if the patient has specific risk factors of methicillin-resistant *Stephylococcus aureus* (MRSA) (eg, MRSA colonization) *S aureus* coverage should be included. Patients should be treated according to the results of microbiological studies performed.

Guided by clinical response and the specific infectious organism, an 8- to 14-day course is recommended for bacterial infections.[44] The approach to pneumonia management in heart and/or lung transplant recipients is summarized in **Fig. 7**.

Mediastinitis

Postsurgical mediastinitis is a rare but a life-threatening complication occurring after heart and lung transplantation. In most series, the reported incidence is between 1% and 2%.[45] The associated mortality is high and varies between 14% and 47%.[46] In comparison to lung transplant, heart transplant patients have a higher risk

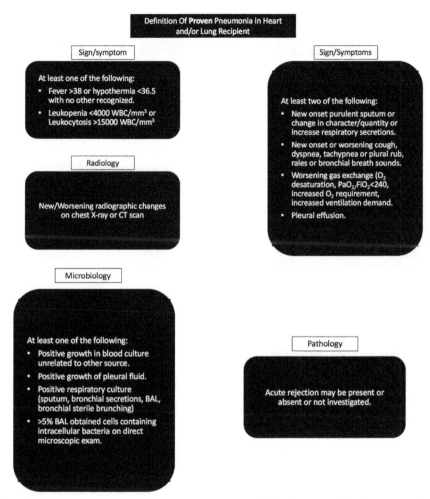

Fig. 5. The diagnostic criteria for proven pneumonia in heart and/or lung transplant recipients.

of developing mediastinitis. Abid and colleagues[47] have reported their 15 years of experience on mediastinitis in heart and lung transplant recipients. Between 1985 and 2000, 776 patients underwent heart and/or lung transplant; 21 (2.7%) developed mediastinitis: 14 hearts, 3 heart-lung, and 4 lungs. There were 6 (28.6%) deaths. In heart transplant patients, the most common organism was *S aureus*, whereas in lung transplant gram-negative rods were the predominant organisms.

Major risk factors associated with mediastinitis include obesity, diabetes mellitus, length of postoperative hospitalization, ventricular assistance device before surgery, and duration of mechanical ventilation after transplantation.

Clinical presentation is frequently not typical. A high index of suspicion is required. The most frequent symptom is pain, disproportionate to sternotomy. Elevated white blood cells, temperature, and erythema are less frequent. Diagnosis is made by computed tomography with sampling mediastinal tissue or fluid collection for culture.[48–50]

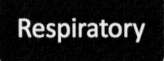

Diagnostic tests for the evaluation of Pneumonia In Heart and/or Lung transplant recipients

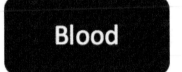

Respiratory

- Viral PCR or Antigen; Influenza, Parainfluenza, RSV, ADV, hMPV, rhinovirus, Coronavirus.
- DFA for PJP.
- Culture; bacterial, fungal and mycobacterial.
- Galactomannan.

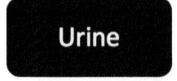

Blood

- Culture; bacterial.
- CMV PCR
- Galactomannan.
- Histoplasma antigen.
- Cryptococcus antigen.
- Blastomycosis antigen.

Urine

- Histoplasma antigen.
- Legionella antigen.
- Pneumococcal antigen

Fig. 6. The diagnostic tests for the evaluation of pneumonia in heart and/or lung transplant recipients.

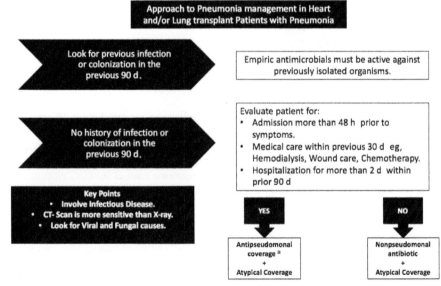

Fig. 7. The approach to pneumonia management in heart and/or lung transplant recipients with pneumonia.

Empirical treatment should include coverage for *S aureus*, *Staphylococcus epidermis*, and gram-negative rods after blood cultures have been obtained. Duration of treatment depends on surgical resection of the sternum. If the sternum is resected, a 2- to 3-week course is sufficient, whereas if only debridement is done then a minimum of 4 to 6 weeks is required.[51]

OPPORTUNISTIC INFECTIONS
Cytomegalovirus Infection

CMV infection is the most prevalent opportunistic infection in both heart and lung transplant recipients.[52] It comes second only to bacterial infections as an overall cause of infections in heart and lung recipients.[53,54] CMV is one of the herpesviruses and can stay latent within the body for life with possible reactivation.[55] Among the multitude of risk factors associated with CMV disease, the serostatus of the donor and recipient is the most important (donor seropositive and recipient seronegative) followed by use of antithymocyte globulins for rejection.[56]

CMV is known to augment the net state of immunosuppression and may result in facilitating the occurrence of other opportunistic bacterial and fungal infections.[57] It may also predispose to acute allograft rejection in both heart and lung transplant recipients. Similarly, it has been reported to be associated with cardiac allograft vasculopathy and bronchiolitis obliterans in lung transplant recipients.[58]

Before the era of universal prophylaxis administration, 30% to 90% of CMV-seropositive patients would have evidence of the virus in their blood and most would progress to disease. The incidence and timing of CMV infection and disease has changed over the last decade. Median time to the onset of CMV disease or infection has significantly increased after the widespread use of universal prophylaxis.[59-61]

The virus is commonly detected in patients admitted to the ICU.[62,63] The presence of CMV in the blood warrants treatment.[64,65] However, the authors do not recommend treatment of CMV if the test is only positive in bronchoalveolar lavage with concomitantly negative CMV in the blood.[66,67]

Patients on CMV treatment should have their viral load assay repeated on a weekly basis using quantitative polymerase chain reaction to monitor response to treatment.[68,69] In CMV pneumonitis, administering intravenous immunoglobulin or CMV-specific immunoglobulin is controversial.[70,71]

Aspergillosis

Invasive aspergillosis is a major cause of morbidity and mortality in patients who had undergone heart and/or lung transplants.[72,73] It is estimated that 9% of deaths after lung transplant is attributed to invasive aspergillosis.[74] In the solid organ population, it mainly affects lung transplant patients. Pappas and colleagues[75] looked into the incidence of invasive fungal infections among 1063 organ transplant recipients in 23 US transplant centers. They found invasive aspergillosis to be the second most common cause in 19% of patients. Almost half (48%) of these cases occurred in lung transplant recipients and 10% in heart transplant recipients. Most of the cases happened in the first 6 months after transplant.

Risks factors for invasive aspergillosis in lung transplant recipients include colonization with *Aspergillus*, CMV disease, airway ischemia, and single lung transplantation, whereas in heart transplant recipients risk factors include CMV disease and posttransplant hemodialysis.[76-80]

Invasive pulmonary aspergillosis should be suspected in heart and/or lung transplant recipients who present with fever and/or respiratory symptoms in the first

3 months after transplantation, have a positive culture result of *Aspergillus* species, and have abnormal radiological findings in particular nodules.[81]

Lung and sinuses are involved in more than 90% of cases of aspergillosis. Singh and colleagues[82] reviewed 159 cases of aspergillosis after lung transplant published in the literature. The most common presentation was tracheobronchitis or bronchial anastomotic infection in 58% of cases, whereas 32% had invasive pulmonary and 22% had disseminated infection.

The diagnosis of invasive aspergillosis in transplant patients is hampered by the lack of specific clinical and radiological signs and low sensitivity of culture-based diagnostic methods.[40,83] Galactomannan has been proposed as surrogate marker for invasive aspergillosis. However, with limited sensitivity of serum galactomannan in transplant patients, bronchoalveolar lavage has been proved to be highly sensitive (approaching 98%). Hence, in pneumonia workup BAL galactomannan should be assessed.[84] Conversely (1,3)-β-D-glucan is very nonspecific in the setting of lung transplant recipients.[85]

Voriconazole is the recommended first-line therapy.[86,87] Liposomal amphotericin B or caspofungin could be considered as an alternative.[88] Duration of therapy depends on extent of disease, clinical response, and immunologic status of the patients.[89,90] To ensure proper exposure of voriconazole treatment, monitoring of serum trough levels should be performed. Regular monitoring of liver enzymes and serum concentration calcineurin inhibitors is required to avoid hepatotoxicity and nephrotoxicity.[91]

Pneumocystis Jirovecii Pneumonia

Pneumocystis jirovecii is an opportunistic fungus that causes life-threatening pulmonary infection in SOT recipients.[92] Before the era of universal prophylaxis, the incidence in heart and/or lung transplant recipients was 10% to 40%.[93] PJP is associated with graft loss, and mortality remains high (up to 60%) despite treatment with trimethoprim-sulfamethoxazole (TMP-SMX).[94] Heart and lung transplant recipients should stay on PJP prophylaxis for life.[95,96]

Critical care physicians should consider PJP as one differential in heart and/or lung transplant recipients admitted with pneumonia to the critical care unit, especially if not on PJP prophylaxis. Lehto and colleagues[97] reviewed 609 bronchoscopies on 40 lung or heart/lung transplant recipients, and they found that 23 (4.9%) of bronchoscopy specimens had PJP. Of these 15 (65%) were on prophylaxis.

Signs and symptoms are nonspecific, mostly presenting with dry cough, fever, and shortness of breath. Imaging is also nonspecific and can show bilateral interstitial infiltrates.[98] Diagnosis is based on direct identification of the organism in respiratory tract or secretions.[99] Serum (1,3)-D-glucan has high sensitivity (up to 95%) and if negative can exclude PJP.[100]

TMP-SMX is the drug of choice for PJP given 15 to 20 mg/kg/d intravenously divided every 6 to 8 hours.[101] Corticosteroids are commonly administered; yet their use is not well substantiated in transplantation.[102] Patients on TMP-SMX should have their cell count, creatinine, and potassium monitored at regular intervals. Intravenous TMP-SMX can be switched to oral once patient is improving to complete 21 days. In patients with sulfa drug allergy and suspected PJP an infectious disease consult should be sought for appropriate management.

Mycoplasma Hominis and Ureaplasma Urealyticum Infection

In lung transplant recipients, hyperammonemia is a rare but fatal condition in the early posttransplant period.[103] Chen and colleagues[104] evaluated 807 lung transplant patients for developing hyperammonemia syndrome and found that only 8 (1%) had developed it, of which 6 (75%) died.

Systemic infection with *M hominis* and *U Urealyticum* is a unique cause of hyperammonemia in lung transplant recipients.[105] Any recent lung transplant recipients with lethargy, seizure, or coma should have their ammonia levels checked and if high a macrolide, fluoroquinolone, or a tetracycline should be started. Combination therapy could be considered, especially with high resistance. Diagnosis is based on special cultures and polymerase chain reaction. Recently there has been a suggestion that this may be a donor-derived infection.[106]

REFERENCES

1. Chambers DC, Yusen RD, Cherikh WS, et al. The Registry of the International Society for Heart and Lung Transplantation: thirty-fourth adult lung and heart-lung transplantation report-2017; focus theme: allograft ischemic time. J Heart Lung Transplant 2017;36(10):1047–59.

2. Yusen RD, Edwards LB, Kucheryavaya AY, et al. The Registry of the International Society for Heart and Lung Transplantation: thirty-second official adult lung and heart-lung transplantation report–2015; focus theme: early graft failure. J Heart Lung Transplant 2015;34(10):1264–77.

3. Fishman JA. Infection in organ transplantation. Am J Transplant 2017;17(4): 856–79.

4. Green M. Introduction: infections in solid organ transplantation. Am J Transplant 2013;13(Suppl 4):3–8.

5. Fishman JA. Infection in solid-organ transplant recipients. N Engl J Med 2007; 357:2601–14.

6. Singer M, Deutschman CS, Seymour CW, et al. The third international consensus definitions for sepsis and septic shock (Sepsis-3). JAMA 2016; 315:801–10.

7. Seymour CW, Liu VX, Iwashyna TJ, et al. Assessment of clinical criteria for sepsis: for the third international consensus definitions for sepsis and septic shock (sepsis-3). JAMA 2016;315(8):762–74.

8. Kalil AC, Dakroub H, Freifeld AG. Sepsis and solid organ transplantation. Curr Drug Targets 2007;8(4):533–41.

9. Donnelly JP, Locke JE, MacLennan PA, et al. Inpatient mortality among solid organ transplant recipients hospitalized for sepsis and severe sepsis. Clin Infect Dis 2016;63(2):186–94.

10. Kalil AC, Sandkovsky U, Florescu DF. Severe infections in critically ill solid organ transplant patients. Clin Microbiol Infect 2018 [pii:S1198-743X(18)30362-8]. [Epub ahead of print].

11. Florescu DF, Sandkovsky U, Kalil AC. Sepsis and challenging infections in the immunosuppressed patient in the intensive care unit. Infect Dis Clin North Am 2017;31(3):415–34.

12. Trzeciak S1, Sharer R, Piper D, et al. Infections and severe sepsis in solid-organ transplant patients admitted from a university-based ED. Am J Emerg Med 2004;22(7):530–3.

13. Pietrantoni C, Minai OA, Yu NC, et al. Respiratory failure and sepsis are the major causes of ICU admissions and mortality in survivors of lung transplants. Chest 2003;123(2):504–9.

14. Kalil AC, Syed A, Rupp ME, et al. Is bacteremic sepsis associated with higher mortality in transplant recipients than in nontransplant patients? A matched case-control propensity-adjusted study. Clin Infect Dis 2015;60(2):216–22.

15. Hamandi B, Holbrook AM, Humar A, et al. Delay of adequate empiric antibiotic therapy is associated with increased mortality among solid-organ transplant patients. Am J Transplant 2009;9(7):1657–65.

16. Rodríguez C, Muñoz P, Rodríguez-Créixems M, et al. Bloodstream infections among heart transplant recipients. Transplantation 2006;81(3):384–91.

17. Palmer SM, Alexander BD, Sanders LL, et al. Significance of blood stream infection after lung transplantation: analysis in 176 consecutive patients. Transplantation 2000;69(11):2360–6.

18. Husain S, Chan KM, Palmer SM, et al. Bacteremia in lung transplant recipients in the current era. Am J Transplant 2006;6(12):3000–7.

19. Baden LR, Swaminathan S, Angarone M, et al. Prevention and treatment of cancer-related infections, version 2.2016, NCCN clinical practice guidelines in oncology. J Natl Compr Canc Netw 2016;14(7):882–913.

20. Mermel LA, Allon M, Bouza E, et al. Clinical practice guidelines for the diagnosis and management of intravascular catheter-related infection: 2009 Update by the Infectious Diseases Society of America. Clin Infect Dis 2009;49(1):1–45.

21. Gadre SK, Koval C, Budev M. Candida blood stream infections post lung transplant. J Heart Lung Transplant 2017;36(4):S241.

22. Pappas PG, Kauffman CA, Andes DR, et al. Clinical practice guideline for the management of candidiasis: 2016 update by the infectious diseases society of America. Clin Infect Dis 2016;62(4):e1–50.

23. Morrell M, Fraser VJ, Kollef MH. Delaying the empiric treatment of candida bloodstream infection until positive blood culture results are obtained: a potential risk factor for hospital mortality. Antimicrob Agents Chemother 2005;49(9):3640–5.

24. Ostrosky-Zeichner L, Shoham S, Vazquez J, et al. MSG-01: a randomized, double-blind, placebo-controlled trial of caspofungin prophylaxis followed by preemptive therapy for invasive candidiasis in high-risk adults in the critical care setting. Clin Infect Dis 2014;58(9):1219–26.

25. Knitsch W, Vincent JL, Utzolino S, et al. A randomized, placebo-controlled trial of preemptive antifungal therapy for the prevention of invasive candidiasis following gastrointestinal surgery for intra-abdominal infections. Clin Infect Dis 2015;61(11):1671–8.

26. Kollef M, Micek S, Hampton N, et al. Septic shock attributed to Candida infection: importance of empiric therapy and source control. Clin Infect Dis 2012;54(12):1739–46.

27. Cisneros JM1, Muñoz P, Torre-Cisneros J, et al. Pneumonia after heart transplantation: a multi-institutional study. Spanish transplantation infection study group. Clin Infect Dis 1998;27(2):324–31.

28. Aguilar-Guisado M1, Givaldá J, Ussetti P, et al, RESITRA cohort. Pneumonia after lung transplantation in the RESITRA Cohort: a multicenter prospective study. Am J Transplant 2007;7(8):1989–96.

29. Olland A, Reeb J, Puyraveau M, et al. Bronchial complications after lung transplantation are associated with primary lung graft dysfunction and surgical technique. J Heart Lung Transplant 2017;36(2):157–65.

30. Ruiz I, Gavaldà J, Monforte V, et al. Donor-to-host transmission of bacterial and fungal infections in lung transplantation. Am J Transplant 2006;6(1):178–82.

31. Maurer JR, Tullis DE, Grossman RF, et al. Infectious complications following isolated lung transplantation. Chest 1992;101(4):1056–9.
32. Mattner F, Fischer S, Weissbrodt H, et al. Post-operative nosocomial infections after lung and heart transplantation. J Heart Lung Transplant 2007;26(3):241–9.
33. Gasink LB, Blumberg EA. Bacterial and mycobacterial pneumonia in transplant recipients. Clin Chest Med 2005;26(4):647–59.
34. Clark NM, Reid GE, AST Infectious Diseases Community of Practice. Nocardia infections in solid organ transplantation. Am J Transplant 2013;13(Suppl 4): 83–92.
35. Avery RK, Michaels MG, AST Infectious Diseases Community of Practice. Strategies for safe living after solid organ transplantation. Am J Transplant 2013; 13(Suppl 4):304–10.
36. Ison MG1, Fishman JA. Cytomegalovirus pneumonia in transplant recipients. Clin Chest Med 2005;26(4):691–705.
37. Kovacs JA, Hiemenz JW, Macher AM, et al. Pneumocystis carinii pneumonia: a comparison between patients with the acquired immunodeficiency syndrome and patients with other immunodeficiencies. Ann Intern Med 1984;100(5): 663–71.
38. Singh N1, Paterson DL. Aspergillus infections in transplant recipients. Clin Microbiol Rev 2005;18(1):44–69.
39. Meije Y, Piersimoni C, Torre-Cisneros J, et al, ESCMID Study Group of Infection in Compromised Hosts. Mycobacterial infections in solid organ transplant recipients. Clin Microbiol Infect 2014;20(Suppl 7):89–101.
40. Husain S, Mooney ML, Danziger-Isakov L, et al, ISHLT Infectious Diseases Council Working Group on Definitions. A 2010 working formulation for the standardization of definitions of infections in cardiothoracic transplant recipients. J Heart Lung Transplant 2011;30(4):361–74.
41. Chakinala MM, Trulock EP. Pneumonia in the solid organ transplant patient. Clin Chest Med 2005;26(1):113–21.
42. Fujii T, Nakamura T, Iwamoto A. Pneumocystis pneumonia in patients with HIV infection: clinical manifestations, laboratory findings, and radiological features. J Infect Chemother 2007;13(1):1–7.
43. Guilinger RA, Paradis IL, Dauber JH, et al. The importance of bronchoscopy with transbronchial biopsy and bronchoalveolar lavage in the management of lung transplant recipients. Am J Respir Crit Care Med 1995;152(6 Pt 1): 2037–43.
44. Kalil AC, Metersky ML, Klompas M, et al. Executive summary: management of adults with hospital-acquired and ventilator-associated pneumonia: 2016 clinical practice guidelines by the infectious diseases society of America and the American Thoracic Society. Clin Infect Dis 2016;63(5):575–82.
45. Karwande SV, Renlund DG, Olsen SL, et al. Mediastinitis in heart transplantation. Ann Thorac Surg 1992;54(6):1039–45.
46. Gummert JF, Barten MJ, Hans C, et al. Mediastinitis and cardiac surgery–an updated risk factor analysis in 10,373 consecutive adult patients. Thorac Cardiovasc Surg 2002;50(2):87–91.
47. Abid Q, Nkere UU, Hasan A, et al. Mediastinitis in heart and lung transplantation: 15 years' experience. Ann Thorac Surg 2003;75(5):1565–71.
48. Sénéchal M, LePrince P, Tezenas du Montcel S, et al. Bacterial mediastinitis after heart transplantation: clinical presentation, risk factors and treatment. J Heart Lung Transplant 2004;23(2):165–70.

49. Misawa Y, Fuse K, Hasegawa T. Infectious mediastinitis after cardiac operations: computed tomographic findings. Ann Thorac Surg 1998;65(3):622–4.
50. Yamaguchi H, Yamauchi H, Yamada T, et al. Diagnostic validity of computed tomography for mediastinitis after cardiac surgery. Ann Thorac Cardiovasc Surg 2001;7(2):94–8.
51. El Oakley RM, Wright JE. Postoperative mediastinitis: classification and management. Ann Thorac Surg 1996;61(3):1030–6.
52. Fisher RA. Cytomegalovirus infection and disease in the new era of immunosuppression following solid organ transplantation. Transpl Infect Dis 2009;11(3): 195–202.
53. Vaska PL. Common infections in heart transplant patients. Am J Crit Care 1993; 2(2):145–54.
54. Zamora MR. Cytomegalovirus and lung transplantation. Am J Transplant 2004; 4(8):1219–26.
55. Fishman JA. Overview: cytomegalovirus and the herpesviruses in transplantation. Am J Transplant 2013;13(Suppl 3):1–8.
56. Harvala H, Stewart C, Muller K, et al. High risk of cytomegalovirus infection following solid organ transplantation despite prophylactic therapy. J Med Virol 2013;85(5):893–8.
57. Snyder LD, Finlen-Copeland CA, Turbyfill WJ, et al. Cytomegalovirus pneumonitis is a risk for bronchiolitis obliterans syndrome in lung transplantation. Am J Respir Crit Care Med 2010;181(12):1391–6.
58. Delgado JF, Reyne AG, de Dios S, et al. Influence of cytomegalovirus infection in the development of cardiac allograft vasculopathy after heart transplantation. J Heart Lung Transplant 2015;34(8):1112–9.
59. Hodson EM, Ladhani M, Webster AC, et al. Antiviral medications for preventing cytomegalovirus disease in solid organ transplant recipients. Cochrane Database Syst Rev 2013;(2):CD003774.
60. Schoeppler KE1, Lyu DM, Grazia TJ, et al. Late-onset cytomegalovirus (CMV) in lung transplant recipients: can CMV serostatus guide the duration of prophylaxis? Am J Transplant 2013;13(2):376–82.
61. Potena L, Solidoro P, Patrucco F, et al. Treatment and prevention of cytomegalovirus infection in heart and lung transplantation: an update. Expert Opin Pharmacother 2016;17(12):1611–22.
62. Papazian L, Hraiech S, Lehingue S, et al. Cytomegalovirus reactivation in ICU patients. Intensive Care Med 2016;42(1):28–37.
63. Lachance P, Chen J, Featherstone R, et al. Impact of cytomegalovirus reactivation on clinical outcomes in immunocompetent critically ill patients: protocol for a systematic review and meta-analysis. Syst Rev 2016;5(1):127.
64. Asberg A, Humar A, Rollag H, et al, VICTOR Study Group. Oral valganciclovir is noninferior to intravenous ganciclovir for the treatment of cytomegalovirus disease in solid organ transplant recipients. Am J Transplant 2007;7(9):2106–13.
65. Kotton CN1, Kumar D, Caliendo AM, et al, Transplantation Society International CMV Consensus Group. Updated international consensus guidelines on the management of cytomegalovirus in solid-organ transplantation. Transplantation 2013;96(4):333–60.
66. Lodding IP, Schultz HH, Jensen JU, et al. Cytomegalovirus viral load in bronchoalveolar lavage to diagnose lung transplant associated CMV pneumonia. Transplantation 2018;102(2):326–32.
67. Coussement J, Steensels D, Nollevaux MC, et al. When polymerase chain reaction does not help: cytomegalovirus pneumonitis associated with very low or

undetectable viral load in both blood and bronchoalveolar lavage samples after lung transplantation. Transpl Infect Dis 2016;18(2):284–7.

68. Caliendo AM, St George K, Allega J, et al. Distinguishing cytomegalovirus (CMV) infection and disease with CMV nucleic acid assays. J Clin Microbiol 2002;40(5):1581–6.

69. Humar A, Kumar D, Boivin G, et al. Cytomegalovirus (CMV) virus load kinetics to predict recurrent disease in solid-organ transplant patients with CMV disease. J Infect Dis 2002;186(6):829–33.

70. Snydman DR. Cytomegalovirus immunoglobulins in the prevention and treatment of cytomegalovirus disease. Rev Infect Dis 1990;12(Suppl 7):S839–48.

71. Haidar G, Singh N. Viral infections in solid organ transplant recipients: novel updates and a review of the classics. Curr Opin Infect Dis 2017;30(6):579–88.

72. Singh N, Husain S, AST Infectious Diseases Community of Practice. Aspergillosis in solid organ transplantation. Am J Transplant 2013;13(Suppl 4):228–41.

73. Neofytos D, Fishman JA, Horn D, et al. Epidemiology and outcome of invasive fungal infections in solid organ transplant recipients. Transpl Infect Dis 2010; 12(3):220–9.

74. Paterson DL, Singh N. Invasive aspergillosis in transplant recipients. Medicine (Baltimore) 1999;78(2):123–38.

75. Pappas PG, Alexander BD, Andes DR, et al. Invasive fungal infections among organ transplant recipients: results of the Transplant-Associated Infection Surveillance Network (TRANSNET). Clin Infect Dis 2010;50(8):1101–11.

76. Montoya JG, Chaparro SV, Celis D, et al. Invasive aspergillosis in the setting of cardiac transplantation. Clin Infect Dis 2003;37(Suppl 3):S281–92.

77. Montoya JG, Giraldo LF, Efron B, et al. Infectious complications among 620 consecutive heart transplant patients at Stanford University Medical Center. Clin Infect Dis 2001;33(5):629–40.

78. Munoz P, Rodriguez C, Bouza E, et al. Risk factors of invasive aspergillosis after heart transplantation: protective role of oral itraconazole prophylaxis. Am J Transplant 2004;4:636–43.

79. Speziali G, McDougall JC, Midthun DE, et al. Native lung complications after single lung transplantation for emphysema. Transpl Int 1997;10:113–5.

80. Husni RN, Gordon SM, Longworth DL, et al. Cytomegalovirus infection is a risk factor for invasive aspergillosis in lung transplant recipients. Clin Infect Dis 1998;26(3):753–5.

81. Muñoz P1, Alcalá L, Sánchez Conde M, et al. The isolation of Aspergillus fumigatus from respiratory tract specimens in heart transplant recipients is highly predictive of invasive aspergillosis. Transplantation 2003;75(3):326–9.

82. Singh N, Husain S. Aspergillus infections after lung transplantation: clinical differences in type of transplant and implications for management. J Heart Lung Transplant 2003;22(3):258–66.

83. Park YS, Seo JB, Lee YK, et al. Radiological and clinical findings of pulmonary aspergillosis following solid organ transplant. Clin Radiol 2008;63(6):673–80.

84. Pasqualotto AC, Xavier MO, Sánchez LB, et al. Diagnosis of invasive aspergillosis in lung transplant recipients by detection of galactomannan in the bronchoalveolar lavage fluid. Transplantation 2010;90(3):306–11.

85. Mutschlechner W, Risslegger B, Willinger B, et al. Bronchoalveolar lavage fluid (1,3)β-D-glucan for the diagnosis of invasive fungal infections in solid organ transplantation: a prospective multicenter study. Transplantation 2015;99(9): e140–4.

86. Fortún J, Martín-Dávila P, Sánchez MA, et al. Voriconazole in the treatment of invasive mold infections in transplant recipients. Eur J Clin Microbiol Infect Dis 2003;22(7):408–13.

87. Denning DW, Ribaud P, Milpied N, et al. Efficacy and safety of voriconazole in the treatment of acute invasive aspergillosis. Clin Infect Dis 2002;34(5):563–71.

88. Wieland T, Liebold A, Jagiello M, et al. Superiority of voriconazole over amphotericin B in the treatment of invasive aspergillosis after heart transplantation. J Heart Lung Transplant 2005;24(1):102–4.

89. Herbrecht R, Denning DW, Patterson TF, et al. Invasive Fungal Infections Group of the European Organisation for Research and Treatment of Cancer and the Global Aspergillus Study Group. Voriconazole versus amphotericin B for primary therapy of invasive aspergillosis. N Engl J Med 2002;347(6):408–15.

90. Patterson TF, Thompson GR, Denning DW, et al. Practice guidelines for the diagnosis and management of aspergillosis: 2016 update by the infectious diseases society of America. Clin Infect Dis 2016;63(4):e1–60.

91. Kulkarni HS, Witt CA. Voriconazole in lung transplant recipients - how worried should we be? Am J Transplant 2018;18(1):5–6.

92. Martin SI, Fishman JA, AST Infectious Diseases Community of Practice. Pneumocystis pneumonia in solid organ transplantation. Am J Transplant 2013; 13(Suppl 4):272–9.

93. Kramer MR, Stoehr C, Lewiston NJ, et al. Trimethoprim-sulfamethoxazole prophylaxis for Pneumocystis carinii infections in heart-lung and lung transplantation–how effective and for how long? Transplantation 1992;53(3):586–9.

94. Rodriguez M, Fishman JA. Prevention of infection due to Pneumocystis spp. in human immunodeficiency virus-negative immunocompromised patients. Clin Microbiol Rev 2004;17(4):770–82.

95. Gordon SM, LaRosa SP, Kalmadi S, et al. Should prophylaxis for Pneumocystis carinii pneumonia in solid organ transplant recipients ever be discontinued? Clin Infect Dis 1999;28(2):240–6.

96. Perez-Ordoño L, Hoyo I, Sanclemente G, et al. Late-onset Pneumocystis jirovecii pneumonia in solid organ transplant recipients. Transpl Infect Dis 2014;16(2): 324–8.

97. Lehto JT, Koskinen PK, Anttila VJ, et al. Bronchoscopy in the diagnosis and surveillance of respiratory infections in lung and heart-lung transplant recipients. Transpl Int 2005;18(5):562–71.

98. Kanne JP, Yandow DR, Meyer CA. Pneumocystis jiroveci pneumonia: high-resolution CT findings in patients with and without HIV infection. AJR Am J Roentgenol 2012;198(6):W555–61.

99. LaRocque RC, Katz JT, Perruzzi P, et al. The utility of sputum induction for diagnosis of Pneumocystis pneumonia in immunocompromised patients without human immunodeficiency virus. Clin Infect Dis 2003;37(10):1380–3.

100. Karageorgopoulos DE, Qu JM, Korbila IP, et al. Accuracy of β-D-glucan for the diagnosis of Pneumocystis jirovecii pneumonia: a meta-analysis. Clin Microbiol Infect 2013;19(1):39–49.

101. Garnacho-Montero J, Olaechea P, Alvarez-Lerma F, et al. Epidemiology, diagnosis and treatment of fungal respiratory infections in the critically ill patient. Rev Esp Quimioter 2013;26(2):173–88.

102. McKinnell JA, Cannella AP, Injean P, et al. Adjunctive glucocorticoid therapy for non-HIV-related pneumocystis carinii pneumonia (NH-PCP). Am J Transplant 2014;14(4):982–3.

103. Lichtenstein GR, Yang YX, Nunes FA, et al. Fatal hyperammonemia after ortho-topic lung transplantation. Ann Intern Med 2000;132(4):283–7.

104. Chen C, Bain KB, Iuppa JA, et al. Hyperammonemia syndrome after lung trans-plantation: a single center experience. Transplantation 2016;100(3):678–84.

105. Bharat A, Cunningham SA, Scott Budinger GR, et al. Disseminated Ureaplasma infection as a cause of fatal hyperammonemia in humans. Sci Transl Med 2015; 7(284):284re3.

106. Fernandez R, Ratliff A, Crabb D, et al. Ureaplasma transmitted from donor lungs is pathogenic after lung transplantation. Ann Thorac Surg 2017;103(2):670–1.

Section II: Liver, Kidney, and Small Bowel

Preface

Caring for the Critically Ill Liver Transplant Patients: A Fifty-Year Journey!

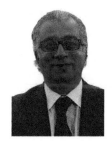

Ali Al-Khafaji, MD, MPH, FCCM
Editor

I am truly excited, honored, and humbled to serve as an editor for this special issue of *Critical Care Clinics* devoted to the care of critically ill liver transplant patients.

The journey of liver transplantation started with the pivotal foundation work of the late Thomas E. Starzl. Although he attempted the first human liver transplant in 1963, the successful liver transplant was not achieved until 1967, more than 50 years ago.

Over the last five decades, there have been extensive improvements in surgical techniques, immunosuppression, and most importantly, the critical care management of these patients that led to an enormous expansion of the transplantation field.

In this issue of *Critical Care Clinics*, we have chosen a number of topics that cover most conditions encountered when caring for patients with liver disease before and after liver transplant.

We intended to present a current practical overview, and we sincerely hope that each review will serve attendings, fellows, residents, nursing, and other medical staff as a handy reference providing rationales and solutions to one of the most challenging patients to care for in the field of transplantation.

Each topic starts with a brief synopsis and key messages followed by an in-depth discussion with an expansive reference list.

I must thank many people who contributed directly or indirectly to this endeavor. First, the authors, who have done a superb job and sacrificed a significant amount of time that they could have spent doing other important things. Second, the outstanding indefatigable editorial and production staff of the *Clinics*. Third, my mother, wife, and three children, who continue to function as my valuable reset button every single day. Finally, and most importantly, our patients, who without them none of this work matters.

We sincerely hope that we have covered all the important clinically relevant issues and that the readers of this issue will benefit from the authors' contributions.

Ali Al-Khafaji, MD, MPH, FCCM
Transplant Intensive Care Unit
University of Pittsburgh School of Medicine
Room 613 Scaife Hall
3550 Terrace Street
Pittsburgh, PA 15261, USA

E-mail address:
alkhafajia2@upmc.edu

Website:
https://www.ccm.pitt.edu

Perioperative Management of the Liver Transplant Recipient

David J. Kramer, MD[a,b,]*, Eric M. Siegal, MD[a,b],
Sarah J. Frogge, DNP, APNP[a], Manpreet S. Chadha, MD[a,c]

KEYWORDS

- Liver failure • Liver transplantation • Critical illness • Critical care medicine
- Perioperative management

KEY POINTS

- The age threshold for liver transplantation is climbing, and these patients have significant comorbidities and increasingly advanced liver disease at the time of transplantation.
- Multidisciplinary medical care with critical care medicine, transplant surgery, anesthesiology, hepatology, and nephrology collaborating provides optimal timing for liver transplantation and perioperative intensive care.
- Recognition of compromised organ perfusion and impending multiple systems organ failure requires ongoing monitoring and rapid resuscitation.

OVERVIEW

The population of solid organ transplant recipients is growing. Although perioperative management remains the purview of subspecialized intensivists, it is increasingly likely that clinicians caring for the critically ill will be called on to address issues in this unique population. This review proposes a framework for clinical evaluation and management of the critically ill transplant recipient that applies in a range of clinical settings. Solid organ transplantation reflects a multifaceted set of responsibilities to the recipient, the donor, and society. The transplant center remains deeply committed to the long-term outcome of the recipient. A team comprising organ-specific subspecialists and transplant intensivists optimally comanages critically ill transplant recipients.

[a] Aurora Critical Care Service, Advocate Aurora Health Care, 2901 W Kinnickinnic River Parkway, Suite 305, Milwaukee, WI 53215, USA; [b] Department of Medicine, University of Wisconsin School of Medicine and Public Health in Madison, 750 Highland Avenue, Madison, WI 53726, USA; [c] Aurora Abdominal Transplant and Hepatobiliary Program, 2801 W Kinnickinnic River Parkway, Suite 580, Milwaukee, WI 53215, USA
* Corresponding author.
E-mail address: David.Kramer@Aurora.org

Crit Care Clin 35 (2019) 95–105
https://doi.org/10.1016/j.ccc.2018.08.012
0749-0704/19/© 2018 Elsevier Inc. All rights reserved.

criticalcare.theclinics.com

PROCESS

Care of the critically ill transplant recipient is increasingly multidisciplinary. Although the number of transplant centers has increased over the past 3 decades, the number of transplants performed at many centers is relatively small. Consequently, clinicians with vast experience are in short supply. Quality-improvement requires ongoing assessment of outcomes and real-time feedback and discussion among the care givers. Handoffs among different care teams should be structured and consistent.

Nursing experience and engagement cannot be overvalued. It affords select patients the opportunity to avoid the ICU entirely.[1] Unfortunately, the average tenure of surgical ICU nurses is decreasing. Over the past 25 years, advanced practice clinicians in the forms of nurse practitioners and physicians assistants have been incorporated into ICU practice and are of particular value for transplant critical care services.[2] These clinicians have more focused experience than many house staff and ensure that transplant candidates and recipients are managed consistently with multidisciplinary guidance from surgeons and physicians.

CANDIDATE SELECTION: TOO SICK FOR TRANSPLANT?

Model for End-Stage Liver Disease (MELD)-driven liver allocation prioritizes sicker patients for transplant and has resulted in many candidates taken to surgery from the ICU. Candidate acuity seems to explain approximately one-third of the variance in outcome with the remainder explained by the characteristics of the organ donor (donor risk index[3]) and operative details, including operative time, red blood cell transfusion requirement, and warm ischemia time. Minimizing the aggregate risk contributed by these 3 domains is ideal but not always possible. At the time of an offer, the potential recipient may accept the attendant risk rather than possibility of clinical deterioration precluding transplantation in the future with a better organ. Recently, the age of the donor has been recognized to have an impact on graft survival in recipients with hepatitis C.[4] The contribution of donor age to poor outcome in the high-MELD recipient is recognized in minimizing product of donor age and recipient MELD (D-MELD) to below 1600.[5] The use of living donor organs for high MELD patients is controversial in the United States but in Asia excellent outcomes are reported.[6]

Candidate selection among the critically ill remains controversial. The combination of acuity (severity of illness) and its duration must be considered before accepting an organ for the ICU patient. Relative acute contraindications to transplantation include the need for high-dose vasopressors (1 µg/kg/min of norepinephrine or equivalent) and pulmonary hypertension with elevated pulmonary vascular resistance or compromised right ventricular function with low cardiac output. Acute lung injury/acute respiratory distress syndrome (ARDS) is common in liver failure.[7] Lung injury worsens with transplant and the resultant hypoxic pulmonary arterial vasoconstriction increases right ventricular pressures and compromises hepatic outflow. Carefully selected patients with liver failure–induced acute lung injury/ARDS improve with successful liver transplantation.[8,9] The authors, however, defer transplantation in mechanically ventilated patients requiring PEEP greater than 12 cm H_2O and/or fraction of inspired oxygen (Fio_2) greater than 50%, particularly when lung injury persists over more than 24 hours to 48 hours.

Frailty and physiologic reserve have an impact on transplant outcomes and require preoperative evaluation. The outcomes in patients who are bed-bound for more than 1 week are poor. Mobilization of the liver transplant candidate and recipient requires minimizing sedation and maximizing physical therapy. When sedation is absolutely necessary, the authors prefer dexmedetomidine or, failing that, propofol. Benzodiazepines, even short-acting ones, have markedly prolonged duration of action in patients with liver disease and are associated with delirium and rarely indicated. Intubation and mechanical ventilation are not absolute contraindications to mobilization and ambulation.

Protein calorie malnutrition is common in liver failure despite increased weight, which often reflects water retention. In addition to anorexia and early satiety, with dysfunctional gastric emptying, muscle weakness begets swallowing dysfunction and increases the risk for aspiration. In the absence of adequate oral intake, tube feedings can be instilled with tubes placed beyond the pylorus and preferably beyond the ligament of Treitz to minimize the risk of aspiration.

GOALS OF CARE

The ICU team becomes deeply invested emotionally and professionally in the outcome of patients for whom death is imminent and transplant is the only hope. The success of a transplant program depends on recognizing when the patient is too sick to transplant, deciding not to proceed, and communicating the rationale for these decisions with both the family and the health care team. The threshold for proceeding with liver transplantation varies across programs and within programs from patient to patient relating to the complexity of disease and resource availability.

The authors formally address goals of care at each stage of the transplant process. These are determined in discussion with the patient and family to identify priorities and define clinical limitations. The authors specifically address resuscitation in the event of cardiac arrest—code status. Although it may be obvious that a patient with liver failure and multiple systems organ failure requiring vasopressor support, mechanical ventilation, and renal replacement therapy does not benefit from attempted cardiac resuscitation, outcomes of cardiopulmonary resuscitation in hospitalized patients are poor. Full code status is appropriate during and after surgery but severe complications may warrant reassessment. Such re-evaluation should be seen as placing a patient's goals at the forefront of consideration for the clinical team.

POSTOPERATIVE MANAGEMENT

Enhanced recovery after liver surgery has recently been reviewed.[10] Similar principles can guide perioperative management for liver transplant recipients.[11] Balanced anesthetic techniques with short-acting neuromuscular blockade and minimal narcotics and benzodiazepines allow many liver transplant recipients to be rapidly liberated form mechanical ventilation. Some programs have refined this process to the point patients can transfer to the ward after surgery and avoid the ICU entirely.[1] More typically, early liberation from mechanical ventilation in the ICU affords minimization of sedation and early mobilization.

After handoff from the anesthesia and surgical teams, the ICU team needs to rapidly assess neurologic, cardiac, respiratory, renal, and hepatic function.

Function of the transplanted liver may be gauged initially by observing coagulation (prothrombin time and factor V), bile quality, and metabolism of tacrolimus. Aminotransferase elevation and area under the curve of enzymes during the first 36 hours seems to correlate with preservation injury. Ischemic injury is mitigated with use of N-acetylcysteine.[12] Although controversy exists as to benefit of N-acetylcysteine in liver transplantation,[13] the authors initiate infusion prior to reperfusion and continue for 72 hours for organs procured after cardiac death.[14,15] Allograft vascular integrity is routinely assessed with Doppler ultrasonography, with angiography considered in patients sonographic abnormalities or with an unusual pattern of aminotransferase elevation. Biliary integrity can be evaluated with cholangiography 72 hours postoperatively.

Liver support with mechanical devices is in a nascent stage. The Molecular Adsorbent Recirculation System does not have an indication for liver failure. It may have utility, however, in the postoperative period by mitigating cholestasis and the risk for cholemic nephropathy.[16] Associated reduction in vasopressor support with improved hemodynamics may be beneficial.[17]

The liver is less susceptible to rejection than other solid organ transplants, and patients who are severely ill, debilitated, or elderly mount a weakened immune response to the allograft. These patients are at markedly elevated risk of infection.[18] The authors, therefore, attenuate immunosuppression. Multimodality immunosuppression is achieved with corticosteroids, mycophenolate mofetil, and tacrolimus, which can be titrated based on underlying disease, such as hepatocellular carcinoma or cholangiocarcinoma. Tacrolimus metabolism is impaired in the setting of moderate to severe preservation injury. Dosing interval can then be extended to 24 hours. Monotherapy with calcineurin inhibitor (CNI) can usually be achieved by the fourth month postoperatively. Mammalian target of rapamycin inhibitors have been associated with thrombosis of the hepatic artery and are deferred in the early postoperative period.

HEMODYNAMICS

The hemodynamics of liver failure are similar to sepsis with systemic vasodilation and elevated cardiac output, but they normalize over the month after transplantation. Postoperative third-spacing and oozing result in volume contraction, which may compromise cardiac output. Appropriate volume resuscitation is indicated with monitoring for worsening anemia. Arterial vasodilation results in splanchnic pooling, and over-aggressive volume resuscitation results in hepatic, mesenteric, and renal congestion and compromised organ function. Judicious use of norepinephrine increases arterial tone and improves perfusion pressure without volume overload and increased critical closing pressures. Its mixed α-adrenergic and β-adrenergic effects maintain cardiac output, which might otherwise fall with an increased afterload resulting in decreased organ perfusion. Controversy surrounds the choice of hemodynamic monitoring in these patients. The authors monitor ventricular filling and function with point-of-care ultrasound[19] and pulmonary arterial pressures directly for the first 24 hours after surgery.

Atrial arrhythmias are common. Patients are often too vasodilated to tolerate calcium channel blockade. Selective β-blockade may be better tolerated and can be titrated for ventricular rate control. Parenteral amiodarone may be administered in the short term with little allograft hepatotoxicity.

NEUROLOGIC

Slow resolution of hepatic encephalopathy may complicate the post-transplant course but delayed recovery from anesthesia, side effects of narcotics and sedative-hypnotics, and neurotoxicity of CNI, corticosteroids, and some cephalosporins should be considered. Allograft preservation injury may severely impair CNI clearance, leading to supratherapeutic levels. Neurotoxicity may be seen at any blood level, however, and potentiate it by hypomagnesemia and hypocholesterolemia. The presentation of CNI neurotoxicity ranges from subtle changes in personality to a unique expressive aphasia, to anomia, to coma. CNIs also lower the seizure threshold and these seizures may be akinetic (nonconvulsive epilepsy). Continuous electroencephalography is particularly useful in patients who fail to wake up after liver transplant.

Structural lesions in the brain are an uncommon etiology of altered sensorium and more typically present with motor or sensory deficits. The transplant recipient population is aging, however, and candidates are more likely to have atherosclerotic cardiovascular disease with attendant risk of ischemic stroke. Intracranial hemorrhage is of particular concern in the patient with uncontrolled hypertension and thrombocytopenia or, less commonly, severe coagulopathy due to factor deficiencies. Hepatocerebral and hepatospinal syndromes are typically recognized prior to transplant and may have lateralizing signs, and resolution is protracted and often incomplete.[20]

Requirements for analgesia are less than what might be expected given the extent of surgery.[21] Intense pain should prompt evaluation for surgical complications, including bleeding, infection, and ischemia of nontransplanted organs. Narcotics remain the mainstay for management. Lower total daily doses of narcotics can be achieved with patient-controlled narcotic analgesia. The authors favor agents, such as fentanyl, hydromorphone, and oxycodone. Adjuncts include low-dose acetaminophen and ketamine infusion (10–20 mg/h). Ketamine metabolism is impaired in liver failure and toxicity may manifest as confusion and hallucinations. Nonpharmacologic approaches include adjustment in patient position, heating pads, music, and transcutaneous electrical neural stimulation. Topical lidocaine in the form of a delayed-release patch may mitigate incisional pain. Pharmacologic approaches may include low-dose acetaminophen (<2000 mg/d in adults) and low-dose infusion of ketamine (20 mg/h). Metabolism of ketamine is prolonged, however, by hepatic dysfunction. Nonsteroidal anti-inflammatory drugs are often contraindicated by existing or acute kidney injury and may potentiate the nephrotoxicity of CNIs. Portal hypertension and concerns for bleeding often preclude epidural anesthesia.

Sleep disturbances are common in advanced liver disease and undoubtedly lower the threshold or even precipitate acute delirium. The authors commonly prescribe melatonin or its synthetic analog, ramelteon. Dexmedetomidine is particularly useful for managing sleep deprivation, because its analgesic properties lower the need for narcotics,[22,23] although acquisition costs may be a factor for some programs. The authors avoid benzodiazepines in the management of insomnia and anxiety. In patients for whom hemodynamic side effects of dexmedetomidine preclude its use, propofol may be titrated safely in patients intubated and mechanically ventilated with less risk of delirium than benzodiazepines.

Neurologic complications in patients with acute liver failure persist in the early postoperative period. Intracranial hypertension may result from cerebral vasodilation and increased blood volume. Cerebral autoregulation is impaired in acute liver failure[24,25] and may be restored by mild hypothermia, which also restores reactivity to carbon dioxide.[26] Postoperative management includes gradual restoration of euthermia, maintenance of mild hypernatremia (145–155 mEq/L), and avoidance of central venous congestion. Intracranial pressure monitoring is center-specific for patients with acute liver failure.[27] Transcranial Doppler is more widely available with cerebral compliance inferred from the velocity-time curve.[28]

RESPIRATORY

Rapid postoperative liberation from mechanical ventilation is the goal. Spontaneous breathing modes can be implemented with recovery from anesthesia and patients should be extubated when protecting their airway, hemodynamically stable and return to operating room is not imminent.

Pulmonary dysfunction related to liver failure comprises abnormalities of the alveolar-capillary interface with acute lung injury/ARDS; pulmonary vascular abnormalities, including capillary dilatation, resulting in hypoxemia with ventilation perfusion mismatch (hepatopulmonary syndrome); and pulmonary hypertension (portopulmonary hypertension). More common complications, such as pneumonia, atelectasis, pleural effusion (hepatic hydrothorax), and even pulmonary embolism.

Liver failure, blood transfusion, and aspiration pneumonitis may singularly or in combination may result in lung injury and ARDS. Lung-protective ventilating strategies targeting tidal volume of 6-mL/kg ideal body weight[29] and appropriate levels of positive end-expiratory pressure (PEEP) should be implemented with induction of anesthesia and continued postoperatively. Chest wall compliance is often reduced by edema and/or obesity. Transpulmonary pressure (Ptp)measurements may be used to guide PEEP titration.[30] If this is unavailable, the authors determine starting PEEP by dividing body mass index by 4 (BMI/4). This formula underestimates PEEP relative to that determined by PtP but is nonetheless consistently higher than the ubiquitous default of 5 cm H_2O.[31,32]

Severe hypoxemia related to the hepatopulmonary syndrome often responds to prolonged high Fio_2. Low levels of PEEP or continuous positive airway pressure may help. Because the anatomic problem is pulmonary capillary dilatation, benefit from inhaled pulmonary vasodilators, such as nitric oxide or epoprostenol, may only infrequently improve oxygenation. Surprisingly, moderate hypoxemia does not impair liver allograft function and is not a reason in itself to continue mechanical ventilation.

Preoperative exercise testing, with measurement of pulmonary hemodynamics, can readily define patients with portopulmonary hypertension who will not survive liver transplantation Even when recognized and treated preoperatively, portopulmonary hypertension may be problematic in the early postoperative period, particularly in the setting of allograft dysfunction with preservation injury. Uncontrolled pulmonary arterial hypertension causes right ventricular dysfunction and hepatic congestion, amplifying liver failure-induced pulmonary hypertension.[33] The authors use transesophageal echocardiography intraoperatively and transthoracic echocardiography in the ICU to monitor right ventricular function and pulmonary artery catheterization to determine pulmonary hemodynamics. Lung volume is optimized to minimize pulmonary vascular resistance. Fluid resuscitation is conservative. The authors continue preoperative intravenous pulmonary vasodilators and often add inhaled nitric oxide. Pulmonary hypertension, however, can accelerate as systemic hemodynamics normalize and right ventricular failure may develop. The authors down-titrate vasodilator therapy over the first year after liver transplantation and recognize that some patients are never weaned off. Recurrence of liver disease may be heralded by a rise in pulmonary artery pressures and manifest by dyspnea and right heart failure.

In patients who require protracted ventilatory support, the authors favor early percutaneous tracheostomy, which is safe[34] and improves patient comfort and ability to communicate while providing more flexibility for weaning from mechanical ventilation and earlier patient mobilization.

RENAL

Renal dysfunction is common in liver failure. Although typically ascribed to hepatorenal syndrome, other causes are frequently identified by careful history, analysis of the urine, determination of kidney size, and renal biopsy.[35,36] Maintenance of perfusion pressure combined with reduction in intra-abdominal pressure and renal venous pressure help maintain renal blood flow. Calcineurin inhibition can be delayed in selected patients with postoperative renal failure. Renal replacement with continuous techniques should be considered in patients with oligo anuria in time to avoid volume overload with pulmonary edema, hepatic congestion, and cardiorenal syndrome.[37]

Electrolyte imbalances are common. Patients often present for surgery with significant hyponatremia. Central pontine myelinolysis is of particular concern. The authors monitor serial sodium levels in target and increase of no more than 12 mEq/L sodium shift over a 24-hour period. This may require infusion of hypotonic fluids during surgery. Although hypokalemia in the immediate preoperative period is often tolerated, because potassium rises with blood product transfusion intraoperatively, it warrants correction in the postoperative period to minimize arrhythmias. Hypomagnesemia has been associated with CNI-induced neurotoxicity. The authors use parenteral replacement to maintain levels in the high normal range. Hypophosphatemia may reflect refeeding syndrome, contribute to muscle weakness and delay liberation from mechanical ventilation. Hypocalcemia is common and ionized calcium should be measured because correction algorithms based on albumin and total calcium are error prone.

GASTROINTESTINAL AND NUTRITION

Although variceal hemorrhage may be acutely controlled by liver transplantation,[38] portal hypertension does not immediately resolve. Esophagitis, gastritis, and gastric and duodenal ulceration occur with increased frequency in portal hypertension and may also be related to corticosteroid use. Upper gastrointestinal bleeding is a concern in the postoperative period. Prophylaxis with H_2-receptor antagonists or proton pump inhibitors mitigates this risk but increases the risk of enteric colonization and infection with Clostridium difficile[39] and vancomycin-resistant enterococci as well as the risk of pneumonia.[40] The risks of stress ulcer prophylaxis may be mitigated by shorter duration correlated with resolution of critical illness, portal hypertension, and corticosteroid use as well as the initiation of enteric feeding.

The etiology of gastrointestinal bleeding is best determined endoscopically and may be particularly difficult to identify if the source is the jejunojejunostomy for patients with a Roux-en-Y biliary reconstruction. Presentation is often with melena, and supportive management with transfusion and correction of coagulopathy and thrombocytopenia suffice. Hemobilia may complicate liver biopsy and also present with melena, which may require upper endoscopy with a pediatric colonoscope to reach the jejunojejunostomy and see blood in the afferent limb. Control may require selective arterial embolization.

Protein calorie malnutrition is common in liver failure and may complicate recovery after liver transplantation. As discussed previously, the authors routinely place nasojejunal feeding tubes for tube feeding because many patients do not develop adequate caloric and protein intake until 10 days to 14 days after surgery. Calculation of nitrogen balance and measurement of resting energy expenditure may be useful to guide nutritional prescription. Prealbumin can be measured serially. Stores of fat-soluble vitamins may also be depleted and warrant supplementation.

INFECTION

Infection is a common and potentially lethal complication after surgery. Surgical site infection, line site infection, and pneumonia are particularly problematic in the early postoperative period. Integrity of the biliary and enteric anastomoses should be sought. Primary bacteremia or fungemia warrants reevaluation of hepatic arterial flow. Invasive catheter management requires balancing competing imperatives: early removal to reduce the risk of infection versus hemodynamic instability, which requires immediate resuscitation. Perioperative antimicrobial prophylaxis might best be stratified according to risk of infection. Patients at low risk include those with isolated liver failure who are admitted from home for the transplant. Patients who are ICU-bound prior to surgery or who have been in the hospital with infectious complications of liver disease, however, should be considered at high risk. Other risk factors for infection include retransplantation, massive blood product transfusion, and prolonged cold ischemia time. Prophylaxis should include antifungals and an antibacterial that reflects prior colonization and the hospital's antibiogram. In the ICU, preoperative chlorhexidine bathing can be performed according to protocol although the extent of benefit is controversial in less controlled settings.[41]

Herpes family viral infections may result from immunosuppression, particularly with administration of T-cell–specific agents, such as thymoglobulin. For herpes simplex, prophylaxis with acyclovir in the early postoperative period is appropriate. Prophylaxis with ganciclovir or valganciclovir may be considered for patients with thymoglobulin induction or treatment of rejection and in cytomegalovirus (CMV) seronegative recipients of CMV-seropositive grafts. Although these agents are effective, myelosuppression is common,[42] and tracking of viral load by serial measurements of CMV DNA polymerase chain reaction is preferable to guide timely initiation of antivirals and monitor response on treatment.

Donor-derived infection is an ongoing concern. Understanding of donor risk factors for infection and monitoring of predonation cultures is essential.

HEMATOLOGIC CONSIDERATIONS

Pretransplant anemia is common. Evaluation of vitamin B_{12} and iron stores as well as supplementation of folic acid is appropriate. In patients with renal insufficiency, erythropoietin analogs may be considered. In the absence of active bleeding, a hemoglobin of 7 g/dL is targeted as for other critically ill patients.[43] Leukopenia and thrombocytopenia may reflect splenic sequestration or myelosuppression from medication. Postoperative thrombocytopenia usually reflects sequestration in the graft and operative field. Autoimmune thrombocytopenia may be associated with positive panel reactive antibody and respond to intravenous immunoglobulin or plasmapheresis. Prolongation of the prothrombin time is common and reflects liver allograft dysfunction rather than the risk of bleeding. Antifibrinolytics are increasingly used empirically during surgery. The authors use whole-blood thromboelastography (TEG, Haemonetics, Braintree, MA) or rotational thromboelastometry (ROTEM, Haemoview, Brisbane Qld, Australia) to guide blood product replacement and assess risk/benefit of continuing antifibrinolytics.

REHABILITATION

Severe deconditioning with muscle wasting in the setting of malnutrition complicates recovery from liver transplantation. Patients should be mobilized early in the postoperative period even if mechanical ventilation, continuous renal replacement therapy, or low-dose to moderate-dose vasopressor support is on-going.[44] This can require several personnel, including the intensivist team, bedside nurse, and physical, occupational, and respiratory therapy teams to ensure that the patient is mobilized safely.

SUMMARY

Perioperative management of the liver transplant recipient is a team sport that increasingly requires critical care management before surgery. Close collaboration among the intensivist, surgeon, anesthesiologist, hepatologist, and nephrologist is essential. Transplant viability must be reassessed regularly and particularly with each donor organ offered. Early discussion with patient and family allow for realistic determination of goals based on patient aspirations and clinical realities. The resolution of multiple organ systems failure with successful liver transplantation is often nothing short of miraculous, but many critically ill recipients have a protracted ICU course. Early attention to hemodynamics with optimal resuscitation and judicious vasopressor support, respiratory care designed to minimize iatrogenic injury, and early renal support are key. Preoperative nutrition support and physical rehabilitation with emphasis on mobility and preserving function should remain a focus of postoperative care. The relative immune tolerance of the liver allograft affords the opportunity to minimize immunosuppression in the early postoperative period with up-titration as physiologic improvement occurs.

REFERENCES

1. Taner CB, Willingham DL, Bulatao IG, et al. Is a mandatory intensive care unit stay needed after liver transplantation? Feasibility of fast-tracking to the surgical ward after liver transplantation. Liver Transpl 2012;18:361–9.
2. Kramer DJ, Arasi LC, Grek AA, et al. Transplant critical care service (TxCCS): role of nurse practitioners. Liver Transpl 2011;17(Suppl 1):S192.
3. Feng S, Goodrich NP, Bragg-Gresham JL, et al. Characteristics associated with liver graft failure: the concept of a donor risk index. Am J Transplant 2006;6(4):783–90.
4. Ghabril M, Dickson R, Wiesner R. Improving outcomes of liver retransplantation: an analysis of trends and the impact of Hepatitis C infection. Am J Transplant 2008;8(2):404–11.
5. Halldorson JB, Bakthavatsalam R, Fix O, et al. D-MELD, a simple predictor of post liver transplant mortality for optimization of donor/recipient matching. Am J Transplant 2009;9(2):318–26.
6. Moon DB, Lee SG, Kang WH, et al. Adult living donor liver transplantation for acute-on-chronic liver failure in high-model for end-stage liver disease score patients. Am J Transplant 2017;17(7):1833–42.
7. Matuschak GM, Rinaldo JE, Pinsky MR, et al. Effect of end-stage liver failure on the incidence and resolution of the adult respiratory distress syndrome. J Crit Care 1987;2:162–73.
8. Matuschak GM, Shaw BW. Adult respiratory distress syndrome associated with acute liver allograft rejection: resolution following a hepatic retransplantation. Crit Care Med 1987;15:878–81.
9. Doyle HR, Marino IR, Miro A, et al. Adult respiratory distress syndrome secondary to end stage liver disease: successful outcome following liver transplantation. Transplantation 1993;55(2):292–6.
10. Song W, Wang K, Zhang RJ, et al. The enhanced recovery after surgery (ERAS) program in liver surgery: a meta-analysis of randomized controlled trials. Springerplus 2016;5:207.
11. Brustia R, Monsel A, Conti F, et al. Enhanced recovery in liver transplantation: a feasibility study. World J Surg 2018. [Epub ahead of print].
12. D'Amico F, Vitale A, Piovan D, et al. Use of N-acetylcysteine during liver procurement: a prospective randomized controlled study. Liver Transplant 2013;19(2):135–44.
13. Hilmi IA, Peng Z, Planinsic RM, et al. N-acetylcysteine does not prevent hepatorenal ischaemia-reperfusion injury in patients undergoing orthotopic liver transplantation. Nephrol Dial Transplant 2010;25(7):2328–33.
14. Taner CB, Canabal JM, Willingham DW, et al. N-Acetylcysteine use and perioperative transfusion requirements in OLT. Liver Transpl 2010;16(6 suppl 1):S247–8.
15. Farrell SJ, Aldag E, Pedersen R, et al. Evaluation of the effects of N-Acetylcysteine treatment in adult liver transplant recipients. J Pharm Soc Wis 2016;19:49–52.

16. Kramer DJ. Renal and liver failure management—ICU perspective. 18th International Symposium on Albumin Dialysis (ISAD). 2017; 18. p. 12–3.
17. Banares R, Nevens F, Larsen FS, et al. Extracorporeal albumin dialysis with the molecular adsorbent recirculating system in acute-on-chronic liver failure: the RELIEF trial. Hepatology 2013;1153–62.
18. Aduen JF, Sujay B, Dickson RC, et al. Outcomes after liver transplant in patients aged 70 years or older compared with those younger than 60 years. Mayo Clin Proc 2009;84(11):973–8.
19. Shokoohi H, Boniface KS, Pourmand A, et al. Bedside ultrasound reduces diagnostic uncertainty and guides resuscitation in patients with undifferentiated hypotension. Crit Care Med 2015;43:2562–9.
20. Lewis M, Howdle PD. The neurology of liver failure. Q J Med 2003;96:623–33.
21. Moretti EW, Robertson KM, Tuttle-Newhall JE, et al. Orthotopic liver transplant patients require less postoperative morphine than do patients undergoing hepatic resection. J Clin Anesth 2002;14(6):416–20.
22. Lu W, Fu Q, Luo X, et al. Effects of dexmedetomidine on sleep quality of patients after surgery without mechanical ventilation in ICU. Medicine 2017;96(23):e7081.
23. Skrobik Y, Duprey MS, Hill NS, et al. Low-dose nocturnal dexmedetomidine prevents icu delirium a randomized, placebo-controlled trial. Am J Respir Crit Care Med 2018;197:1147–56.
24. Larsen FS, Ejlersen E, Clemmesen JO, et al. Preserved cerebral oxidative metabolism in fulminant hepatic failure: an autoregulation study. Liver Transpl Surg 1996;2:348–53.
25. Strauss G, Hansen BA, Kirkegaard P, et al. Liver function, cerebral blood flow autoregulation and hepatic encephalopathy in fulminant hepatic failure. Hepatology 1997;25:837–9.
26. Jalan R, Olde Damink SWM, Deutz NEP, et al. Restoration of cerebral blood flow autoregulation and reactivity to carbon dioxide in acute liver failure by moderate hypothermia. Hepatology 2001;34:50–4.
27. Stravitz RT, Kramer AH, Davern T, et al, for the Acute Liver Failure Study Group. Recommendations of the US acute liver failure study group. Crit Care Med 2007; 35:2498–508.
28. Aggarwal S, Brooks DM, Kang Y, et al. Noninvasive monitoring of cerebral perfusion pressure in patients with acute liver failure using transcranial Doppler ultrasonography. Liver Transpl 2008;14:1048–57.
29. The Acute Respiratory Distress Syndrome Network. Ventilation with lower tidal volumes as compared with traditional tidal volumes for acute lung injury and the acute respiratory distress syndrome. N Engl J Med 2000;342:1301–8.
30. Talmor D, Sarge T, Malhorta A, et al. Mechanical ventilation guided by esophageal pressure in acute lung injury. N Engl J Med 2008;359:2095–104.
31. Reindl L, Peterson LM, Manansala R, et al. Non-invasive estimation of optimal positive end-expiratory pressure (PEEP) for mechanically ventilated obese patients. Respiratory Care, in press.
32. Nezami B, Peterson LM, Klumph M, et al. Impact of obesity on ventilator-associated events. Abstract submitted for presentation on Society of Critical Care Medicine Annual Congress. San Francisco (CA), February 2019.
33. Ramsay M. Portopulmonary hypertension and right heart failure in patients with cirrhosis. Curr Opin Anesthesiol 2010;23:145–50.
34. Waller EA, Aduen JF, Kramer DJ, et al. Safety of percutaneous dilatational tracheostomy with direct bronchoscopic guidance for solid organ allograft recipients. Mayo Clin Proc 2007;82(12):1502–8.

35. Wadei HM, Geiger XJ, Cortese C, et al. Kidney allocation to liver transplant candidates with renal failure of undetermined etiology: role of percutaneous renal biopsy. Am J Transplant 2008;8(12):2618–26.
36. Nadim MK, Durand F, Kellum JA, et al. Management of the critically ill patient with cirrhosis: a multidisciplinary perspective. Hepatol 2016;64:717–35.
37. Gambardella L, Gaudino M, Ronco C, et al. Congestive kidney failure in cardiac surgery: the relationship between central venous pressure and acute kidney injury. Interact Cardiovasc Thorac Surg 2016;23(5):800–5.
38. Iwatsuki S, Starzl TE, Todo S, et al. Liver transplantation in the treatment of bleeding esophageal varices. Surgery 1988;104(4):697–705.
39. Dial S, Delaney JA, Barkun AN, et al. Use of gastric acid-suppressive agents and the risk of community-acquired Clostridium difficile-associated disease. JAMA 2005;294:2989–95.
40. Laheij RJ, Sturkenboom MC, Hassing RJ, et al. Risk of community-acquired pneumonia and use of gastric acid-suppressive drugs. JAMA 2004;292:1955–60.
41. Chlebicki MP, Safdar N, O'Horo JC, et al. Preoperative chlorhexidine shower or bath for prevention of surgical site infection: a meta-analysis. Am J Infect Control 2013;41(2):167–73.
42. Kusne S, Blair JE. Viral and fungal infections after liver transplantation — part II. Liver Transplant 2006;12:2–11.
43. Hebert PC, Wells G, Blajchman MA, et al. A multicenter, randomized, controlled clinical trial of transfusion requirements in critical care. Transfusion requirements in critical care investigators, Canadian critical care trials group. N Engl J Med 1999;340:409–17.
44. Bailey P, Thomsen GE, Spuhler VJ, et al. Early activity is feasible and safe in respiratory failure patients. Crit Care Med 2007;35:139–45.

Critical Care Management of Living Donor Liver Transplants

Kristina Lemon, MD, FRCSC[a], Ali Al-Khafaji, MD, MPH, FCCM[b],*,
Abhinav Humar, MD, FRCSC[a]

KEYWORDS

- Hepatic artery thrombosis (HAT) • Postoperative bleeding
- Enhanced recovery after surgery (ERAS) • Bile leak • Acute kidney injury (AKI)
- Immunosuppression • Postoperative prophylaxis

KEY POINTS

- Living donor liver transplantation is a valuable option for patients in the era of significant organ donor shortage.
- Enhanced recovery after surgery protocols may be valuable. These patients should be managed like other elective surgical patients, and every effort should be made to expedite their recovery and minimize their time in hospital.
- Live donor transplant recipients have higher rates of vascular and biliary complications compared with deceased organ recipients and it is important to be vigilant for early signs and symptoms of these complications.
- Donors are generally young and healthy and, although the risk of complications is low, it is important to monitor these patients very carefully because complications can have dire consequences.
- Patients are best managed using a multidisciplinary team approach that includes nursing staff, surgeons, intensivists, respiratory therapists, clinical pharmacists, nutritionists, and physical therapists.

INTRODUCTION

Despite efforts to increase organ donation, there is a critical shortage of organ donors, leading to an increase number of patients waiting on the liver transplant (LT) list.[1]

Disclosures or Conflict of Interest: None.
Financial Support: None.
[a] Department of Surgery, University of Pittsburgh Medical Center, Thomas E. Starzl Transplantation Institute, 3459 Fifth Avenue, Pittsburgh, PA 15213, USA; [b] Department of Critical Care Medicine, University of Pittsburgh Medical Center, The CRISMA (Clinical Research, Investigation and Systems Modeling of Acute Illness) Center, 3550 Terrace Street, Scaife 613, Pittsburgh, PA 15261, USA
* Corresponding author.
E-mail address: alkhafajia2@upmc.edu

Crit Care Clin 35 (2019) 107–116
https://doi.org/10.1016/j.ccc.2018.08.001
0749-0704/19/© 2018 Elsevier Inc. All rights reserved.

In addition, many available donors donate marginal livers due to advanced age and obesity. Therefore, other options, such as living donor LT, should be considered as alternatives to expand the donor pool. In North America, live donor LT (LDLT) makes up a small percentage of the total number of LTs carried out each year. However, in other areas of the world, such as the Middle East and Asia, it makes up the most of the LTs performed. Although the management of LDLT recipients is often similar to the management of deceased donor LT recipients, this review focuses on the unique challenges presented by LDLT patients, both the transplant recipient and the donor. Patients are best managed using a multidisciplinary team approach that includes nursing staff, surgeons, intensivists, respiratory therapists, clinical pharmacists, nutritionists, and physical therapists.

THE SURGICAL PROCEDURE

It is helpful for anyone involved in the care of LDLT patients to be aware of what the surgical procedure entails. The LDLT process begins with an extensive medical, surgical, and psychosocial evaluation of the potential donor. If the recipient is an adult, the right lobe of the donor's liver is generally used. If the recipient is a child who weighs less than 25 kg, the left lateral segment of the donor's liver is generally used.

The donor hepatectomy operation generally takes 6 to 8 hours and recovery after the operation takes 5 to 7 days of hospitalization. The overall incidence of complications after a donor hepatectomy ranges from 30% to 40%.[2] If the recipient is an adult, the risk of complications may be higher because a larger portion, usually the right lobe, is removed. Complications include bleeding, bile leaks, vascular thrombosis, infections, and incisional hernias, with less than 1% risk of death.[3] The recipient operation consists of total hepatectomy to remove the diseased liver and then implantation of the donor's liver segment. The key principles are to achieve adequate outflow (via the hepatic venous anastomosis) and sufficient inflow via the hepatic artery and portal vein, and, finally, biliary anastomosis.

THE DONOR

At the authors' center, most donors will arrive in the intensive care unit (ICU) extubated and generally hemodynamically stable. They often leave the ICU within 24 hours of their arrival.

The Immediate Postoperative Period

Donors are managed according to an enhanced recovery after surgery (ERAS) protocol. The basic principles of an ERAS protocol include early postoperative enteral nutrition, early ambulation, and narcotic-sparing pain control regimens.

Monitoring

Most donors will arrive in the ICU directly from the operating room (OR) with standard cardiac and respiratory monitors in place, including a central line, arterial line, and pulse oximetry. Whether continued monitoring with the arterial line and central line is needed is a decision that must be made on an individual patient basis according to the stability of the patient.

Immediate postoperative laboratory tests, including a complete blood count, basic metabolic profile, liver function tests, and lactate, provide baseline values. Elevations in the transaminases, bilirubin, international normalized ratio (INR), and lactate are to be expected and generally should not be considered concerning or require intervention in isolation. For example, the donor's ability to clear lactate will be impaired initially secondary to the decreased liver volume. Generally, elevated lactate level may not be interpreted as a marker of decreased intravascular volume in the absence of other signs of hypovolemia, such as tachycardia or oliguria, and should not be overtreated with fluid resuscitation, especially if the lactate level is downtrending.

Nutrition

Preoperative nutrition should be continued, including permitting consumption of clear fluids such as electrolyte-rich drinks, up to 2 hours before the operation. Postoperative early removal of nasogastric tubes and early initiation of enteral nutrition decreases the time to return of bowel function and leads to earlier discharge from hospital.[4] Typically, we remove the nasogastric tube on the evening of postoperative day (POD) 0 and initiate a clear liquid diet on the morning of POD 1. Patients are advanced to a soft diet as soon as they begin passing flatus.

Ambulation

Early ambulation should begin as early as POD 1 and most patients will not need significant intervention from physical therapy. Often, the use of an abdominal binder can provide support and ease some of the discomfort with ambulation.

Pain Control

Although many narcotic-sparing pain control regimens exist part of an ERAS protocol, all include a preoperative component, an intraoperative component, and a postoperative component.

Preoperative regimens often involve the use of a long-acting opioid; an antiinflammatory medication; and, often, additional analgesics such as gabapentin. Intraoperatively, the use of either spinal or epidural analgesia, as well as long-acting local anesthetics injected into the incision itself, can have a significant impact on postoperative pain, especially in the initial 48 hours. Postoperatively, the authors use both intravenous ketamine and lidocaine infusions. With appropriate dosing, we have been able to achieve good pain control with minimal side effects, allowing minimum use of opioids and leading to the earlier return of bowel function. In addition, ketorolac, cyclobenzaprine, and intravenous acetaminophen are used.

Complications

Live donor hepatectomy is among the very few procedures in which a completely healthy patient is put at risk with no benefit to their own physical health. As such, donor safety should always be considered the primary concern in LDLT.

Biliary complications is the most common complication, with a reported incidence between 2% to 18%. The Adult-to-Adult Living Donor Liver Transplantation Cohort study reported an overall donor morbidity of 38%, with infections accounting for 12% of the complications and bile leaks accounting for 9%.[3] A recent systematic review found a pooled biliary complication rate of 6.6%, with 9% of these patients requiring operative intervention.[3] Most surgical complications are reported using Clavien grading (**Box 1**). Most biliary complications reported are Clavien grade I or II, and include bile leaks or bilomas that resolve without further interventions.[3] Complications of biliary strictures seem to be significantly less common than bile leaks in this population and are usually treated with endoscopic retrograde cholangiopancreatography (ERCP).[3] Persistent leaks from the cut surface of the liver and damage to the biliary tree requiring reoperation have been reported. There has only been a single reported death secondary to biliary complications in a living donor.[3] Several studies have compared the biliary complication rate in left lobe versus right lobe donors and it

---

Box 1
Clavien classification of surgical complications

Grade I: Any deviation from the normal postoperative course without the need for pharmacologic treatment or surgical, endoscopic, and radiological interventions

Grade II: Requiring pharmacologic treatment with drugs other than those allowed for grade I complications

Grade III: Requiring surgical, endoscopic, or radiological intervention
   Grade IIIa: Intervention not under general anesthesia
   Grade IIIb: Intervention under general anesthesia

Grade IV: Life-threatening complication
   Grade IVa: Single-organ dysfunction
   Grade IVb: Multiorgan dysfunction

Grade V: Death of a patient

---

does seem that there are more complications associated with right lobe donation.[3] Other factors that may contribute to biliary complications include donor age, length of the donor operation, and the techniques used to confirm biliary anatomy before bile duct division.[3] Although bile leaks are the most common surgical complication in LDLT donors, these patients are also at risk for liver dysfunction or failure related to a small liver remnant. In most adult-to-adult LDLTs, approximately 60% to 70% of the donor liver is removed. Although this is safe in almost all healthy donors, it may lead to the so-called small-for-size syndrome. As the liver remnant regenerates, most patients will show recovery and normalization of their liver function tests. If the remnant liver fails to regenerate, the donor can progress to liver failure and require transplantation; this has never been reported in North America. Finally, in addition to liver-specific complications, these patients are at risk for other postoperative complications, such as pneumonia, thromboembolic events, paralytic ileus, bowel obstruction, and bleeding.

THE RECIPIENT

It is important to remember that this was a scheduled surgery and the patient has usually been optimized as much as possible before the operation.

The Handover

Effective communication between the surgical, anesthetic, and ICU team concerning the current status of the patient is essential, including hemodynamic stability, use of vasopressors, amount of fluids, and blood products used during the procedure.

During the handover, a brief history of the patient, events that occurred during the operation, and any specific goals over the next 12 to 24 hours should be communicated.

Most patients arrive in the ICU intubated with varying degrees of sedation on board.

It is not uncommon to have preexisting cardiac or respiratory issues in this patient population that may require a more cautious approach to extubation. In addition to portopulmonary hypertension and hepatopulmonary syndrome, it is common for these patients to have cardiorespiratory problems that are unrelated to their underlying liver disease. For example, obstructive sleep apnea is common, especially in patients with an underlying diagnosis of nonalcoholic steatohepatitis, and should be considered when deciding on extubation. Barring any unexpected complications, most patients are extubated within the first 12 hours after surgery.

The gastrointestinal system should be assessed to determine the state of the intestinal tract, what surgical anastomoses may be present, and if and when the intestinal tract can be used for nutrition. Finally, it is important to discuss the renal function and determine if there were preexisting problems such as hepatorenal syndrome or chronic renal disease. Renal function, specifically urine output (UO), during the procedure and immediately postoperatively should be assessed, along with the possible need for renal support therapies in the early posttransplant period. Although most recipients will have good renal function, it is important to remember that, despite the controlled nature of these cases, this is a major operative procedure with all the potential for multisystem problems that are associated with transplantation and ischemia or reperfusion injuries. The significance of decreased UO in patients with liver disease has been studied recently.[5,6] Incorporating UO into the diagnostic criteria of acute kidney injury (AKI) dramatically increases the measured incidence of AKI.[5] In addition, the presence of oliguria, even without serum creatinine increase, was shown to be significantly associated with adverse outcomes in patients with chronic liver disease and in LDLT recipients.[6]

In LDLT, some of the usual markers of volume status can be deceiving and should not be used in isolation to make management decisions. For example, a patient's ability to clear lactate from their circulation depends on their liver function and a patient who receives a small graft may clear lactate levels very slowly despite being euvolemic. It is important to take individual values such as the serum lactate into consideration, along with clinical parameters such as heart rate and UO.

Monitors and Lines

Most patients will arrive at the ICU with arterial line, central line, a pulmonary artery catheter, Foley catheter, nasogastric tube, and at least 1 surgically placed abdominal drain. In general, invasive hemodynamic parameters are measured for the first 12 to 24 hours, or until the patient reaches a state of hemodynamic stability. Most of these invasive monitors are discontinued on the morning of POD 1 as the patient is transitioned to a lower-acuity level of care.

Initial laboratory tests include a complete blood count; a complete metabolic profile, including blood urea nitrogen (BUN), creatinine, electrolytes, and liver enzymes; and liver function tests, including coagulation parameters and serum lactate. Concerns with any of these values should prompt close monitoring over the course of the first night, with repeat bloodwork testing and urgent ultrasound as needed. In the authors' center, all LDLT recipients are monitored with continuous hepatic arterial pulse monitoring with an implantable Doppler probe placed in the OR for the first 24 hours, as well as routine bedside Doppler ultrasound on the first POD and repeat ultrasounds as needed after that. After the first 24 hours, the implantable Doppler monitor is checked by both nursing staff and the surgical team with each routine vitals check. An alternate approach is to conduct daily bedside ultrasounds for several days after the transplant.

Nutrition

Removing the nasogastric tube on the first POD is usually safe and most patients will be able to begin clear fluids at that time. The patients' diet should include nutritional supplements as early as possible. For patients who are not able to be extubated quickly or have a prolonged ICU course, there should be no hesitation to place a feeding tube and start enteral feeds. At the authors' center, we obtain a bedside swallowing evaluation by speech therapy before initiation of oral nutrition.

Immunosuppression or Prophylaxis

LDLT recipients are placed on bacterial, viral, and fungal prophylaxis in the postoperative period. The duration of these regimens will vary by institution but, generally, they will all extend past the patients' time in the ICU. Common protocols include trimethoprim or sulfamethoxazole for prophylaxis against pneumocystis pneumonia, acyclovir for prophylaxis against viruses such as herpesvirus, and fluconazole for fungal prophylaxis.

Common immunosuppression regimens usually involve triple therapy, including a calcineurin inhibitor such as tacrolimus, an antimetabolite such as mycophenolate mofetil, and a steroid taper. The authors generally use induction therapy with basiliximab as a means to delay the introduction of calcineurin inhibitors in patients with preexisting renal dysfunction. The ICU team should be aware of the common side effects associated with these medications; for example, tacrolimus is commonly associated with neurotoxicity, renal dysfunction, and (on a more minor level) tremors. Mycophenolate mofetil can be associated with significant myelosuppression and (more commonly) gastrointestinal upset and diarrhea.

Complications

Early recognition, diagnosis, and treatment of complications are essential to prevent clinical deterioration.

Hemorrhage

Hemorrhage is often the most immediately apparent and life-threatening complication of liver transplantation. Although a slow bleed can sometimes be subtle, a bleed from any of the large vessel anastomoses will present as hemodynamic instability, decreasing hemoglobin, and increasing bloody surgical drain output. However, it is common for these drains to clot, leading to no drainage at all. A lack of surgical drain output should not be considered reassuring in the presence of these other clinical signs. It is important for the ICU team to quickly recognize the problem, contact the surgical team, optimize the patient's coagulation parameters, and maintain hemodynamic stability with transfusions of blood products as needed until the patient is able to be returned to the OR. In those patients who show evidence of generalized oozing; that is, slowly drifting hemoglobin, bloody drain output, and abnormal coagulation parameters but without hemodynamic instability, bleeding is usually a multifactorial problem relating to underlying coagulopathy, fibrinolysis, and platelet dysfunction. This should be managed medically by optimizing the coagulation parameters with the transfusion of blood products. An additional potential source of bleeding is gastrointestinal from the jejunojejunal bowel anastomosis if a Roux-en-Y limb was created for reconstruction of the biliary tree. This presents similarly to other sources of upper gastrointestinal tract bleeding, with a slowly dropping hemoglobin, rising BUN, and melena. Usually, this type of bleeding can be managed conservatively with transfusion and octreotide infusion to decrease portal pressures. If the bleeding is severe or persistent, operative exploration may be required because endoscopic therapy is generally difficult.

Vascular complications

The overall incidence of vascular complications after LT ranges from 8% to 12%, with thrombosis being an early postoperative complication, and stenosis and pseudoaneurysm developing at a later stage.[7] The incidence of vascular complications is higher in the LDLT recipients than in the deceased donor transplant recipients. This is thought to be secondary to a combination of the increased complexity of vascular reconstruction required and the smaller size of the donor vessels. If vascular complication is suspected, Doppler ultrasound and contrast-enhanced ultrasound remain the diagnostic tests of choice in this patient population.[8]

Although the overall incidence of hepatic artery thrombosis (HAT) in all LTs ranges from 3% to 5%, the early living donor experience is reported as having an incidence as high as 28%.[9] HAT can be classified as either early (occurring within 30 days of transplant) or late (occurring >30 days from transplant). Early HAT may present with pain, fever, ascites, and a sudden increase in serum transaminases. Early HAT is associated with ABO-incompatible transplants, increased cold ischemic time of the allograft, acute rejection, and technical factors. These include the small caliber of the vessels, use of an arterial graft for reconstruction, spasm or kinking of the hepatic artery, an intimal injury, or a hematoma causing compression of the artery itself. In contrast, late HAT can present in a much more subtle manner because the body has had a chance to develop collateral circulation. It is often related to chronic rejection and sepsis. Previously, early retransplantation was the only possible treatment of HAT and was associated with a mortality rate approaching 50%.[9] As the ability to diagnose HAT earlier has improved, the possibility to revascularize these patients has also improved, with a reported incidence of approximately 75% of patients who can be salvaged with multimodality treatment.[9] Sometimes the first sign of a problem with the hepatic artery is an abnormality on the implantable Doppler signal or ultrasound imaging study. When the problem is recognized at this stage, before there are clinical or laboratory signs of graft dysfunction, the likelihood of salvaging the allograft without the need for retransplantation is significantly improved.

Hepatic artery stenosis (a chronic complication), hepatic artery pseudoaneurysm (exceedingly rare with a reported rate of 0.3%–1%), and splenic artery steal syndrome (seen in 3%–8% of patients and prevented with ligation of the splenic artery intraoperatively) are other forms of hepatic artery complications.[9]

The incidence of portal vein complications is significantly lower than that of HAT; however, the consequences of this complication can be devastating because the liver receives approximately 70% of its blood flow form the portal vein. The incidence of portal vein thrombosis (PVT) in all LTs is reported as less than 2%.[10] However, in the living donor population, the incidence is 1% to 12.5%.[10] PVT is best diagnosed on ultrasound and has been found to be more common in those patients who had preoperative PVT, especially if a vein graft was required for reconstruction of the portal vein. Early presentation is often associated with severe graft dysfunction, including portal hypertension, intestinal edema, bleeding varices, and massive ascites. In contrast, late PVT may be relatively asymptomatic because collaterals are usually present. If PVT is recognized early, thrombectomy, either operatively or with mechanical or chemical thrombolysis, can often salvage the graft, avoiding the need for retransplantation.

Hepatic vein stenosis is uncommon in living donor transplant recipients, occurring in 0.5% of patients.[10] Stenosis of the hepatic veins can lead to liver congestion, resulting in ascites and laboratory values similar to those seen in a small-for-size syndrome. This is due to the inadequate drainage of areas of the liver, resulting in a smaller volume of functional liver. As with the other types of vascular complications, hepatic venous stenosis (HVS) is best diagnosed with Doppler ultrasound. Early HVS is usually caused by technical factors, whereas late HVS is usually caused by intimal hyperplasia or perianastomotic fibrosis.[10]

Biliary complications
As with vascular complications, biliary complications are more common in LDLT recipients when compared with cadaveric donor recipients. Biliary reconstruction in the

LDLT recipient often involves multiple small bile ducts. Biliary complications in the immediate postoperative period include bile leaks and cholangitis; biliary stricture is a more common late complication.

LDLT recipients have 2 potential sources for a postoperative bile leak. There is a risk of leak from the anastomosis itself if biliary reconstruction was performed using duct-to-duct anastomosis. This usually is treated endoscopically with ERCP and stent placement. In the setting of a hepaticojejunostomy, however, it is best to manage these leaks operatively with surgical repair of the anastomosis if possible. In addition, the LDLT recipient also has the potential to have bile leakage from the cut surface of the liver itself. Most leaks will resolve on their own with conservative management and adequate drainage. If signs of sepsis develop, a computed tomography scan of the abdomen should be done to rule out undrained bilomas. Undrained collection should be treated with adequate drainage, either percutaneously or operatively.

It is important to have a high index of suspicion for cholangitis when an LDLT recipient presents with signs and symptoms of sepsis but no other obvious source of infection. As with all patients presenting with cholangitis, patients should have blood cultures drawn and be treated with broad-spectrum antibiotics as soon as possible to prevent progressing to septic shock. Risk factors include the presence of biliary stricture, hepatic arterial complications such as stenosis or thrombosis, and biliary reconstruction with a hepaticojejunostomy. If any of these risk factors are present, interventions should be carried out to prevent recurrence cholangitis.

Graft complications

Despite the large number of LDLT and split LTs that have been done worldwide, it is unclear what the minimum graft volume necessary to ensure an optimal outcome in LDLT recipients is. If the graft is too small to meet the metabolic demands of the recipient, it will lead to small-for-size syndrome, possibly leading to graft failure. In most centers, a ratio of graft weight to recipient weight of greater than 0.8 is used as a cutoff to prevent small-for-size syndrome. Factors that predispose to small-for-size syndrome include poor pretransplant condition of the recipient, prolonged ischemia times, high portal flow rates, and graft steatosis.

Small-for-size syndrome is defined as dysfunction or failure of the small partial liver graft occurring within the first postoperative week in the absence of technical, immunologic, or infectious causes. Graft dysfunction is defined as the presence of 2 of the following 3 features: total bilirubin greater than 5.8 mg/dL, INR greater than 2, and grade 3 or 4 encephalopathy on 3 consecutive days.[11] To give the small graft time to hypertrophy, the management is supportive and usually includes an octreotide infusion to decrease portal flow, maintenance of a euvolemic state with albumin replacement of large volume ascites, and good nutrition. Fresh frozen plasma should be considered in patients with significantly elevated INR; however, there is no exact INR value at which fresh frozen plasma transfusion is universally recommended. Most of these patients will recover with time and support as the liver hypertrophies. A small percentage, however, will progress to liver failure and will require retransplantation.

Medical complications

There is a long list of medical complications that can arise postoperatively in the LDLT recipient. Complications range from minor wound complications to life-threatening events.

Postoperative delirium is not uncommon in this patient population and can be seen more frequently in patients who have a history of encephalopathy pretransplant. As in other postoperative patients, the workup for postoperative delirium should include an infectious workup for sources of sepsis and a review of the medications looking for a likely culprit. In the transplant population, the most common offender is usually the calcineurin inhibitor. It is important to ensure that infectious causes are ruled out before attributing the delirium to medications alone.

Pulmonary complications in LDLT recipients include pulmonary edema, pleural effusions, atelectasis, acute lung injury, and pneumonia. Rates of hospital-acquired or ventilator-acquired pneumonia range from 5% to 48% in LT recipients.[12] The general LT literature has shown an increased incidence of postoperative pneumonia associated with higher pretransplant Model for End-Stage Liver Disease (MELD) scores of greater than 25.[12] In patients who develop pneumonia, hospital stays were longer and mortality is higher. Early extubation has been shown to be a protective factor and should be attempted whenever possible.[12]

AKI is very common in the LT population, in both the preoperative and postoperative period, and is commonly associated with prolonged hospital stays, high health care costs, and increased morbidity and mortality. Preoperative renal dysfunction is often due to hepatorenal syndrome or hypovolemia secondary to diuretic treatment of ascites. Postoperative dysfunction in the living donor population is less common than in deceased donor transplant recipients.[13] It can be caused by many factors, including the presence of preoperative hepatorenal syndrome, long OR times, hypovolemia, or drug toxicity. Severity of liver disease before LT represented by high MELD scores is associated with increased risk of post-LT AKI.[14–16] Many patients with MELD score greater than 30 will require post-LT renal replacement therapy.[17,18] It is important to optimize fluid status, minimize insults to the kidneys from all sources (eg, medications, intravenous contrast dye, hemodynamic instability), support with renal replacement therapy, and give the kidneys a chance to recover. Most patients will recover to a point at which they no longer need dialysis support. Even those who require relatively short-term (<6 weeks) dialysis before transplant will likely recover enough renal function to discontinue dialysis dependence given enough time.

SUMMARY

As the rates of LDLT continue to increase, it is essential to have a multidisciplinary team familiar with the unique challenges presented by these patients. Although patients are optimized before transplant and their operations are often more controlled, they are still at risk for major complications.

REFERENCES

1. Al-Khafaji A, Murugan R, Kellum JA. What's new in organ donation: better care of the dead for the living. Intensive Care Med 2013;39:2031–3.
2. Ghobrial RM, Freise CE, Trotter JF, et al. Donor morbidity after living donation for liver transplantation. Gastroenterology 2008;135:468–76.
3. Braun HJ, Ascher NL, Roll GR, et al. Biliary complications following living donor hepatectomy. Transplant Rev (Orlando) 2016;30:247–52.
4. King AB, Kensinger CD, Shi Y, et al. Intensive care unit enhanced recovery pathway for patients undergoing orthotopic liver transplants recipients: a prospective, observational study. Anesth Analg 2018;126:1495–503.
5. Amathieu R, Al-Khafaji A, Sileanu FE, et al. Significance of oliguria in critically ill patients with chronic liver disease. Hepatology 2017;66:1592–600.

6. Mizota T, Minamisawa S, Imanaka Y, et al. Oliguria without serum creatinine increase after living donor liver transplantation is associated with adverse post-operative outcomes. Acta Anaesthesiol Scand 2016;60(7):874–81.

7. Humar A, Payne W. Critical care of liver and intestinal transplant recipients. In: Irwin R, Rippe J, editors. Critical care medicine. 6th edition. Philadelphia: Lippin-cott Williams and Wilkins; 2008. p. 2133–49.

8. Abdelaziz O, Attia H. Doppler ultrasonography in living donor liver transplantation recipients: intra- and post-operative vascular complications. World J Gastroen-terol 2016;22:6145–72.

9. Ikegami T, Hashikura Y, Nakazawa Y, et al. Risk factors contributing to hepatic artery thrombosis following living-donor liver transplantation. J Hepatobiliary Pan-creat Surg 2006;13:105–9.

10. Rather SA, Nayeem MA, Agarwal S, et al. Vascular complications in living donor liver transplantation at a high-volume center: evolving protocols and trends observed over 10 years. Liver Transpl 2017;23:457–64.

11. Julka KD, Chen CL, Vasavada B. Liver lobe graft side and outcomes in living-donor liver transplant with small-for-size grafts. Exp Clin Transplant 2014;12: 343–50.

12. Prieto Amorin J, Lopez M, Rando K, et al. Early bacterial pneumonia after hepatic transplantation: epidemiologic profile. Transplant Proc 2018;50:503–8.

13. Hilmi IA, Damian D, Al-Khafaji A, et al. Acute kidney injury after orthotopic liver transplantation using living donor versus deceased donor grafts: a propensity score-matched analysis. Liver Transpl 2015;21:1179–85.

14. Kundakci A, Pirat A, Komurcu O, et al. Rifle criteria for acute kidney dysfunction following liver transplantation: incidence and risk factors. Transplant Proc 2010; 42:4171–4.

15. O'Riordan A, Wong V, McQuillan R, et al. Acute renal disease, as defined by the RIFLE criteria, post-liver transplantation. Am J Transplant 2007;7:168–76.

16. Tinti F, Umbro I, Mecule A, et al. RIFLE criteria and hepatic function in the assess-ment of acute renal failure in liver transplantation. Transplant Proc 2010;42: 1233–6.

17. Schlegel A, Linecker M, Kron P, et al. Risk assessment in high- and Low-MELD liver transplantation. Am J Transplant 2017;17:1050–63.

18. Utsumi M, Umeda Y, Sadamori H, et al. Risk factors for acute renal injury in living donor liver transplantation: evaluation of the RIFLE criteria. Transpl Int 2013;26: 842–52.

Graft Dysfunction and Management in Liver Transplantation

Beverley Kok, MBBS, Victor Dong, MD,
Constantine J. Karvellas, MD, SM, FRCPC, FCCM*

KEYWORDS

- Graft dysfunction • Cholestasis • Rejection • Liver transplantation

KEY POINTS

- Graft dysfunction post liver transplantation can range from mild transient biochemical derangement to acute liver failure potentially leading to graft loss.
- Hepatic artery thrombosis can present early or late, resulting in biliary complications such as ischemic cholangiopathy, which may progress to secondary biliary cirrhosis and eventual graft failure.
- Acute cellular rejection is a T-cell–mediated inflammatory response to donor HLA antigens presenting to host T cells.
- In chronic rejection, progressive damage to the bile ducts causes a predominantly cholestatic graft dysfunction that may eventually result in graft loss.
- As grafts from marginal donors (eg, deceased cardiac donors) have increased, there are greater risks of posttransplant complications.

INTRODUCTION

Liver allograft dysfunction manifests across a spectrum in both timing and clinical presentation. Although hepatic graft function can be assessed by dynamic investigations, such as indocyanine green clearance,[1] lidocaine metabolism,[2] or LiMAx test,[3] these tests are not widely available. Immediately post transplantation, bile flow is one of the first indications of graft function,[4] although external biliary tubes for monitoring bile flow posttransplant are no longer the routine practice, potentially related to increased risk of cholangitis.[5] Although nonspecific, liver biochemistry abnormalities are still the mainstay investigation used in monitoring for dysfunction. This review

Disclosures/Conflict of Interest: None.
Financial Support: None.
Division of Gastroenterology (Liver Unit), Department of Critical Care Medicine, University of Alberta, 1-40 Zeidler Ledcor Building, Edmonton, Alberta T6G-2X8, Canada
* Corresponding author.
E-mail address: dean.karvellas@ualberta.ca

Crit Care Clin 35 (2019) 117–133
https://doi.org/10.1016/j.ccc.2018.08.002
0749-0704/19/© 2018 Elsevier Inc. All rights reserved.

provides a summary of the main causes and management strategies for liver graft dysfunction in the early through late posttransplant stages (**Table 1**).

VASCULAR ISSUES
Hepatic Artery Thrombosis (Early Versus Late)

Hepatic artery thrombosis (HAT) is the commonest vascular complication following liver transplantation (LT).[6,7] It presents significant detriment to graft function, to the extent of rapid graft failure and death.[8] Although incidence is variable, with higher incidences reported in the pediatric population at 20%, incidence in the adult population has been reported at up to 6.8%.[8] It is unclear whether reduced sized grafts (such as split grafts or living-related LT) may be associated with increased occurrence of HAT, although most series have reported no association.[8–11]

After transplantation, the hepatic artery continues to contribute to approximately 50% of oxygenated blood flow to the liver. Compromise results in hypoperfusion of the graft and particularly to the biliary tree as the post-LT bile ducts are entirely dependent on blood flow from the hepatic artery.[7] Even if HAT resolves, there is substantial risk that biliary ischemia will have occurred, resulting in biliary complications, such as biloma or ischemic cholangiopathy, which may progress to secondary biliary cirrhosis and eventual graft failure.[12]

HAT may usually be classified into early HAT and late HAT. However, definitions for early HAT vary, and range from within 2 weeks post-LT[8] to within 100 days post-LT.[13] Most studies differentiate early versus late HAT at 4 weeks post-LT.[8] Early HAT is associated with higher rates of graft loss and mortality as compared with late HAT.[14,15] Early HAT is usually apparent in the first week post-LT,[8,16] and may present more obviously with acute graft dysfunction manifesting with massive aspartate transaminase (AST)/alanine transaminase (ALT) elevations (usually >1000 U/L), coagulopathy, fever, biliary leaks, and signs of acute liver failure such as hepatic encephalopathy.[14,17–19] Early HAT may also be clinically and biochemically silent[16]; most centers carry out protocol Doppler ultrasounds in the early post-LT period for this reason,[8] although in the absence of guidelines, intensity and duration of monitoring during the early postoperative phase varies widely from

Table 1
Causes of graft dysfunction and management strategies

Cause	Management Pointers
Primary graft nonfunction/ Early graft dysfunction	Conservative, manage organ failures (particularly acute kidney injury), may need to consider retransplantation, particularly in primary nonfunction.
Hepatic artery thrombosis	Revascularization (surgical vs radiological), may require retransplantation depending on degree of graft damage, consider antiplatelet agents.
Venous complications	Radiological vs surgical intervention. Consider anticoagulation.
Graft rejection	Histologic confirmation is required. Immunosuppression should be optimized, may frequently necessitate steroid bolus and taper. Graft loss may occur with chronic rejection, necessitating retransplantation.
Biliary complications (ie, strictures)	Imaging and endoscopic intervention as appropriate. May require surgical refashioning of anastomosis if refractory to endoscopic therapy.

center to center. Conversely, late HAT may be identified years following LT and tends to manifest more insidiously with gradual worsening of graft function, hepatic abscesses, and recurrent cholangitis or may be detected incidentally on imaging.[14] Although duplex Doppler ultrasound is an appropriate first step on suspicion of HAT, diagnosis is usually confirmed by computed tomography (CT) or MRI angiography.[7,16]

Although there are no evidence-based guidelines toward managing HAT post-LT, management options include revascularization, retransplant, and observation. Success rate of surgical revascularization is inconsistent and reported between 10% and 55%.[6,8,15] Interventional radiology–assisted attempts at revascularization and thrombolysis have reported success rates of 46% to 68%.[20,21] As such, in the case of early HAT, and especially if acute liver failure has developed with irreversible graft damage, most transplant centers will allow relisting of the patient with urgent status,[22] as early retransplant (<30 days post-LT) is associated with better outcomes.[23] However, revascularization in asymptomatic early HAT may be associated with improved outcomes and graft survival with avoidance of retransplant.[24] Success rates from revascularization may also depend on timing, with better outcomes seen if performed early post-LT.[15]

In late HAT, due to the development of collateral blood supply, graft dysfunction tends to be chronic and slowly progressive, with less risk of developing acute liver failure (ALF).[7] Although revascularization attempts may still be pursued, management strategies revolve around optimizing biliary issues, such as ischemic cholangiopathy (with endoscopic dilatations/antibiotic therapy). These patients are likely to develop recurrent cholangitis and liver abscesses, and may require retransplant. In a study using United Network for Organ Sharing data in 623 LT recipients, retransplant for HAT was associated with better graft and patient survival compared with retransplant for other reasons.[23] HAT patients who underwent retransplantation at more than 30 days post-LT had increased risk of early graft loss and overall graft survival compared with those who underwent retransplant within 30 days post-LT.[23]

Portal Vein Thrombosis/Stenosis

Portal vein thrombosis (PVT) has been reported in up to 7% of grafts.[16] PVT can cause graft dysfunction or failure, acutely presenting with elevated AST/ALT, although may also manifest with symptoms of portal hypertension, such as ascites; graft failure may occur with significant hepatic necrosis.[6] The risk of PVT is higher if PVT was present pre-LT and if a portal vein graft was used.[6] Portal vein stenosis may also present with a similar clinical picture.[16] Anticoagulation, surgical exploration, or radiologically assisted thrombectomy can be pursued, but if significant hepatic necrosis has occurred, retransplant may be required. PVT is usually diagnosed with duplex Doppler ultrasound and cross-sectional imaging.[16]

Venous Congestion

Venous outflow complications are uncommon and may occur at a rate of 1% to 2%, presenting initially with delayed graft function, hepatomegaly, ascites, and variceal bleeding.[25] Doppler examination is usually the first investigation, although transjugular venography with pressure measurements may be required for definitive diagnosis. Although success rates with angioplasty are high,[26] restenosis occurs frequently and may necessitate stent placement.[27] Although venous anastomosis may influence development of hepatic venous outflow obstruction, with previous series reporting higher incidence with piggy-back venous anastomosis (3%–4%)[28,29] as compared with caval replacement (<2%),[30,31] more contemporary large series have reported low incidence of venous complications (<1%) with piggy-back in whole grafts,[32] or far improved incidence (<4%), even if using reduced sized grafts,[33] which may reflect improvement in overall technique.

PRIMARY NONFUNCTION (AND PRIMARY GRAFT DYSFUNCTION)

Primary nonfunction (PNF) is a term that is used to describe a hepatic graft that does not perform metabolic functions following LT. There is no universally accepted definition for PNF, although its characteristics include progressive severe deranged liver enzymes (within 48 hours post-LT), severe coagulopathy, inability of the liver to produce bile, lactic acidosis, hypoglycemia, and multiorgan failure with a clinical picture similar to ALF.[34–36] The diagnosis is achieved retrospectively, with most of the definitions incorporating "retransplant within 7 days post-LT" as a criterion.[37] True PNF is the most extreme form of early primary graft dysfunction and the only treatment is immediate retransplant.[34,35] The reported incidence for PNF ranges from 0.9% to 7.2%.[37]

Milder forms of primary graft dysfunction/early graft dysfunction may be completely reversible without requirement for retransplant, although full recovery may take up to 28 days.[37] The reported incidence of this ranges from 5.2% to 36.3%.[37] Clinically, patients with primary graft dysfunction differ from those with PNF in that apart from abnormal liver biochemistry tests, they may not be overtly symptomatic. The management is supportive. The relevance of noting primary graft dysfunction is due to the association with inferior long-term outcomes for graft and patient survival.[38,39] Other factors found to be associated with primary graft dysfunction include use of extended criteria grafts with associated long warm ischemic time,[40] older donors,[41,42] grafts with steatosis,[43,44] and prolonged cold ischemic time.[45] Additionally, it has now been found that ischemia-reperfusion injury (IRI) is a risk factor for acute kidney injury,[46] and early graft dysfunction has been associated with development of new-onset acute kidney injury requiring renal replacement therapy within the first month post-LT, as well as risk factors for developing end-stage renal disease within the first year post-LT.[47]

A proposed definition for primary graft dysfunction defines this by the presence of 1 or more of the following variables: (1) bilirubin greater than 10 mg/dL on postoperative day 7, (2) international normalized ratio >1.6 on postoperative day 7, and[18] alanine aminotransferase or aspartate aminotransferase >2000 IU/L within 7 postoperative days.[37,38] A novel continuous score using the same parameters, known as the "model for early allograft function (MEAF)," is obtainable within the first 3 postoperative days and may be more useful in grading severity of dysfunction, and has been shown to be predictive of short-term and long-term survival.[48,49]

The underlying pathophysiology behind early allograft dysfunction is thought to be related to IRI, which is discussed later in this article in the section "Ischemia-Reperfusion Injury."

Aside from repeat LT for PNF, numerous strategies have been investigated to optimize graft recovery with limited benefit. A meta-analysis investigating effects of prostaglandin administration in the perioperative period demonstrated no risk reduction in either incidence of PNF, requirement for retransplant, or mortality.[50] At present, there is no conclusive evidence to support the use of PGI2,[51] nitric oxide,[52] polyethylene glycol,[53] or molecular adsorbent recirculating system[36,54] in the treatment of primary graft dysfunction. Despite a previous randomized controlled study showing potential for N acetyl-cysteine in improving graft survival (from postulated modulation on IRI),[55] these findings were not borne out in subsequent studies.[56,57]

REJECTION

Despite the liver being considered "immunotolerant," rejection occurs commonly. Most rejection cases would be due to acute cellular rejection at an estimated 10% to 30%,[58] followed by chronic rejection, which takes place in 3% to 17%,[59] and finally hyperacute rejection, which is rare. The mechanisms behind each form of rejection differ.[60]

Hyperacute Rejection

Hyperacute rejection (HAR) develops due to formation of antibodies against the donor's major histocompatibility complex and although rare, will ultimately lead to destruction of the graft. The pathophysiology behind HAR is complex, but can be summarized by ischemic necrosis of the graft from occlusion of the major vessels due to deposition of antibodies in the sinusoids and endothelium of the graft, as well as thrombosis formation from the activated complement cascade.[60] Hence, the presentation is usually early post-LT with extreme elevated transaminases, consumptive thrombocytopenia, and subsequent development of ALF. The 2 situations in which HAR may occur are donor-recipient ABO incompatibility, and lymphocytotoxic antibodies directed against the donor.[61] However, ABO-incompatible LT is possible with preemptive circumvention of HAR with B-cell desensitization techniques and plasma exchange pre-LT.[62,63]

Acute Cellular Rejection

Acute cellular rejection (ACR) occurs in up to 66% of LT recipients,[58,64] most commonly within the 6 weeks post-LT.[58,65] It is a T-cell–mediated inflammatory response to donor HLA antigens presenting to host T cells.[60] Patients may experience pyrexia, tenderness to the liver, and nonspecific malaise, although they are usually asymptomatic with abnormal hepatic biochemistry tests and often, peripheral eosinophilia.[66] The liver test abnormalities arise as a result of portal inflammation, bile duct inflammation, and endothelial inflammation, characteristics that form the histologic criteria for diagnosing ACR in liver grafts.[67] Liver tests may, however, remain entirely normal despite ACR.[68]

The diagnosis of ACR requires histologic confirmation,[67] although in practice this is oftentimes clinically diagnosed on the exclusion of other potential causes for abnormal liver tests, and managed by optimization of immunosuppression, especially if liver tests are only mildly abnormal. Otherwise, high-dose intravenous methylprednisolone (followed by a quick oral taper) are usually used for biopsy-proven moderate-severe ACR with good success.[69] ACR occurring within 3 months post-LT is not associated with decrease in graft loss or survival.[70] However, ACR occurring more than 3 to 6 months post-LT, referred to as "late ACR" is associated with decreased graft loss and survival.[71]

Chronic (Ductopenic) Rejection

In chronic rejection, progressive damage to the bile ducts causes a predominantly cholestatic graft dysfunction that may eventually result in graft loss.[72] Chronic rejection is associated with number of prior ACR episodes and degree of severity of ACR, donor-recipient sex mismatch, use of extended criteria donors, as well as autoimmune etiology to primary LT.[59] Significant escalation of immunosuppression may reverse chronic rejection, such as with use of lymphocyte-depleting medication; however, retransplantation is often required.[73]

POST–LIVER TRANSPLANT CHOLESTASIS

Cholestasis is a common occurrence after LT and is due to impairment of bile production in the grafted liver or bile flow. Blood tests show variable elevations in serum bilirubin, serum alkaline phosphatase (ALP), and serum gamma-glutamyl transpeptidase with serum transaminases being normal or elevated.[74] Post-LT cholestasis can be categorized as intrahepatic (due to injury of liver cells and problems with bile production) or extrahepatic (due to mechanical obstruction of bile flow).[75] Intensive care unit (ICU) management focuses on early cholestatic conditions, defined as occurring less than 6 months post LT[76] (**Table 2**).

INTRAHEPATIC CHOLESTASIS

Post-LT intrahepatic cholestasis occurs because of impaired production and secretion of bile due to hepatocyte and microscopic intrahepatic bile duct injury.[74] It is reported in 25% to 53% of patients after LT.[77] Risk factors include receipt of platelets and cryoprecipitate intraoperatively, suboptimal graft appearance, incompatible blood grouping, being an inpatient before transplant, and bacteremia during the first 30 days after LT.[74] Most patients remain subclinical, but a subset develops severe cholestasis, which may lead to graft failure and retransplantation, along with increased mortality within the first year after LT.[74] Etiologies include primary graft nonfunction, ischemia and reperfusion injury, infections, drug toxicity, small-for-size graft, and ACR.[78]

Ischemia-Reperfusion Injury

IRI occurs in 17% to 50% of transplants.[79] It is due to damage during the organ procurement process, storage of the graft, and transplantation itself.[80] Two forms of IRI are warm IRI (injury during organ procurement and transplantation with interruption and restoration of hepatic circulation) and cold IRI (injury during graft storage).[81] Warm IRI leads to hepatocellular damage through Kupffer cell–mediated release of cytotoxic substances, whereas cold IRI causes hepatic sinusoidal endothelial cell and microcirculation disruptions.[82] In both forms, the first stage involves ischemic injury, which is a local process of cellular metabolic derangement due to hypoxia and lack of ATP production. This is followed by reperfusion injury, where significant inflammatory immune responses lead to cytotoxic damage of the graft.[83]

Severe IRI diagnosed on a time-zero biopsy of the graft during LT was a significant predictor of poor post-LT outcomes with 50% graft loss 1 year post-LT.[84] Up to 25% of patients need retransplant within the first 3 months post-LT.[85] IRI has also been

Table 2 Etiologies of post–liver transplant cholestasis	
Intrahepatic Cholestasis	**Extrahepatic Cholestasis**
Primary graft nonfunction	Biliary stricture
Ischemia and reperfusion injury	Biliary leak
Infections	Choledocholithiasis
Small-for-size graft	Biliary cast formation
Drug toxicity	Cholangitis
Acute cellular rejection	

suggested as a determinant in development of acute kidney injury post-LT leading to longer ICU and hospital stays along with reduced 1-year survival.[46] Risk factors include both donor and transplant factors. Donor properties increasing susceptibly to IRI include poor donor nutritional status, advanced donor age (age >70 years), and donor liver steatosis.[86] Transplant factors include prolonged cold and warm ischemic times.[77]

Normally post-LT, serum transaminases begin to improve rapidly, usually within several hours and normalize within 1 week.[87] IRI is reflected by persistently elevated or rising serum transaminases and may also result delayed decline in serum gamma-glutamyltransferase (GGT) and bilirubin. Cholestasis can persist for up to 17 days.[88] Liver biopsy may be required to make a definitive diagnose and shows steatosis, cholestasis, and ballooning degeneration of hepatocytes.[89]

Once IRI occurs, the only treatment option is supportive management. Mild injury usually spontaneously resolves. However, more severe cases can result in graft dysfunction and may require retransplant.[79] Different medications have been investigated as potential preventive agents. These have included antioxidants, vasopressors, renin-angiotensin system modulators, beta-blockers, growth factors, calcium channel blockers, and protease inhibitors.[90] Given the donor-related risk factors of IRI, careful selection of donor grafts may decrease the chance of IRI. However, due to graft shortages, candidate donors may not be perfectly ideal. Graft preservation through ex vivo perfusion and surgical optimization through minimizing cold and warm ischemic times may be the best option.

Infections

Infectious complications are a frequent cause of cholestasis immediately post-LT. Bacterial infections occur in up to 70% of patients.[91] The most frequent sources of infection are intra-abdominal, nosocomial, chest, surgical site, and catheter-related infections. *Pseudomonas aeruginosa* and enteric gram-negative organisms (*Enterobacter*) are most commonly seen.[92] Bacteremia during the first 30 days post-LT is significantly associated with intrahepatic cholestasis.[74] Proinflammatory cytokines and endotoxins during sepsis disrupt bile acid transport at the sinusoidal and canalicular membranes leading to cholestasis.[93]

Viral infections occur in 30% to 50% of patients, with cytomegalovirus (CMV) being most common as either a new or reactivated infection.[94] The highest risk of CMV infection is during the first 3 to 4 months post-LT and in seronegative recipients with a seropositive graft.[77] CMV damages hepatocytes and causes injury to the biliary epithelium, leading to cholestasis.[95]

Risk factors for post-LT infections involve donor, recipient, surgical, and post-LT factors. Donor factors include prolonged ICU stay, infection, and marginal graft.[96] Recipient factors include elderly age, model for end-stage liver disease (MELD) score greater than 30, ALF, poor nutritional status, prolonged ICU stay, infection, and diabetes.[97] Surgical factors include surgical time greater than 12 hours, retransplantation, transfusion of greater than 15 units of blood, and Roux-en-Y biliary anastomosis.[97] Post-LT factors include prolonged mechanical ventilation, type and amount of immunosuppression, and development of post-LT complications (primary nonfunction, HAT, biliary strictures).[97] Broad-spectrum antibiotics should be initiated as early as possible, along with antivirals if a viral infection such as CMV is suspected. If required, source control should be attempted. Regarding surgical site infections, there is no evidence to suggest benefit or harm to antibiotic prophylaxis post-LT.[98] However, regarding CMV infection, prophylaxis is recommended for all patients who are seronegative at the time of transplantation.[77]

Small-for-Size Graft

Small-for-size syndrome complicates live donor LT if partial liver graft hepatocyte cellular mass is inadequate to meet functional demands of the recipient.[99] Typical adult live donor LT grafts should encompass 30% to 40% of the recipient's liver volume.[100] If the graft size is too small, portal hyperperfusion and arterial hypoperfusion lead to inadequate supply of oxygen and growth factors for liver regeneration and sinusoidal microcirculatory dysfunction.[99] Subsequently, portal hypertension, graft inflammation, and graft injury develop.

Small-for-size syndrome presentations are variable. In mild cases, minor hepatic dysfunction and isolated elevated serum bilirubin occur. In severe cases, coagulopathy, ascites, variceal bleeding, encephalopathy, and irreversible graft failure occur, necessitating the need for urgent retransplantation.[99] Liver biopsy may be required, and shows ischemic changes, ballooning hepatocytes, and cholestasis.[101] Most treatment options have focused on decreasing the portal hyperperfusion and flow. Surgical procedures, such as splenic artery ligation, splenectomy, and portosystemic shunts have been used, along with medications like octreotide, nonselective B-blockers aimed at constricting splanchnic circulation.[76] If recovery does not occur, retransplantation is required.

Drug Toxicity

Drug-induced liver toxicity post-LT may occur due to immunosuppressive medications to prevent rejection as well as antibiotics and antiviral agents needed to treat infections. The most common presentation is an increase in serum ALP with or without the presence of jaundice or pruritis.[102] Liver biopsy may be necessary if the diagnosis is uncertain and may show acute cholestatic hepatitis, cholestasis with bile duct injury, or vanishing duct syndrome.[102] Most frequently encountered drugs that can lead to toxicity are cyclosporine, azathioprine, tacrolimus, trimethoprim-sulfamethoxazole, and fluconazole.[77] Treatment involves immediate discontinuation of the suspected medication and supportive management.

EXTRAHEPATIC CHOLESTASIS

Post-LT extrahepatic cholestasis occurs in up to 50% and necessitates retransplantation in up to 12.5% of LT recipients.[103] Risk factors for biliary complications include HAT, prolonged cold and warm graft ischemic time, use of partial grafts (live donor liver grafts), duct-to-duct anastomosis, and tense anastomosis suturing.[104] Treatment entails endoscopic management with endoscopic retrograde cholangiopancreatography (ERCP) and biliary stenting, radiologic management with percutaneous drainage or surgical management with biliary revision.

Biliary Stricture

Biliary strictures are common post-LT.[105] They are divided into anastomotic strictures (AS) and nonanastomotic strictures (NAS) (single or multiple narrowings proximal to the site of biliary anastomosis).[106] AS incidence is close to 10%.[107] Early-occurring AS is due to technical surgical issues (injury to the bile ducts, small-caliber bile ducts, donor-recipient bile duct size mismatch) and postoperative bile leak.[108] NAS occurs in 10% of patients.[106] These strictures are secondary to ischemic and immunologic events. Risk factors include HAT, ductopenic rejection, blood type incompatibility, underlying liver disease of primary sclerosing cholangitis or autoimmune hepatitis, prolonged cold and warm ischemic times, and donation after cardiac death (DCD).[109] NAS is associated with biliary sludge, stones, and cast formation secondary to biliary epithelium sloughing from the ischemic or immunologic injury.

Clinically, patients may be asymptomatic with biochemistry showing elevated serum bilirubin, ALP, and GGT along with mild to moderately elevated serum transaminases.[110] Patients may display jaundice if the obstruction is severe or prolonged. Patients may develop cholangitis and present with fever, abdominal pain, and hemodynamic instability. Initial evaluation involves liver ultrasound with Doppler to study hepatic vasculature, including the flow of the hepatic artery. Reduced flow may suggest ischemic biliary stricture formation when coupled with cholestatic rise in liver enzymes. Ultrasound can also detect changes in bile duct caliber. However, ultrasound has poor sensitivity in detecting biliary stricture and obstruction.[108] Scintigraphy of the biliary tract may provide insight into biliary obstruction due to strictures and has better sensitivity compared with ultrasound.[108] Magnetic resonance cholangiopancreatography, however, is considered the best noninvasive diagnostic tool for investigating biliary strictures with both a sensitivity and specificity of 90%.[111] The gold standard for biliary stricture diagnosis involves invasive analysis of the biliary tract through ERCP or percutaneous transhepatic cholangiography (PTC), but given the risk of procedural complications, these techniques are reserved for therapeutics.[108]

Management of post-LT biliary strictures can be accomplished endoscopically, radiologically, or surgically. Endoscopic therapy through ERCP is the first-line approach when technically feasible. ERCP options include stricture dilation and stenting.[106] Radiologic therapy involves PTC-guided biliary dilation and stenting. This is a second-line option for complex cases in which ERCP therapy has failed because of the increased invasiveness of PTC-guided therapies and risks of hemorrhage, bile leaks, and infection.[106] Finally, surgical treatments include biliary revision and retransplantation. These options are used only as a last resort in cases refractory to both endoscopic and radiologic management.[106] Success rates are higher for treating AS compared with NAS given the diffuse nature of NAS. NAS also reduces graft survival and leads to retransplantation in 30% to 50% of patients.[112]

Bile Leak

Bile leaks occur commonly post-LT with an incidence of up to 25%.[113] They are categorized as anastomotic, cystic duct–related, T-tube–related, or cut-surface–related (in the case of live donor grafts).[113] The main risk factors include anastomotic site disruption from surgical technique or complication, bile duct ischemia from hepatic artery flow disruption, prolonged cold and warm ischemia times, and use of live donor grafts.[114] Bile leaks increase the development of biliary strictures and also reduce graft and patient survival post-LT.[115]

Bile leaks usually present 2 to 14 days post-LT.[116] It is usually suspected when there is persistent bilious output through operative drains, presence of bilious ascites, or presence of a biloma.[116] Patients may also have elevated liver enzymes in a cholestatic pattern. Once a bile leak is suspected, diagnosis is confirmed with CT imaging or ERCP.[116]

Small bile leaks and T-tube–related bile leaks can be managed expectantly and generally heal spontaneously. Up to one-half of T-tube–related bile leaks close within 24 hours.[117] For leaks that require therapy, ERCP with papillotomy and biliary stenting is the treatment of choice. The aim is to reduce pressure at the leak site by diverting away bile flow.[114] Rates of resolution with stenting are close to 90%[113]; however, in patients with persistent bile leaks despite ERCP therapy or who develop structuring, surgical management with biliary reconstruction may be required.[118]

DONOR FACTORS AFFECTING GRAFT FUNCTION

Given the shortage of supply of donor organs, increased used of extended criteria/marginal grafts (eg, DCD) as well as new techniques (ex vivo perfusion of the graft) to better preserve marginal grafts have been implemented to increase organ availability. DCD and ex vivo graft perfusion are 2 major factors that can affect the graft function.

Donation After Cardiac Death

DCD has allowed greater graft availability for liver transplants. It can be associated with significant warm ischemia time and differs from donation after brain death (DBD) as DBD grafts usually do not experience warm ischemia.[119] Warm ischemia has the potential to negatively affect graft quality and function. Multiple studies have found that graft survival using DCD grafts was lower compared with DBD grafts.[119] Along these lines, several studies have also shown reduced patient survival in those who receive DCD grafts.[119] Complications associated with DCD LT include primary nonfunction, HAT, and biliary stricture. These complications are seen in greater proportions of DCD compared with DBD.[119]

Because of greater potential for post-LT complications and worse clinical outcomes that can be seen with DCD transplants, optimal donors and recipients have been extensively evaluated. Currently both donor-related and recipient-related factors may worsen post-LT outcomes for DCD transplants. Donor-related factors include age older than 50, warm ischemia greater than 30 minutes, and cold ischemia greater than 8 hours.[120] Recipient-related factors include high MELD score and presence of hepatocellular carcinoma.[120]

Ex Vivo Liver Perfusion

As grafts from DCD and marginal donors have increased, it has been increasingly recognized that there is greater risk of post-LT complications. As a result, ex vivo liver perfusion (EVLP) has been widely studied as a way to decrease preservation injury and IRI.[121] With EVLP, a nutrient solution is used to perfuse the liver through the portal vein with collection through the inferior vena cava. The principle is to provide the graft with substrates for cellular energy production along with removal of toxic metabolites. Currently the 2 major EVLP strategies are hypothermic and normothermic.[121]

Hypothermic EVLP is intended to use the protective effects of hypothermia while still supplying the liver with oxygen and nutrients. This has been shown to cause less oxidative damage and inflammatory response.[122] Several studies have shown improved graft survival and less post-LT complications using this technique.[123] DCD grafts treated with hypothermic EVLP have been shown to have better outcomes compared with untreated DCD grafts as well.[123]

Normothermic EVLP aims to mimic normal conditions of the human body, maintain functional integrity of the donor liver, and reduce the effects of ischemia and reperfusion injury.[124] It is thought that normothermic perfusion helps support a healthy endothelium and restores normal levels of ATP.[124] Multiple studies have shown greater synthetic liver function, reduced biliary injury, and improved survival in porcine DCD transplant models.[124] There has also been a study demonstrating improved early biochemical function in DCD transplant patients receiving normothermic EVLP grafts compared with untreated grafts.[124]

REFERENCES

1. Vos JJ, Wietasch JK, Absalom AR, et al. Green light for liver function monitoring using indocyanine green? An overview of current clinical applications. Anaesthesia 2014;69:1364–76.
2. Conti F, Dousset B, Cherruau B, et al. Use of lidocaine metabolism to test liver function during the long-term follow-up of liver transplant recipients. Clin Transplant 2004;18:235–41.
3. Stockmann M, Lock JF, Malinowski M, et al. How to define initial poor graft function after liver transplantation? A new functional definition by the LiMAx test. Transpl Int 2010;23:1023–32.
4. Shiffman ML, Carithers RL Jr, Posner MP, et al. Recovery of bile secretion following orthotopic liver transplantation. J Hepatol 1991;12:351–61.
5. Sun N, Zhang J, Li X, et al. Biliary tract reconstruction with or without T-tube in orthotopic liver transplantation: a systematic review and meta-analysis. Expert Rev Gastroenterol Hepatol 2015;9:529–38.
6. Duffy JP, Hong JC, Farmer DG, et al. Vascular complications of orthotopic liver transplantation: experience in more than 4,200 patients. J Am Coll Surg 2009; 208:896–903 [discussion: 903–5].
7. Wozney P, Zajko AB, Bron KM, et al. Vascular complications after liver transplantation: a 5-year experience. AJR Am J Roentgenol 1986;147:657–63.
8. Bekker J, Ploem S, de Jong KP. Early hepatic artery thrombosis after liver transplantation: a systematic review of the incidence, outcome and risk factors. Am J Transplant 2009;9:746–57.
9. Silva MA, Jambulingam PS, Gunson BK, et al. Hepatic artery thrombosis following orthotopic liver transplantation: a 10-year experience from a single centre in the United Kingdom. Liver Transpl 2006;12:146–51.
10. Yang Y, Zhao JC, Yan LN, et al. Risk factors associated with early and late HAT after adult liver transplantation. World J Gastroenterol 2014;20:10545–52.
11. Heffron TG, Welch D, Pillen T, et al. Low incidence of hepatic artery thrombosis after pediatric liver transplantation without the use of intraoperative microscope or parenteral anticoagulation. Pediatr Transplant 2005;9:486–90.
12. Fujiki M, Hashimoto K, Palaios E, et al. Probability, management, and long-term outcomes of biliary complications after hepatic artery thrombosis in liver transplant recipients. Surgery 2017;162:1101–11.
13. Abbasoglu O, Levy MF, Testa G, et al. Does intraoperative hepatic artery flow predict arterial complications after liver transplantation? Transplantation 1998; 66:598–601.
14. Mourad MM, Liossis C, Gunson BK, et al. Etiology and management of hepatic artery thrombosis after adult liver transplantation. Liver Transpl 2014;20:713–23.
15. Scarinci A, Sainz-Barriga M, Berrevoet F, et al. Early arterial revascularization after hepatic artery thrombosis may avoid graft loss and improve outcomes in adult liver transplantation. Transplant Proc 2010;42:4403–8.
16. Kok T, Slooff MJ, Thijn CJ, et al. Routine Doppler ultrasound for the detection of clinically unsuspected vascular complications in the early postoperative phase after orthotopic liver transplantation. Transpl Int 1998;11:272–6.
17. Abou-Alfa GK, Schwartz L, Ricci S, et al. Phase II study of sorafenib in patients with advanced hepatocellular carcinoma. J Clin Oncol 2006;24:4293–300.
18. Shaked A, McDiarmid SV, Harrison RE, et al. Hepatic artery thrombosis resulting in gas gangrene of the transplanted liver. Surgery 1992;111:462–5.

19. Drazan K, Shaked A, Olthoff KM, et al. Etiology and management of symptomatic adult hepatic artery thrombosis after orthotopic liver transplantation (OLT). Am Surg 1996;62:237–40.

20. Kogut MJ, Shin DS, Padia SA, et al. Intra-arterial thrombolysis for hepatic artery thrombosis following liver transplantation. J Vasc Interv Radiol 2015;26: 1317–22.

21. Singhal A, Stokes K, Sebastian A, et al. Endovascular treatment of hepatic artery thrombosis following liver transplantation. Transpl Int 2010;23:245–56.

22. European Association for the Study of the Liver. EASL clinical practice guidelines: liver transplantation. J Hepatol 2016;64:433–85.

23. Lui SK, Garcia CR, Mei X, et al. Re-transplantation for hepatic artery thrombosis: a national perspective. World J Surg 2018. https://doi.org/10.1007/s00268-018-4609-7.

24. Sheiner PA, Varma CV, Guarrera JV, et al. Selective revascularization of hepatic artery thromboses after liver transplantation improves patient and graft survival. Transplantation 1997;64:1295–9.

25. Darcy MD. Management of venous outflow complications after liver transplantation. Tech Vasc Interv Radiol 2007;10:240–5.

26. Wang SL, Sze DY, Busque S, et al. Treatment of hepatic venous outflow obstruction after piggyback liver transplantation. Radiology 2005;236:352–9.

27. Cheng YF, Chen CL, Huang TL, et al. Angioplasty treatment of hepatic vein stenosis in pediatric liver transplants: long-term results. Transpl Int 2005;18: 556–61.

28. Parrilla P, Sánchez-Bueno F, Figueras J, et al. Analysis of the complications of the piggy-back technique in 1,112 liver transplants. Transplantation 1999;67: 1214–7.

29. Navarro F, Le Moine MC, Fabre JM, et al. Specific vascular complications of orthotopic liver transplantation with preservation of the retrohepatic vena cava: review of 1361 cases. Transplantation 1999;68:646–50.

30. Lerut J, Tzakis AG, Bron K, et al. Complications of venous reconstruction in human orthotopic liver transplantation. Ann Surg 1987;205:404–14.

31. Settmacher U, Nüssler NC, Glanemann M, et al. Venous complications after orthotopic liver transplantation. Clin Transplant 2000;14:235–41.

32. Khorsandi SE, Athale A, Vilca-Melendez H, et al. Presentation, diagnosis, and management of early hepatic venous outflow complications in whole cadaveric liver transplant. Liver Transpl 2015;21:914–21.

33. Koc S, Akbulut S, Soyer V, et al. Hepatic venous outflow obstruction after living-donor liver transplant: single center experience. Exp Clin Transplant 2017. https://doi.org/10.6002/ect.2017.0045.

34. Pokorny H, Gruenberger T, Soliman T, et al. Organ survival after primary dysfunction of liver grafts in clinical orthotopic liver transplantation. Transpl Int 2000;13(Suppl 1):S154–7.

35. Uemura T, Randall HB, Sanchez EQ, et al. Liver retransplantation for primary nonfunction: analysis of a 20-year single-center experience. Liver Transpl 2007;13:227–33.

36. Novelli G, Morabito V, Lai Q, et al. Glasgow coma score and tumor necrosis factor alpha as predictive criteria for initial poor graft function. Transplant Proc 2012;44:1820–5.

37. Chen XB, Xu MQ. Primary graft dysfunction after liver transplantation. Hepatobiliary Pancreat Dis Int 2014;13:125–37.

38. Olthoff KM, Kulik L, Samstein B, et al. Validation of a current definition of early allograft dysfunction in liver transplant recipients and analysis of risk factors. Liver Transpl 2010;16:943–9.
39. Heise M, Settmacher U, Pfitzmann R, et al. A survival-based scoring-system for initial graft function following orthotopic liver transplantation. Transpl Int 2003;16: 794–800.
40. D'Alessandro AM, Fernandez LA, Chin LT, et al. Donation after cardiac death: the University of Wisconsin experience. Ann Transplant 2004;9:68–71.
41. Mathe Z, Paul A, Molmenti EP, et al. Liver transplantation with donors over the expected lifespan in the model for end-staged liver disease era: is Mother Nature punishing us? Liver Int 2011;31:1054–61.
42. Johnson SR, Alexopoulos S, Curry M, et al. Primary nonfunction (PNF) in the MELD Era: an SRTR database analysis. Am J Transplant 2007;7:1003–9.
43. Kulik U, Lehner F, Klempnauer J, et al. Primary non-function is frequently associated with fatty liver allografts and high mortality after re-transplantation. Liver Int 2017;37:1219–28.
44. Urena MA, Ruiz-Delgado FC, González EM, et al. Assessing risk of the use of livers with macro and microsteatosis in a liver transplant program. Transplant Proc 1998;30:3288–91.
45. Cameron AM, Ghobrial RM, Yersiz H, et al. Optimal utilization of donor grafts with extended criteria: a single-center experience in over 1000 liver transplants. Ann Surg 2006;243:748–53 [discussion: 53–5].
46. Jochmans I, Meurisse N, Neyrinck A, et al. Hepatic ischemia/reperfusion injury associates with acute kidney injury in liver transplantation: prospective cohort study. Liver Transpl 2017;23:634–44.
47. Wadei HM, Lee DD, Croome KP, et al. Early allograft dysfunction after liver transplantation is associated with short- and long-term kidney function impairment. Am J Transplant 2016;16:850–9.
48. Pareja E, Cortes M, Hervás D, et al. A score model for the continuous grading of early allograft dysfunction severity. Liver Transpl 2015;21:38–46.
49. Jochmans I, Fieuws S, Monbaliu D, et al. "Model for early allograft function" outperforms "early allograft dysfunction" as a predictor of transplant survival. Transplantation 2017;101:e258–64.
50. Cavalcanti AB, De Vasconcelos CP, Perroni de Oliveira M, et al. Prostaglandins for adult liver transplanted patients. Cochrane Database Syst Rev 2011;(11):CD006006.
51. Barthel E, Rauchfuss F, Hoyer H, et al. Impact of stable PGI(2) analog iloprost on early graft viability after liver transplantation: a pilot study. Clin Transplant 2012; 26:E38–47.
52. Lang JD Jr, Teng X, Chumley P, et al. Inhaled NO accelerates restoration of liver function in adults following orthotopic liver transplantation. J Clin Invest 2007; 117:2583–91.
53. Pasut G, Panisello A, Folch-Puy E, et al. Polyethylene glycols: an effective strategy for limiting liver ischemia reperfusion injury. World J Gastroenterol 2016;22: 6501–8.
54. Pocze B, Fazakas J, Zádori G, et al. MARS therapy, the bridging to liver retransplantation—three cases from the Hungarian liver transplant program. Interv Med Appl Sci 2013;5:70–5.
55. D'Amico F, Vitale A, Piovan D, et al. Use of N-acetylcysteine during liver procurement: a prospective randomized controlled study. Liver Transpl 2013;19: 135–44.

56. Jegatheeswaran S, Siriwardena AK. Experimental and clinical evidence for modification of hepatic ischaemia-reperfusion injury by N-acetylcysteine during major liver surgery. HPB (Oxford) 2011;13:71–8.

57. Hilmi IA, Peng Z, Planinsic RM, et al. N-acetylcysteine does not prevent hepatorenal ischaemia-reperfusion injury in patients undergoing orthotopic liver transplantation. Nephrol Dial Transplant 2010;25:2328–33.

58. Rodriguez-Peralvarez M, Rico-Juri JM, Tsochatzis E, et al. Biopsy-proven acute cellular rejection as an efficacy endpoint of randomized trials in liver transplantation: a systematic review and critical appraisal. Transpl Int 2016;29:961–73.

59. Choudhary NS, Saigal S, Bansal RK, et al. Acute and chronic rejection after liver transplantation: what a clinician needs to know. J Clin Exp Hepatol 2017;7: 358–66.

60. Hale DA. Basic transplantation immunology. Surg Clin North Am 2006;86: 1103–25, v.

61. Ratner LE, Phelan D, Brunt EM, et al. Probable antibody-mediated failure of two sequential ABO-compatible hepatic allografts in a single recipient. Transplantation 1993;55:814–9.

62. Honda M, Sugawara Y, Kadohisa M, et al. Long-term outcomes of ABO-incompatible pediatric living donor liver transplantation. Transplantation 2018. https://doi.org/10.1097/tp.0000000000002197.

63. Lee EC, Kim SH, Shim JR, et al. A comparison of desensitization methods: rituximab with/without plasmapheresis in ABO-incompatible living donor liver transplantation. Hepatobiliary Pancreat Dis Int 2018;17:119–25.

64. Shaked A, Ghobrial RM, Merion RM, et al. Incidence and severity of acute cellular rejection in recipients undergoing adult living donor or deceased donor liver transplantation. Am J Transplant 2009;9:301–8.

65. Wiesner RH, Demetris AJ, Belle SH, et al. Acute hepatic allograft rejection: incidence, risk factors, and impact on outcome. Hepatology 1998;28:638–45.

66. Nagral A, Quaglia A, Sabin CA, et al. Blood and graft eosinophils in acute cellular rejection of liver allografts. Transplant Proc 2001;33:2588–93.

67. Banff schema for grading liver allograft rejection: an international consensus document. Hepatology 1997;25:658–63.

68. Bartlett AS, Ramadas R, Furness S, et al. The natural history of acute histologic rejection without biochemical graft dysfunction in orthotopic liver transplantation: a systematic review. Liver Transpl 2002;8:1147–53.

69. Volpin R, Angeli P, Galioto A, et al. Comparison between two high-dose methylprednisolone schedules in the treatment of acute hepatic cellular rejection in liver transplant recipients: a controlled clinical trial. Liver Transpl 2002;8:527–34.

70. Seiler CA, Renner EL, Czerniak A, et al. Early acute cellular rejection: no effect on late hepatic allograft function in man. Transpl Int 1999;12:195–201.

71. Nacif LS, Pinheiro RS, Pécora RA, et al. Late acute rejection in liver transplant: a systematic review. Arq Bras Cir Dig 2015;28:212–5 [in English, Portuguese].

72. Demetris A, Adams D, Bellamy C, et al. Update of the International Banff Schema for Liver Allograft Rejection: working recommendations for the histopathologic staging and reporting of chronic rejection. An international panel. Hepatology 2000;31:792–9.

73. Blakolmer K, Seaberg EC, Batts K, et al. Analysis of the reversibility of chronic liver allograft rejection implications for a staging schema. Am J Surg Pathol 1999;23:1328–39.

74. Fusai G, Dhaliwal P, Rolando N, et al. Incidence and risk factors for the development of prolonged and severe intrahepatic cholestasis after liver transplantation. Liver Transpl 2006;12:1626–33.
75. Ben-Ari Z, Pappo O, Mor E. Intrahepatic cholestasis after liver transplantation. Liver Transpl 2003;9:1005–18.
76. Ponziani FR, Bhoori S, Pompili M, et al. Post-liver transplant intrahepatic cholestasis: etiology, clinical presentation, therapy. Eur Rev Med Pharmacol Sci 2017; 21:23–36.
77. Corbani A, Burroughs AK. Intrahepatic cholestasis after liver transplantation. Clin Liver Dis 2008;12:111–29, ix.
78. Harnois DM, Watt KDS. Cholestasis post-liver transplantation. In: Carey EJ, Lindor KD, editors. Cholestatic liver disease. New York: Humana Press; 2014. p. 189–99.
79. Lee YM, O'Brien CB, Yamashiki N, et al. Preservation injury patterns in liver transplantation associated with poor prognosis. Transplant Proc 2003;35: 2964–6.
80. Zhai Y, Petrowsky H, Hong JC, et al. Ischaemia-reperfusion injury in liver transplantation—from bench to bedside. Nat Rev Gastroenterol Hepatol 2013;10: 79–89.
81. Zhai Y, Busuttil RW, Kupiec-Weglinski JW. Liver ischemia and reperfusion injury: new insights into mechanisms of innate-adaptive immune-mediated tissue inflammation. Am J Transplant 2011;11:1563–9.
82. Ikeda T, Yanaga K, Kishikawa K, et al. Ischemic injury in liver transplantation: difference in injury sites between warm and cold ischemia in rats. Hepatology 1992;16:454–61.
83. Fondevila C, Busuttil RW, Kupiec-Weglinski JW. Hepatic ischemia/reperfusion injury—a fresh look. Exp Mol Pathol 2003;74:86–93.
84. Ali JM, Davies SE, Brais RJ, et al. Analysis of ischemia/reperfusion injury in time-zero biopsies predicts liver allograft outcomes. Liver Transpl 2015;21: 487–99.
85. Azoulay D, Linhares MM, Huguet E, et al. Decision for retransplantation of the liver: an experience- and cost-based analysis. Ann Surg 2002;236:713–21 [discussion: 21].
86. Peralta C, Jiménez-Castro MB, Gracia-Sancho J. Hepatic ischemia and reperfusion injury: effects on the liver sinusoidal milieu. J Hepatol 2013;59:1094–106.
87. Totsuka E, Fung JJ, Ishii T, et al. Influence of donor condition on postoperative graft survival and function in human liver transplantation. Transplant Proc 2000; 32:322–6.
88. Cutrin JC, Cantino D, Biasi F, et al. Reperfusion damage to the bile canaliculi in transplanted human liver. Hepatology 1996;24:1053–7.
89. Neil DA, Hubscher SG. Are parenchymal changes in early post-transplant biopsies related to preservation-reperfusion injury or rejection? Transplantation 2001;71:1566–72.
90. Siniscalchi A, Gamberini L, Laici C, et al. Post reperfusion syndrome during liver transplantation: from pathophysiology to therapy and preventive strategies. World J Gastroenterol 2016;22:1551–69.
91. Wade JJ, Rolando N, Hayllar K, et al. Bacterial and fungal infections after liver transplantation: an analysis of 284 patients. Hepatology 1995;21:1328–36.
92. Singh N. Infectious diseases in the liver transplant recipient. Semin Gastrointest Dis 1998;9:136–46.

93. Moseley RH, Wang W, Takeda H, et al. Effect of endotoxin on bile acid transport in rat liver: a potential model for sepsis-associated cholestasis. Am J Physiol 1996;271:G137–46.
94. Mutimer D. CMV infection of transplant recipients. J Hepatol 1996;25:259–69.
95. Martelius T, Krogerus L, Höckerstedt K, et al. Cytomegalovirus infection is associated with increased inflammation and severe bile duct damage in rat liver allografts. Hepatology 1998;27:996–1002.
96. van Hoek B, de Rooij BJ, Verspaget HW. Risk factors for infection after liver transplantation. Best Pract Res Clin Gastroenterol 2012;26:61–72.
97. Fishman JA, Issa NC. Infection in organ transplantation: risk factors and evolving patterns of infection. Infect Dis Clin North Am 2010;24:273–83.
98. Almeida RA, Hasimoto CN, Kim A, et al. Antibiotic prophylaxis for surgical site infection in people undergoing liver transplantation. Cochrane Database Syst Rev 2015;(12):CD010164.
99. Dahm F, Georgiev P, Clavien PA. Small-for-size syndrome after partial liver transplantation: definition, mechanisms of disease and clinical implications. Am J Transplant 2005;5:2605–10.
100. Kawasaki S, Makuuchi M, Matsunami H, et al. Living related liver transplantation in adults. Ann Surg 1998;227:269–74.
101. Demetris AJ, Kelly DM, Eghtesad B, et al. Pathophysiologic observations and histopathologic recognition of the portal hyperperfusion or small-for-size syndrome. Am J Surg Pathol 2006;30:986–93.
102. Chalasani N, Fontana RJ, Bonkovsky HL, et al. Causes, clinical features, and outcomes from a prospective study of drug-induced liver injury in the United States. Gastroenterology 2008;135:1924–34, 1934.e1-4.
103. Thethy S, Thomson BNj, Pleass H, et al. Management of biliary tract complications after orthotopic liver transplantation. Clin Transplant 2004;18:647–53.
104. Mejía GA, Olarte-Parra C, Pedraza A, et al. Biliary complications after liver transplantation: incidence, risk factors and impact on patient and graft survival. Transplant Proc 2016;48:665–8.
105. Forrest EA, Reiling J, Lipka G, et al. Risk factors and clinical indicators for the development of biliary strictures post liver transplant: significance of bilirubin. World J Transplant 2017;7:349–58.
106. Villa NA, Harrison ME. Management of biliary strictures after liver transplantation. Gastroenterol Hepatol (N Y) 2015;11:316–28.
107. Sharma S, Gurakar A, Jabbour N. Biliary strictures following liver transplantation: past, present and preventive strategies. Liver Transpl 2008;14:759–69.
108. Ryu CH, Lee SK. Biliary strictures after liver transplantation. Gut Liver 2011;5:133–42.
109. Guichelaar MM, Benson JT, Malinchoc M, et al. Risk factors for and clinical course of non-anastomotic biliary strictures after liver transplantation. Am J Transplant 2003;3:885–90.
110. Mahajani RV, Cotler SJ, Uzer MF. Efficacy of endoscopic management of anastomotic biliary strictures after hepatic transplantation. Endoscopy 2000;32:943–9.
111. Fulcher AS, Turner MA. Orthotopic liver transplantation: evaluation with MR cholangiography. Radiology 1999;211:715–22.
112. Graziadei IW, Benson JT, Malinchoc M, et al. Long-term outcome of endoscopic treatment of biliary strictures after liver transplantation. Liver Transpl 2006;12:718–25.

113. Sendino O, Fernández-Simon A, Law R, et al. Endoscopic management of bile leaks after liver transplantation: an analysis of two high-volume transplant centers. United European Gastroenterol J 2018;6:89–96.

114. Lee HW, Shah NH, Lee SK. An update on endoscopic management of post-liver transplant biliary complications. Clin Endosc 2017;50:451–63.

115. Gondolesi GE, Varotti G, Florman SS, et al. Biliary complications in 96 consecutive right lobe living donor transplant recipients. Transplantation 2004;77: 1842–8.

116. Simoes P, Kesar V, Ahmad J. Spectrum of biliary complications following live donor liver transplantation. World J Hepatol 2015;7:1856–65.

117. Shuhart MC, Kowdley KV, McVicar JP, et al. Predictors of bile leaks after T-tube removal in orthotopic liver transplant recipients. Liver Transpl Surg 1998;4: 62–70.

118. Shah SA, Grant DR, McGilvray ID, et al. Biliary strictures in 130 consecutive right lobe living donor liver transplant recipients: results of a Western center. Am J Transplant 2007;7:161–7.

119. Eren EA, Latchana N, Beal E, et al. Donations after circulatory death in liver transplant. Exp Clin Transplant 2016;14:463–70.

120. Lee KW, Simpkins CE, Montgomery RA, et al. Factors affecting graft survival after liver transplantation from donation after cardiac death donors. Transplantation 2006;82:1683–8.

121. Barbas AS, Goldaracena N, Dib MJ, et al. Ex-vivo liver perfusion for organ preservation: recent advances in the field. Transplant Rev (Orlando) 2016;30: 154–60.

122. Schlegel A, Graf R, Clavien PA, et al. Hypothermic oxygenated perfusion (HOPE) protects from biliary injury in a rodent model of DCD liver transplantation. J Hepatol 2013;59:984–91.

123. Schlegel A, Muller X, Dutkowski P. Hypothermic machine preservation of the liver: state of the art. Curr Transplant Rep 2018;5:93–102.

124. Ceresa CDL, Nasralla D, Jassem W. Normothermic machine preservation of the liver: state of the art. Curr Transplant Rep 2018;5:104–10.

Extracorporeal Devices

Prem A. Kandiah, MD[a,b], Ram M. Subramanian, MD[c],*

KEYWORDS

- Extracorporeal liver support • Acute liver failure • ALF
- Acute-on-chronic liver failure • ACLF • Bioartificial liver support

KEY POINTS

- Extracorporeal liver support (ECLS) systems support detoxification and synthetic functions of the failing liver.
- The Molecular Adsorbents Recirculating System (MARS) and the Prometheus device are artificial ECLS albumin dialysis systems that have demonstrated detoxification capabilities and biochemical improvement in patients with acute liver failure (ALF) and acute-on-chronic liver failure (ACLF) without improvement in mortality.
- The MARS has consistently demonstrated improvement in grade of hepatic encephalopathy in ACLF.
- Bioartificial ECLS (B-ECLS) systems incorporate a bioreactor containing various forms of hepatocytes to provide synthetic functions in addition to detoxification. There is insufficient evidence to support the clinical use of B-ECLS at this time.
- High-volume plasmapheresis is the only therapy that has demonstrated a statistically significant benefit in transplant-free survival in ALF patients.

INTRODUCTION

Extracorporeal liver support (ECLS) emerged from the need to hemodynamically and biochemically stabilize the higher acuity liver failure patients who have the highest risk of death (**Tables 1–4**). The goal of ECLS in these patients is to optimize the hemodynamic, neurologic, and biochemical parameters in preparation for transplantation, or to facilitate spontaneous recovery in a small subset of patients. In liver failure, patient populations that stand to benefit the most from this therapy can be allotted into 2 main syndromes: (1) acute liver failure (ALF) and (2) acute-on-chronic liver failure (ACLF). In

Disclosure Statement: The authors have no disclosures.
[a] Division of Neuro Critical Care & co appt. in 5E Surgical/Transplant Critical Care, Department of Neurosurgery, Emory University Hospital, 1364 Clifton Road Northeast, 2nd Floor, 2D ICU-D264, Atlanta, GA 30322, USA; [b] Department of Neurology, Emory University Hospital, 1364 Clifton Road Northeast, 2nd Floor, 2D ICU- D264, Atlanta, GA 30322, USA; [c] Critical Care and Hepatology, Emory University, 1364 Clifton Road Northeast, 2nd Floor, 2D ICU- D264, Atlanta, GA 30322, USA
* Corresponding author.
E-mail address: RMSUBRA@emory.edu

Table 1
Comparison of apparatus and components of artificial extracorporeal liver dialysis devices

ECLS Features	Albumin Dialysis		Plasma Adsorption		
	SPAD	MARS	Prometheus	HVPE	HFCHDF
Albumin source	Exogenous with large volume albumin	Exogenous and albumin-sparing	Endogenous and albumin-sparing	Exogenous low albumin content in FFP	NA
Dialytic circuit and filter	1 circuit, 1 filter 1. Standard dialysis filter	2 circuits, 2 filters 1. Standard dialysis filter 2. MARS FLUX 2.1 (Baxter Inc, Deerfield, IL)	2 circuit, 2 filters 1. Fresenius Polysulfone (Fresenius Medical, Waltham, MA) high-flux dialyzer 2. Standard dialysis filter	NA	2 circuits 1. High-flow hemodialysis 2. HVPE (optional)
Separation method	Standard CRRT filter	Albumin-impregnated high-flux dialysis membrane, MARS FLUX 2.1 Sieving coefficients for albumin <0.001	Albumin filter (AlbuFlow AF 01 [Fresenius Medical, Waltham, MA]), Sieving coefficient of albumin is 0.6	Centrifugal plasma exchange or membrane plasma separation	PMM filter
Filter cut off	60 kDa	50 kDa	250 kDa	NA for centrifuge 1000 kDa for filter	70 kDa
Dialysate or substitution fluid	4.4% albumin	1. 20% human albumin dialysate (600 mL) 2. Standard CRRT dialysate	1. Standard renal dialysate	FFP	Standard dialysate ± FFP
Adsorber columns	NA	1. Vapor-activated carbon adsorber 2. Ion-exchanger resin adsorber	1. Neutral resin adsorber 2. Anion exchange adsorber	NA	PMM filter (cytokine-adsorbing)

Abbreviations: FFP, fresh frozen plasma; HFCHDF, high-flow dialysate continuous hemodiafiltration; HVPE, high-volume plasma exchange; NA, not assessed; PMM, polymethyl methacrylate; SPAD, single-pass albumin dialysis.

Table 2
Pertinent studies on artificial extracorporeal liver support and respective outcomes in acute-on-chronic liver failure

ACLF Study	Number of Subjects	Device	Biochemical Improvement	Decreased Plasma Cytokine Levels	Improved Hemodynamics	Improved HE Grade	Survival
Mitzner et al,[32] 2000	13	MARS	Yes	No	Yes	No	Yes (37.5% vs 0% at 7 d)
Heemann et al,[25] 2002	23	MARS	Yes	No	Yes	Yes	Yes (92% vs 55% at 30 d)
Sen et al,[55] 2004	18	MARS	Yes	No	No	Yes	No (45% in both)
Krisper et al,[56] 2005	8	MARS vs Prometheus	Yes MARS Yes[a] Prometheus	No	NA	NA	NA
Laleman et al,[30] 2006	18	MARS or Prometheus	Yes	No	No Prometheus Yes MARS	NA	NA
Hassanein et al,[24] 2007	70	MARS	Yes	No	NA	Yes	NA
Kribben et al,[27] 2012	143	Prometheus	Yes	No	NA	-	No effect on 28/90 d survival[b]
Banares et al,[26] 2013 (RELIEF)	189	MARS	Yes	No	NA	Yes	No effect on 28 d survival

Biochemical improvements: statistically significant reduction in bilirubin, bile acids, creatinine, and ammonia.

[a] Enhanced clearance of unconjugated bilirubin and cholic acid (bile acid).

[b] Patients may have had acute liver injury (ischemic hepatitis) and not ALF.

Modified from Karvellas CJ, Subramanian RM. Current evidence for extracorporeal liver support systems in acute liver failure and acute-on-chronic liver failure. Crit Care Clin 2016;32(3):439–51; with permission.

Table 3
Pertinent studies and on artificial extracorporeal liver support in and respective outcomes in acute liver failure

ALF Study	Number of Subjects	Device	Biochemical Improvement	Decreased Plasma Cytokine Levels	Improved Hemodynamics	Reduction in Intracranial Pressure or Coma	Survival
Schmidt et al,[57] 2003	13	MARS	Yes	No	Yes	NA	No
El Banayosy et al,[18] 2004	27	MARS	No	No	NA	NA	Yes (50% vs 32%)[a]
Yokoi et al,[47] 2009	90	HFCHDF vs plasmapheresis	Yes	Yes	NA	Yes	NA
Bergis et al,[29] 2012	20	Prometheus	Yes[b]	NA	NA	NA	NA
Saliba et al,[12] 2013	102	MARS	Yes	No	NA	NA	No effect on survival
Larsen et al,[42] 2016	182	HVP	Yes	Yes	NA	No	Yes
Komardina et al,[28] 2017[c]	39	Prometheus	Yes	NA	Yes	NA	NA

Biochemical improvements: statistically significant reduction in bilirubin, bile acids, creatinine, and ammonia.
[a] Patients with a MELD score greater than 30 (n = 48, 24 subjects in each group) treated with Prometheus had better survival compared with that of subjects treated with SMT only (28-d survival probability: 57% vs 42%, respectively; 90-d survival probability: 48% vs 9%, respectively; log-rank test, $P = .02$).
[b] Evaluating Prometheus in *Amanita phalloides* poisoning versus historical controls. Significant reduction in urinary amanitin level before and after therapy.
[c] Postcardiac surgery patients with ischemic hepatitis.
Modified from Karvellas CJ, Subramanian RM. Current evidence for extracorporeal liver support systems in acute liver failure and acute-on-chronic liver failure. Crit Care Clin 2016;32(3):439–51; with permission.

Table 4
Clinical studies in acute liver failure and acute-on-chronic liver failure using bioartificial extracorporeal liver support

Study	Number of Subjects	Device	Cell Type	Cell Quantity	Survival
ALF					
Ellis et al,[51] 1996 • Small RCT	24	ELAD	Human hepatoblastoma-derived HepG2/C3A (cultured)	800 g (50 billion cells) 4 hollow-fiber cartridges of 200 mg of cells	No difference in low or high risk
Demetriou et al,[53] 2004 • RCT	171	HepatAssist	Porcine (cryopreserved)	100 g (7 billion) 1 hollow-fiber cartridge 100g	No difference 30-d survival 71%vs 62% P = .26
Mazariegos et al,[10] 2001 • Phase 1	4	BLSS	Porcine (cryopreserved)	100 g (7 billion) 1 hollow-fiber cartridge 100g	Safe
Van de Kerkhove et al,[8] 2002 • Phase 1	7	AMC-BAL	Porcine (cryopreserved)	10 billion in nonwoven polyester matrix	Bridged 6 out of 7 to LT 1 transplant-free survival. PERV DNA detected[a]
Sauer et al,[7] 2003 • Phase 1	8	MELS (hybrid)	Porcine (cryopreserved)	18–44 billion in multilaminated hollow-fiber bundles	Safe Bridged 8 out of 8 to LT Alive at 3 y
ACLF					
Thompson et al,[52] 2018 • RCT	203	ELAD	Human hepatoblastoma-derived HepG2/C3A (cultured)	800 g (50 billion cells) 4 hollow-fiber cartridges of 200 mg of cells	No difference 90-d overall survival (51.0% vs 49.5%, P = .9)

Abbreviations: LT, liver transplant; PERV, porcine endogenous retroviral DNA.

[a] PERV detected in patient's plasma immediately after treatment attributable to porcine liver cell lysis. PERV DNA cleared within 2 weeks post-treatment and no PERV RNA was subsequently detected. Porcine hepatocyte cell line has since been replaced with a human hepatoma cell line (HepaRG).

ALF and ACLF, circulating toxins, multiorgan failure, and hemodynamic instability generate an unfavorable environment for hepatic regeneration and reduce the probability of survival to transplant when hepatic regeneration is improbable.

CRITICAL CARE RATIONAL FOR EXTRACORPOREAL LIVER SUPPORT DEVICES
Hepatic Encephalopathy and Intracranial Hypertension

Hepatic encephalopathy (HE), cerebral edema, intracranial hypertension (IH), and brain herniation in ALF remain major challenges despite the reported reduction in associated mortality from 80% to 20%.[1] The risk of using intracranial monitoring devices is not benign. The associated intracranial hemorrhage rate approaches 10%. Inflammatory cytokines, ammonia, aromatic amino acids, and endogenous benzodiazepines have been implicated in HE. Inflammation, blood-brain-barrier breakdown, and cerebral hyperemia play major roles in the development of cerebral edema and IH, specifically in ALF. ECLS is designed to mitigate these insults has the potential to be neuroprotective.

Common to both ALF and ACLF, pretransplant encephalopathy is shown to correlate with posttransplant encephalopathy and neurologic dysfunction.[2,3] The obtunded transplant recipient needs to overcome delirium, deconditioning, generalized weakness, respiratory muscle weakness, dependence on artificial respiration, risk of aspiration, and infection to thrive during the posttransplant period. ECLS that can prevent high grades of HE would potentially improve recovery and functional status in the posttransplant period. This, in turn, could decrease the duration of ventilatory support and reduce intensive care unit length-of-stay.

Hemodynamic Instability

Although mortality from IH in ALF has declined, most deaths in ALF and ACLF are attributable to shock. The dominant physiology of shock in liver failure is distributive in nature. Increased nitric oxide production, overwhelming production of inflammatory cytokines, and infection have been implicated as the main contributors of circulatory failure. Distributive shock in ALF and ACLF can be refractory to current vasopressors and frequently leads to further end-organ damage.

End-Organ Damage

Other end-organ damage in ALF and ACLF includes acute kidney injury, adrenal insufficiency, disseminated intravascular coagulation, immune dysregulation, and respiratory failure with acute respiratory distress syndrome (ARDS). Heterogeneous effects of proinflammatory cytokines and damage-associated molecular proteins include increased capillary permeability, vasodilatory shock, modulating cell death, and immune dysregulation.[4] An ECLS device with the capacity to decrease the inflammatory response during critical periods may be effective in averting end-organ damage.

Bridge-to-Transplant and Spontaneous Recovery

Transplant teams are preferential to candidates who are most likely to survive and thrive after a liver transplant, and are deterred by candidates with refractory distributive shock, IH, and other severe end-organ damage. ECLS stands to improve candidacy of a patient for liver transplantation by reversing or preventing these problems. Especially true for acetaminophen toxicity, the liver possesses the unique capacity to regenerate when not besieged by complete fibrosis. ECLS may also create a more suitable metabolic environment to facilitate liver regeneration, which may, in turn, improve transplant-free survival.

EXTRACORPOREAL LIVER SUPPORT SYSTEMS

Primary functions of the liver include detoxification of circulating endogenous and exogenous substances, manufacturing circulating proteins, secreting bile, and storing energy as glycogen. ECLS systems are designed to mimic some of these functions and can be classified into 2 broad functional categories:

1. Artificial ECLS (A-ECLS)
2. Bioartificial ECLS (B-ECLS).

A-ECLS systems are designed primarily to replace some of the detoxification functions of the native liver through principles of adsorption and filtration. Types of adsorbent columns and filters, as well as varying filter pore sizes, determine the detoxification capacity of the device. Although conventional hemodialysis or continuous renal replacement therapies are efficient at removal of ammonia, neither eliminates protein-bound toxins. To overcome this problem, A-ECLS exploits the physiology of either endogenous or exogenous albumin as a toxin-binding and scavenging molecule. In addition to removing protein-bound toxin, albumin administration has been shown to be beneficial in spontaneous bacterial peritonitis and hepatorenal syndrome. Four existing A-ECLS systems include

1. The Molecular Adsorbent Recirculating System, trade name MARS (Teraklin AG, Rostock, Germany)
2. The fractionated plasma separation and adsorption device, trade name Prometheus (Fresenius, Hamburg, Germany)
3. Single-pass albumin dialysis (SPAD)
4. High-volume plasma exchange (HVPE)
5. Standard and advanced dialytic renal replacement modes.

B-ECLS systems are hybrid devices designed to perform detoxification and synthetic function using a platform containing artificial hepatocyte cell lines. Currently used cell lines include immortalized human hepatocytes and porcine hepatocytes. Only 2 devices have been studied extensively in humans. Owing to the level of complexity in B-ECLS devices, the logistics of deploying,[5] training, and cost remain major hurdles. B-ECLS devices include

1. Devices with phase II or III studies in humans (not US Food and Drug Administration [FDA] approved)
   • The HepatAssist device, with porcine hepatocytes
   • The ELAD system, with human hepatoblastoma C3A hepatocyte cell line
2. Devices with phase 1 studies in humans (Not FDA approved)
   • Modular ECLS (MELS)[6,7]
   • Amsterdam Medical Center Bioartificial Liver (AMC-BAL)[8]
   • Bioartificial Liver Support System (BLSS).[9,10]

Artificial Extracorporeal Liver Support Devices

MARS: molecular adsorbent recirculating system

The MARS device, developed in 1993, consists of a blood circuit, an albumin circuit, and a renal circuit.[11] The MARS device functions by removing circulating toxins using an albumin-impregnated membrane with adsorbent columns and a recirculating albumin dialysate in series with a continuous renal replacement therapy (CRRT) circuit. Blood is dialyzed against 20% human albumin dialysate across the high-flux dialysis membrane. Then the albumin dialysate is purified as it traverses the 2 sequential adsorbent columns containing activated charcoal and anion exchange resin to remove water-soluble and albumin-bound toxins. Hormones and albumin-bound substances greater than 50 kDa are not removed by the filter membrane. The MARS device does not replace critical aspects of hepatic function such as synthesis of liver-derived proteins or clotting factors, metabolism, or immunologic functions of the liver.

MARS in acute liver failure Several randomized controlled studies (RCTs) have failed to demonstrate mortality reduction associated with MARS therapy in ALF. FULMAR,[12] the largest of studies, demonstrated a nonsignificant difference between the MARS plus standard medical therapy (SMT) versus SMT alone. However, results of this negative study remain difficult to interpret given that, of the 68 subjects who underwent liver transplantation, 75% were transplanted in less than 24 hours. The median listing-to-transplant time was only 16.2 hours. Moreover, 26% of subjects in the MARS group did not complete at least 5 hours of MARS therapy before liver transplant or death. The impact of the MARS on mortality was inadequately assessed given the short duration of intervention in the treatment arm. This study was also underpowered to evaluate transplant-free survival in subjects with acetaminophen overdose. Four subsequent metaanalyses[13–16] have reported opposing conclusions.

A closer look at surrogate markers of clinical improvement reveals some encouraging findings. Schmidt and colleagues[17] conducted a study to assess the effects of a single 6-hour MARS treatment on hemodynamics, oxygen consumption, and biochemical profile in 13 ALF subjects (acetaminophen [APAP], $n = 10$) with HE grade III or IV. Eight subjects received MARS therapy and 5 received SMT. The systemic vascular resistance index increased significantly by 46% in the MARS group during the 6-hour run treatment versus a 6% increase in the controls. Increase in the mean arterial pressure (MAP) was observed in the MARS group, whereas the MAP was unchanged in controls. A significant reduction in bilirubin and creatinine has clearly been demonstrated by the MARS in 2 ALF studies.[18,19] The MARS device may continue to have a role in bridging ALF patients to transplantation and recovery. The contribution of the MARS compared with CRRT for toxin clearance in vivo remains equivocal. Ammonia, blood urea nitrogen, and creatinine are freely cleared by CRRT. The contribution from the MARS device may focus on improving HE; clearing copper, bilirubin, and bile salts; and augmenting hemodynamic stability. Beyond ammonia, there are numerous neurotoxic or neuroactive substances that contribute to HE, such as mercaptans, inflammation, false neurotransmitters and benzodiazepines, manganese, aromatic amino acids, phenols, and short-chain fatty acids. Many of these substances are difficult to detect and study but may provide an explanation for the improvement in the grade of HE observed in subjects receiving MARS treatment.

MARS in fulminant Wilson disease The fatality rate of acute decompensated Wilson disease (WD) approaches 90% if transplantation cannot be performed in time.[20,21] Considerable copper is released from the necrotic hepatocytes. In small studies of this rare disease, the MARS device was shown to reduce excess copper in acute decompensated WD.[22] In a recent study, analysis of the albumin dialysate circuit in 1 subject revealed that copper removal through the MARS occurred mainly in the first few hours, through adsorption by albumin and by the MARS flux membrane, with no substantial removal by the albumin regeneration process.[23] Significant reduction in serum copper level was observed after each MARS session.

MARS in acute-on-chronic liver failure Two small MARS studies reported significant improvement in mortality and reduction of bilirubin and creatinine in subjects with ACLF.[24,25] In subjects with ACLF and type 1 hepatorenal syndrome, Mitzer and colleagues reported a 37.5% absolute survival benefit at day 7 versus 0% in controls. Heemann and colleagues[25] evaluated 30-day survival in ACLF subjects with hyperbilirubinemia, grade greater than or equal to 2 HE, and acute kidney injury. Thirty-day mortality was 92% in the MARS group versus 55% in controls. A significant improvement in the MAP, reduction in bile acid, and reduction of HE grade was noted in the MARS group.[26]

Two subsequent larger studies were designed to evaluate efficacy of the MARS on HE.[24,26] Hassanein and colleagues, randomized 70 ACLF subjects to the MARS or SMT to evaluate the efficacy of the MARS device in treating HE. The study was not powered to assess mortality. The MARS group received 6 hours of therapy daily for 5 days or until a 2-grade improvement in HE. With a comparable acuity of illness in both groups, a 2-grade improvement in HE was achieved in 34% of the MARS group compared with 19% in the SMT group.

The RELIEF study on the therapeutic impact of albumin dialysis with the MARS randomized subjects to the MARS device plus SMT or SMT alone.[26] The RELIEF study demonstrated a reduction in HE in the MARS device plus SMT arm compared with SMT-alone arm. No difference in 28-day survival or adverse events was observed between groups.

Prometheus: fractionated plasma separation and adsorption

Prometheus in acute-on-chronic liver failure In comparison with the 50 kDa filter in the MARS, the Prometheus device uses as a 250 kDa albumin-permeable filter to fractionate plasma. Albumin and other proteins that traverse the filter membrane are purified in tandem through an anion-exchange column and a neutral resin adsorber. The purified plasma is returned to the blood in circuit, which subsequently undergoes conventional high-flux hemodialysis before returning to the patient.

The HELIOS study group published a prospective randomized study involving 145 ACLF subjects randomly assigned to receive either the Prometheus device plus SMT or SMT alone.[27] The primary endpoint of the study was survival at day 28 and day 90 irrespective of liver transplant. Serum bilirubin levels decreased significantly in the Prometheus group but not with the SMT-alone group. There was no statistically significant survival benefit for subjects undergoing fractionated plasma separation and adsorption therapy at either 28 days or 30 days. However, in subjects with hepatorenal syndrome (type I) or a model for end stage liver disease (MELD) score greater than 30, the Prometheus device showed a significant survival benefit in a predefined subgroup analysis.

Prometheus in acute liver failure There are no RCTs and only a few small retrospective studies evaluating the Prometheus device in ALF. The largest of these is a recent uncontrolled single-center retrospective study in subjects with ischemic ALF after cardiac surgery with cardiopulmonary bypass[28] that demonstrated statistically significant stabilization of hemodynamics whereby the MAP increased by 13%.

Bergis and colleagues[29] evaluated the Prometheus device in 20 subjects with *Amanita phalloides* intoxication. Nine consecutive subjects were treated with SMT plus 6 hours of Prometheus therapy and were compared with matched historical controls. Mean urinary amanitin levels were significantly reduced by the Prometheus device, with 42.5 ng/mL before and 1.2 ng/mL after treatment. No hemodynamic, respiratory, or hematological complications were observed. None of the subjects had to undergo liver transplantation. All subjects in the treatment group survived and were discharged fully recovered. One subject in the control group died due to shock and lactic acidosis, and 1 subject remained dialysis-dependent. Mean duration of hospital stay was 7.1 days in the treatment group and 11.7 days in the control group.

MARS versus Prometheus In a small study, subjects with biopsy-proven alcoholic cirrhosis and superimposed alcoholic hepatitis were either treated with SMT plus the MARS or the Prometheus device, or were treated with SMT alone, on 3 consecutive days in 6-hour sessions.[30] Although both the MARS and the Prometheus device demonstrated a reduction in bilirubin levels, the Prometheus device proved more effective than the MARS device in this function. Only the MARS, however, showed significant improvement in MAP and systemic vascular resistance. The hemodynamic improvements in the MARS group accompanied by a decrease in plasma renin activity, aldosterone, norepinephrine ($P<.05$), vasopressin, and nitrate or nitrite levels was not observed in the Prometheus group.

The Prometheus device seems to provide a better in vivo clearance of protein-bound substances compared with the MARS device, evidenced by its ability to more efficiently clear unconjugated bilirubin.[31] The Prometheus device has thus far not demonstrated improvement in hemodynamics or HE, which are important benchmarks in the management of patients with liver failure. Although the RELIEF study did not investigate hemodynamics as an endpoint, 2 smaller studies demonstrated improvement in blood pressure.[25,32] The exact mechanism driving the improvement in hemodynamics by the MARS device remains unknown. The RELIEF study demonstrated that cytokine levels were not effectively cleared by the MARS device, making modulation of inflammation an unlikely mechanism. A theory that the MARS device clears nitric oxide or its intermediary metabolites that are hemodynamically active has been postulated; however, this is difficult to confirm experimentally due to the complex metabolism and short half-life of nitric oxide.

Neither device thus far has shown a mortality benefit. Both devices are predicated on albumin-binding. ACLF patients, however, have significantly lower albumin levels and decreased functional quality of albumin.[33] Reliance on decreased quality and quantity of albumin may impede the detoxification capacity of both devices.

Single-pass albumin dialysis

Unlike the MARS or Prometheus device, SPAD uses a standard CRRT system without any additional columns or circuits. Standard CRRT dialysate is replaced with a 4.4% albumin dialysate. SPAD has been evaluated in a case-control fashion in APAP-ALF but failed to demonstrate mortality improvements.[34] A small crossover RCT study compared SPAD versus the MARS device in 32 subjects using 69 crossovers.[35] The systems significantly reduced plasma bilirubin levels to a similar extent. Only the MARS device, however, reduced plasma bile acids, creatinine, and urea levels while simultaneously increasing the albumin-binding capacity. Cytokine levels of interleukin (IL)-6 and IL-8 and HE were not altered by the MARS device or SPAD. During SPAD treatment, higher rates of metabolic derangement (increase in pH, base excess, and lactate values), and electrolyte disturbances (decreasing calcium levels and increasing sodium levels) were noted.

High-volume plasmapheresis in acute liver failure

Lepore and Martel[36] first reported their experience plasmapheresis in 5 subjects with hepatic coma in 1970. Since then, plasmapheresis has been widely used, especially in Japan, for managing ALF.[37] In Japan, artificial liver support with plasmapheresis and/or hemodiafiltration is used in almost 90% of ALF subjects, in part driven by previously restricted practices in organ donation. Plasmapheresis with albumin or fresh frozen plasma (FFP) is an established therapy for immunologically driven disorders, with FFP being used predominantly in thrombotic thrombocytopenia or preexisting coagulopathy. The predominant method used for plasmapheresis in the United States is centrifugation, although there are apheresis devices that rely on filters for separation. In these apheresis devices, whole blood is pumped into a rapidly rotating separation chamber. Components separate into layers based on their density, with the densest element consisting of cells. The least dense layer, the plasma layer, is removed and discarded. The remaining cellular elements are mixed with a replacement fluid of albumin or FFP and returned to the patient. Standard plasmapheresis requires an exchange of 1 to 1.5 plasma volume, which clears the blood of approximately 60% to 70% of substances present in plasma. In ALF, HVPE with FFP has been evaluated in multiple case series and has been demonstrated to be safe, to decrease severity of HE, and to decrease vasopressor requirements.[38–41]

Recently, the first A-ECLS study in ALF demonstrated a statistically significant benefit to transplant-free survival.[42] The cause of ALF in most subjects in this study was acetaminophen toxicity. Between 1998 and 2010, 183 ALF subjects in 3 European centers were randomized to receive HVPE versus SMT. Subjects were recruited into the study within 24 hours of developing grade II HE. Volume exchanged in HVPE was defined as 15% ideal body weight (8–12 L FFP) with individual runs lasting approximately 9 hours per treatment. Subjects in the study received a mean of 2.4 exchanges (23 L per treated subject). In an intention-to-treat analysis, survival to hospital discharge was 58.7% for subjects treated with HVPE vs 47.8% for the subjects who received SMT alone. Biochemical markers, including international normalized ratio, bilirubin, and ammonia, improved significantly in the HVPE group compared with controls. No statistically significant difference in adverse events, including cardiac arrhythmia, pancreatitis, worsening gas exchange, ARDS, transfusion-related acute lung injury, culture positive infection, or hemorrhage, were noted in either group.

Standard and advanced dialytic renal replacement modes

Continuous renal replacement therapy Debatably, CRRT may be single most important intervention that has serendipitously contributed to the improved outcomes in patients with ALF over the last 2 decades.[1,43] CRRT is a form of extracorporeal renal support that is the standard of care in most liver transplant centers. Continuous venovenous hemofiltration with high filtration volume (90 mL/kg/h) is an effective method for rapidly lowering serum plasma ammonia levels.[44,45] Ammonia clearance, in turn, is closely associated with the ultrafiltration rate.

High-flow dialysate continuous hemodiafiltration with cytokine-adsorbing hemofilter With the established use of plasmapheresis in Japan, concerns of looming cost and side effects associated with large doses of FFP sparked an innovative approach to FFP-sparing dialytic modes. In 1996, a team at Chiba University in Japan trialed the use of high-flow dialysate continuous hemodiafiltration (HFCHDF) to enhance reversal of hepatic coma in subjects with ALF.[46] In a study involving 90 subjects, Yokoi and colleagues[47] reported that the rate of recovery from coma was significantly higher in the HFCHDF group (70.2%) than in the non-HFCHDF group (44.2%). The non-HFCHDF group received either plasma exchange alone or slow plasma exchange in addition to standard continuous hemodiafiltration. HFCHDF allows for a dialysate flow rate approaching 500 mL per minute and blood flow of 250 mL per minute, far exceeding what is capable by CRRT.[48] Subsequent modifications include the use of a polymethyl methacrylate (PMM) hemofilter membrane and setting the filtration flow rate at 5 to 10 mL per minute to maximize cytokine removal. A PMM hemofilter is used for the management of sepsis in Japan.[49,50] To date, cytokine-adsorbing filters, including PMM, have not been FDA approved for clinical use.

BIOARTIFICIAL EXTRACORPOREAL LIVER SUPPORT IN ACUTE LIVER FAILURE
Extracorporeal Cellular Therapy

The ELAD system uses human hepatoblastoma-derived C3A cells nurtured in a bioreactor to detoxify and provide synthetic liver in an extracorporeal circuit. The 2 existing ELAD system studies have yielded negative outcomes. First, a small study in ALF randomizing subjects to the ELAD system plus SMT versus SMT alone failed to demonstrate an outcome difference.[51]

Thompson and colleagues[52] evaluated the ELAD system in a study population of severe alcoholic hepatitis in an international multicenter RCT. Subjects were randomized to receive either SMT or 3 to 5 days of continuous ELAD system treatment plus SMT. In the intention-to-treat analysis, there was no difference in 90-day overall survival. In the prespecified analysis of subjects with MELD, less than 28% ($n = 120$), the ELAD system was associated with a trend toward higher overall survival at 91 days. A new trial investigating a potential benefit of the ELAD system in younger subjects with sufficient renal function and less severe coagulopathy has just been concluded but the results are not available.

HepatAssist

The HepatAssist is a B-ECLS device that uses 7 billion primary porcine-purified hepatocytes from healthy pig donors housed in a bioreactor and has been evaluated in a large-scale, randomized, multicenter clinical trial. The HepatAssist device was evaluated by Demetriou and colleagues[53] in subjects with ALF or with primary nonfunction after liver transplant who were randomized to receive SMT or SMT plus the HepatAssist device. One to 9 HepatAssist device treatments were performed in the intervention group with a mean of 2.9 treatments. No difference in primary endpoint of 30-day survival was reported. At the time of the predetermined interim safety analysis, the trial was prematurely terminated due to futility.

SUMMARY AND CHALLENGES

Artificial liver support devices that rely on endogenous albumin are functionally limited by the quality and quantity of albumin in the patient with liver failure. Although improvement in hemodynamics has been reported, this has not translated to improved outcomes. Serious adverse events were not observed in the larger MARS or Prometheus studies despite concerns of thrombocytopenia and bleeding. Cytokine clearance was not observed with the MARS or Prometheus device, which may explain the limited efficacy of both devices. The consistent finding of improvement in HE and hemodynamics with the MARS device continues drive its utility in clinical practice. In exogenous and endogenous toxidromes, especially pertaining to *A phalloides* poisoning and WD, these devices continue to be very appealing. The development of a process of filtration or an ideal membrane that eliminates cytokines without severely depleting endogenous proteins and coagulation factors remains unattained.

With the encouraging finding by Larsen and colleagues[42] pertaining to HVPE, there is an ongoing shift toward apheresis techniques in management of ALF. Although a high side-effect profile pertaining the exposure to large volumes of FFP was anticipated, this was not evident in the study. Lower volumes of plasma replacement could arguably produce the same desired effects. Consideration of extending the dose and duration of plasmapheresis should be negotiated with caution because immune response is critical to the process of regeneration and preventing infection at later phases of ALF. The use of hybrid devices could leverage the physiologic benefits of multimodal ECLS devices. This concept is already widely practiced with the use of dia-lytic methods either simultaneously or in tandem with HVPE.[48,54]

The heterogeneity in the etiologic factors of liver failure, severity of illness at presen-tation, concomitant infections, and the extent of multiorgan failure collectively renders this patient population exceedingly difficult to study. Although the developments have been slow, mortality in ALF and ACLF has improved over the last 2 decades through the advent of transplantation and the collective critical care interventions deployed. The advancement in ECLS devices will continue to drive the need to understand un-solved facets in the disease process, which will fuel innovation in this arena.

REFERENCES

1. Bernal W, Hyyrylainen A, Gera A, et al. Lessons from look-back in acute liver fail-ure? A single centre experience of 3300 patients. J Hepatol 2013;59(1):74–80.

2. DiMartini A, Chopra K. The importance of hepatic encephalopathy: pre-transplant and post-transplant. Liver Transpl 2009;15(2):121–3.

3. Sotil EU, Gottstein J, Ayala E, et al. Impact of preoperative overt hepatic enceph-alopathy on neurocognitive function after liver transplantation. Liver Transpl 2009; 15(2):184–92.

4. Possamai LA, Thursz MR, Wendon JA, et al. Modulation of monocyte/macro-phage function: a therapeutic strategy in the treatment of acute liver failure. J Hepatol 2014;61(2):439–45.

5. van de Kerkhove MP, Poyck PP, Deurholt T, et al. Liver support therapy: an over-view of the AMC-bioartificial liver research. Dig Surg 2005;22(4):254–64.

6. Sauer IM, Gerlach JC. Modular extracorporeal liver support. Artif Organs 2002; 26(8):703–6.

7. Sauer IM, Kardassis D, Zeillinger K, et al. Clinical extracorporeal hybrid liver sup-port–phase I study with primary porcine liver cells. Xenotransplantation 2003; 10(5):460–9.

8. van de Kerkhove MP, Di Florio E, Scuderi V, et al. Phase I clinical trial with the AMC-bioartificial liver. Int J Artif Organs 2002;25(10):950–9.

9. Patzer IJ, Lopez RC, Zhu Y, et al. Bioartificial liver assist devices in support of pa-tients with liver failure. Hepatobiliary Pancreat Dis Int 2002;1(1):18–25.

10. Mazariegos GV, Kramer DJ, Lopez RC, et al. Safety observations in phase I clin-ical evaluation of the Excorp Medical Bioartificial Liver Support System after the first four patients. ASAIO J 2001;47(5):471–5.

11. Stange J, Mitzner S, Ramlow W, et al. A new procedure for the removal of protein bound drugs and toxins. ASAIO J 1993;39(3):M621–5.

12. Saliba F, Camus C, Durand F, et al. Albumin dialysis with a noncell artificial liver support device in patients with acute liver failure: a randomized, controlled trial. Ann Intern Med 2013;159(8):522–31.

13. Stutchfield BM, Simpson K, Wigmore SJ. Systematic review and meta-analysis of survival following extracorporeal liver support. Br J Surg 2011;98(5):623–31.

14. He GL, Feng L, Duan CY, et al. Meta-analysis of survival with the molecular adsor-bent recirculating system for liver failure. Int J Clin Exp Med 2015;8(10): 17046–54.

15. Vaid A, Chweich H, Balk EM, et al. Molecular adsorbent recirculating system as artificial support therapy for liver failure: a meta-analysis. ASAIO J 2012;58(1): 51–9.

16. Khuroo MS, Khuroo MS, Farahat KL. Molecular adsorbent recirculating system for acute and acute-on-chronic liver failure: a meta-analysis. Liver Transpl 2004; 10(9):1099–106.

17. Schmidt LE, Tofteng F, Strauss GI, et al. Effect of treatment with the molecular adsorbents recirculating system on arterial amino acid levels and cerebral amino acid metabolism in patients with hepatic encephalopathy. Scand J Gastroenterol 2004;39(10):974–80.

18. El Banayosy A, Kizner L, Schueler V, et al. First use of the molecular adsorbent recirculating system technique on patients with hypoxic liver failure after cardiogenic shock. ASAIO J 2004;50(4):332–7.

19. Hanish SI, Stein DM, Scalea JR, et al. Molecular adsorbent recirculating system effectively replaces hepatic function in severe acute liver failure. Ann Surg 2017; 266(4):677–84.

20. Schilsky ML. Wilson disease: current status and the future. Biochimie 2009; 91(10):1278–81.

21. Walshe JM, Dixon AK. Dangers of non-compliance in Wilson's disease. Lancet 1986;1(8485):845–7.

22. Sen S, Felldin M, Steiner C, et al. Albumin dialysis and Molecular Adsorbents Recirculating System (MARS) for acute Wilson's disease. Liver Transpl 2002;8(10): 962–7.

23. Rustom N, Bost M, Cour-Andlauer F, et al. Effect of molecular adsorbents recirculating system treatment in children with acute liver failure caused by Wilson disease. J Pediatr Gastroenterol Nutr 2014;58(2):160–4.

24. Hassanein TI, Tofteng F, Brown RS Jr, et al. Randomized controlled study of extracorporeal albumin dialysis for hepatic encephalopathy in advanced cirrhosis. Hepatology 2007;46(6):1853–62.

25. Heemann U, Treichel U, Loock J, et al. Albumin dialysis in cirrhosis with superimposed acute liver injury: a prospective, controlled study. Hepatology 2002;36(4 Pt 1):949–58.

26. Banares R, Nevens F, Larsen FS, et al. Extracorporeal albumin dialysis with the molecular adsorbent recirculating system in acute-on-chronic liver failure: the RELIEF trial. Hepatology 2013;57(3):1153–62.

27. Kribben A, Gerken G, Haag S, et al. Effects of fractionated plasma separation and adsorption on survival in patients with acute-on-chronic liver failure. Gastroenterology 2012;142(4):782–9.e3.

28. Komardina E, Yaroustovsky M, Abramyan M, et al. Prometheus therapy for the treatment of acute liver failure in patients after cardiac surgery. Kardiochir Torakochirurgia Pol 2017;14(4):230–5.

29. Bergis D, Friedrich-Rust M, Zeuzem S, et al. Treatment of *Amanita phalloides* intoxication by fractionated plasma separation and adsorption (Prometheus(R)). J Gastrointestin Liver Dis 2012;21(2):171–6.

30. Laleman W, Wilmer A, Evenepoel P, et al. Effect of the molecular adsorbent recirculating system and Prometheus devices on systemic haemodynamics and vasoactive agents in patients with acute-on-chronic alcoholic liver failure. Crit Care 2006;10(4):R108.

31. Evenepoel P, Laleman W, Wilmer A, et al. Prometheus versus molecular adsorbents recirculating system: comparison of efficiency in two different liver detoxification devices. Artif Organs 2006;30(4):276–84.

32. Mitzner SR, Stange J, Klammt S, et al. Improvement of hepatorenal syndrome with extracorporeal albumin dialysis MARS: results of a prospective, randomized, controlled clinical trial. Liver Transpl 2000;6(3):277–86.

33. Jalan R, Schnurr K, Mookerjee RP, et al. Alterations in the functional capacity of albumin in patients with decompensated cirrhosis is associated with increased mortality. Hepatology 2009;50(2):555–64.
34. Karvellas CJ, Bagshaw SM, McDermid RC, et al. A case-control study of single-pass albumin dialysis for acetaminophen-induced acute liver failure. Blood Purif 2009;28(3):151–8.
35. Sponholz C, Matthes K, Rupp D, et al. Molecular adsorbent recirculating system and single-pass albumin dialysis in liver failure–a prospective, randomised cross-over study. Crit Care 2016;20:2.
36. Lepore MJ, Martel AJ. Plasmapheresis with plasma exchange in hepatic coma. Methods and results in five patients with acute fulminant hepatic necrosis. Ann Intern Med 1970;72(2):165–74.
37. Fujiwara K, Mochida S, Matsui A, et al, Intractable Liver Diseases Study Group of Japan. Fulminant hepatitis and late onset hepatic failure in Japan. Hepatol Res 2008;38(7):646–57.
38. Kondrup J, Almdal T, Vilstrup H, et al. High volume plasma exchange in fulminant hepatic failure. Int J Artif Organs 1992;15(11):669–76.
39. Nakamura T, Ushiyama C, Suzuki S, et al. Effect of plasma exchange on serum tissue inhibitor of metalloproteinase 1 and cytokine concentrations in patients with fulminant hepatitis. Blood Purif 2000;18(1):50–4.
40. Larsen FS, Ejlersen E, Hansen BA, et al. Systemic vascular resistance during high-volume plasmapheresis in patients with fulminant hepatic failure: relationship with oxygen consumption. Eur J Gastroenterol Hepatol 1995;7(9):887–92.
41. Larsen FS, Hansen BA, Ejlersen E, et al. Cerebral blood flow, oxygen metabolism and transcranial Doppler sonography during high-volume plasmapheresis in fulminant hepatic failure. Eur J Gastroenterol Hepatol 1996;8(3):261–5.
42. Larsen FS, Schmidt LE, Bernsmeier C, et al. High-volume plasma exchange in patients with acute liver failure: an open randomised controlled trial. J Hepatol 2016;64(1):69–78.
43. Cardoso FS, Gottfried M, Tujios S, et al. Continuous renal replacement therapy is associated with reduced serum ammonia levels and mortality in acute liver failure. Hepatology 2017. [Epub ahead of print].
44. Slack AJ, Auzinger G, Willars C, et al. Ammonia clearance with haemofiltration in adults with liver disease. Liver Int 2014;34(1):42–8.
45. Cordoba J, Blei AT, Mujais S. Determinants of ammonia clearance by hemodialysis. Artif Organs 1996;20(7):800–3.
46. Nitta M, Hirasawa H, Oda S, et al. Long-term survivors with artificial liver support in fulminant hepatic failure. Ther Apher 2002;6(3):208–12.
47. Yokoi T, Oda S, Shiga H, et al. Efficacy of high-flow dialysate continuous hemodiafiltration in the treatment of fulminant hepatic failure. Transfus Apher Sci 2009;40(1):61–70.
48. Shinozaki K, Oda S, Abe R, et al. Blood purification in fulminant hepatic failure. Contrib Nephrol 2010;166:64–72.
49. Hirasawa H, Oda S, Matsuda K. Continuous hemodiafiltration with cytokine-adsorbing hemofilter in the treatment of severe sepsis and septic shock. Contrib Nephrol 2007;156:365–70.
50. Nakada TA, Oda S, Matsuda K, et al. Continuous hemodiafiltration with PMMA Hemofilter in the treatment of patients with septic shock. Mol Med 2008;14(5–6):257–63.
51. Ellis AJ, Hughes RD, Wendon JA, et al. Pilot-controlled trial of the extracorporeal liver assist device in acute liver failure. Hepatology 1996;24(6):1446–51.

52. Thompson J, Jones N, Al-Khafaji A, et al. Extracorporeal cellular therapy (ELAD) in severe alcoholic hepatitis: a multinational, prospective, controlled, randomized trial. Liver Transpl 2018;24(3):380–93.

53. Demetriou AA, Brown RS Jr, Busuttil RW, et al. Prospective, randomized, multi-center, controlled trial of a bioartificial liver in treating acute liver failure. Ann Surg 2004;239(5):660–7 [discussion: 667–70].

54. Akcan Arikan A, Srivaths P, Himes RW, et al. Hybrid extracorporeal therapies as a bridge to pediatric liver transplantation. Pediatr Crit Care Med 2018;19(7): e342–9.

55. Sen S, Davies NA, Mookerjee RP, et al. Pathophysiological effects of albumin dialysis in acute-on-chronic liver failure: a randomized controlled study. Liver transplantation: official publication of the American Association for the Study of Liver Diseases and the International Liver Transplantation Society 2004;10(9):1109–19.

56. Krisper P, Haditsch B, Stauber R, et al. In vivo quantification of liver dialysis: comparison of albumin dialysis and fractionated plasma separation. Journal of hepatology 2005;43(3):451–7.

57. Schmidt LE, Wang LP, Hansen BA, et al. Systemic hemodynamic effects of treatment with the molecular adsorbents recirculating system in patients with hyperacute liver failure: a prospective controlled trial. Liver transplantation: official publication of the American Association for the Study of Liver Diseases and the International Liver Transplantation Society 2003;9(3):290–7.

Infectious Complications Following Solid Organ Transplantation

Alexis Guenette, DO[a], Shahid Husain, MD, MS, FECMM, FRCP[b],*

KEYWORDS

- Infections • Solid organ transplant • Critical care • Intensive care unit (ICU) • Sepsis

KEY POINTS

- Solid organ transplant recipients are a complex group of patients who require a low threshold of suspicion regarding infection, and given their underlying immunosuppression, mortality and morbidity are high.
- Individually they require assessment of their net state of immunosuppression and subsequent thorough evaluation of infectious causes.
- Early diagnosis is key along with appropriate, tailored treatment.

INTRODUCTION

Immunosuppression plays an integral role in solid organ transplant (SOT) recipients because it increases graft survival; however, there are unintended consequences, such as infectious complications. One strategy aimed at assessing the functionality of the immune system consists of non-pathogen-specific immune monitoring, consisting of serum immunoglobulins, serum complement factors, peripheral blood lymphocyte subpopulations, soluble CD30, and iATP in CD4$^+$ T cells.[1] Ideally, these would help to demonstrate one aspect of the overall "net state of immunosuppression." The "net state of immunosuppression" comprises all factors that may contribute to the risk of infection; this includes preexisting immune deficits, colonization with antimicrobial-resistant pathogens, immunosuppressive agents, acquired immunodeficiency, prior antimicrobial therapies, mucocutaneous barrier integrity, fluid collections, neutropenia, lymphopenia, and viral coinfections.[2]

Disclosure Statement: A. Guenette has no relationships with a commercial company that has a direct financial interest in subject matter or materials discussed in article or with a company making a competing product. S. Husain has received grants from Astellas, Pfizer, and Merck.
^a Division of Infectious Disease, University Health Network, University of Toronto, 585 University Avenue, 11 PMB 138, Toronto, Ontario M5G 2N2, Canada; ^b Division of Infectious Disease, Multi-Organ Transplant Program, University Health Network, University of Toronto, 585 University Avenue, 11 PMB 138, Toronto, Ontario M5G 2N2, Canada
* Corresponding author.
E-mail address: Shahid.Husain@uhn.ca

Crit Care Clin 35 (2019) 151–168
https://doi.org/10.1016/j.ccc.2018.08.004
0749-0704/19/© 2018 Elsevier Inc. All rights reserved.

Vaccinations, surgical prophylaxis, universal prophylaxis, preemptive or presymptomatic therapy, targeted prophylaxis, and education avoidance are preventative strategies that have been implemented in SOT recipients. Trimethoprim/sulfamethoxazole prophylaxis is given in most institutions for 3 months to a lifetime to prevent *Pneumocystis* pneumonia along with *Toxoplasma gondii*, *Cyclospora cayetanensis*, and many *Nocardia* and *Listeria* species. Antiviral prophylaxis along with nucleic acid–based assays to prevent cytomegalovirus (CMV) and other herpesvirus infections has also transformed posttransplant care.[2]

Infections in SOT recipients reflect the net balance between the recipient's epidemiologic exposures and immunosuppression.[2] Alterations to the balance can be seen with antimicrobial prophylaxis, immunosuppression, and improved graft survival.[2] This balance is also affected during a period of graft rejection or intensification of immunosuppression (**Fig. 1**).[2] In this article, the authors review infectious syndromes encountered in intensive care units among SOT recipients.

BLOODSTREAM INFECTIONS/SEPSIS

Bloodstream infections (BSIs) are associated with poor outcomes along with being the leading cause of mortality and morbidity in SOT.[3–5] Mortality as high as 24%[4,6,7] has been described, and in fact, once septic shock develops, mortality can reach 50%,[4,8] although Kalil and colleagues[9] demonstrated that there may be a decrease in mortality of transplant patients compared with nontransplant patients. It is thought that SOT recipients do not necessarily clinically behave in the same manner due to underlying immunosuppression, and in fact, tend to present with organ failure and thrombocytopenia during sepsis.[10] Universal risk factors for sepsis, regardless of transplanted organ, are CMV serology mismatch, particularly positive donor to negative recipient, CMV disease, which inherently demonstrates an immunomodulatory effect predisposing recipients to higher rates of bacterial and fungal sepsis, prolonged duration of graft cold ischemia, prolonged duration of surgical transplantation procedure, and requirement of large amounts of blood transfusion.[10,11] Management should consist of rapid initiation of intravenous antibiotics, rapid diagnosis, source control, aggressive search

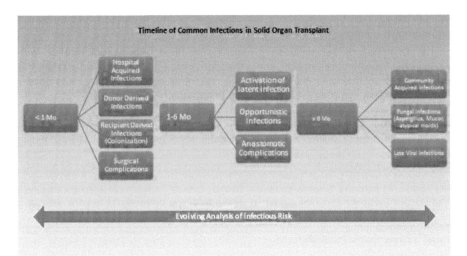

Fig. 1. Timeline of common infections in SOT. (*Adapted from* Fishman JA. From the classic concepts to modern practice. Clin Microbiol Infect 2014;20(suppl 7):4–9; with permission.)

for pathologic condition that mimics severe sepsis, and reduction in immunosuppressive drugs.[10]

Nosocomial BSIs are associated with an even increased risk of septic shock and failure of cure when compared with other BSIs in SOT patients.[3–5,8,12] Gram-positive bacteria are the most frequent source of BSIs and are likely to be associated with intravascular catheters, especially in the nosocomial setting.[3,4] However, with kidney transplant recipients (KTRs), gram-negative bacteria likely related to urinary tract infections (UTIs) are the primary source, regardless of the time period.

The overall incidence of multidrug-resistant organisms (MDRO) is increasing. MDRO gram-negative organisms accounted for about 14% of isolates.[4] Fluconazole-resistant *Candida* spp accounted for up to 46% of cases of candidemia according to Moreno and colleagues.[4,13] Vancomycin-resistant enterococci (VRE) have become an emerging pathogen with studies documenting an incidence of up to 20.5% of nosocomial *Enterococcal* spp BSIs consistent with VRE. These findings along with previous microbiological history and local antibiotic resistance patterns should be considered when determining empiric antimicrobial therapy.

Overall, there are limited studies on infective endocarditis (IE) in sold organ transplant recipients. The incidence of IE in a single center was 1%, with an estimated 171-fold higher incidence as compared with the general population,[14] with an overall mortality up to 57%.[15] There are limited data on the mode of infection and predisposing factors in SOT recipients. Underlying structural abnormalities may not appear to be a risk factor for IE as compared with the general population.[14,15] According to Paterson and colleagues,[15] 50% of infections were due to *Aspergillus fumigatus* or *Staphylococcus aureus*, and 4% were due to viridans streptococci, which is in contrast to the general population. A combination of antibiotic therapy as described in Infectious Diseases Society of America (IDSA) Guidelines, Infective Endocarditis in Adults: Diagnosis, Antimicrobial Therapy, and Management of Complications and surgical management, if warranted, is the current management.

Empiric management of suspected sepsis/BSI should include gram-positive coverage, in the presence of intravascular catheters, and broad gram-negative coverage. The choice of the antibiotic is dependent on the local epidemiology and previous microbiological data. Empiric *Candida* or antifungal coverage is not required, because the early initiation of antifungal has not been shown to improve the outcome in randomized controlled trials of mostly immunocompetent patients.[16,17]

RESPIRATORY TRACT INFECTIONS

Bacterial pneumonia is the most common cause of lower respiratory tract infections.[18–24] According to Giannella and colleagues,[25] community-acquired pneumonia (CAP) was found in 40.7% and hospital-acquired pneumonia (HAP) was found in 59.3% of SOT recipients treated for pneumonia. In lung transplant recipients, bacterial pneumonia or bronchitis accounts for 32% to 63% of all infections with the incidence of bacterial pneumonia peaking in the first 4 to 8 postoperative weeks and then declines by the fourth month. Perioperative antibiotics, which are focused on preoperative cultures from the recipient and donor, reduce the incidence of early bacterial pneumonia to less than 10%.[20,21] Regarding cardiac, hepatic, and renal transplants, the incidence of early bacterial pneumonia is 15%, 9%, and 4% to 6%, respectively,[18–20,26,27] with a mortality of 21% to 35% in liver and kidney transplant recipients. However, mortality between nosocomial and community-acquired infection was extreme at 58% compared with 8%[20–22] with mechanical ventilation and nosocomial infections at a higher increased risk for death.[18,20–22,24] In the initial perioperative period, nosocomial pathogens, such as *Pseudomonas aeruginosa, Escherichia coli, Klebsiella* species, *Acinetobacter* species, and *S aureus*, including methicillin-resistant *S aureus* (MRSA), should be considered in the immediate perioperative period; however, prolonged mechanical ventilation following transplant increases the risk for nosocomial pneumonia.[20–22] Community-acquired pathogens, such as *Haemophilus influenzae, Streptococcus pneumoniae,* and *Legionella* species, may be seen. With the implementation of trimethoprim-sulfamethoxazole prophylaxis, the incidence of *Nocardia* pneumonia has decreased; however, it is still reported.[20,28] Empiric treatment should take into consideration previous microbiological data, local epidemiology, and recent clinical history with regards to empiric antibiotic coverage.

Respiratory viral infections are a significant cause of mortality and morbidity among transplant recipients, including influenza, respiratory syncytial virus, parainfluenza virus, rhinovirus, human metapneumovirus, and coronavirus. The seasonal pattern usually follows that of the general public.[29–31] Disease can consist of mild congestion and rhinorrhea to more severe tracheobronchitis, bronchiolitis, and pneumonia. Clinical manifestation can range from mild or atypical symptoms, including absence of fever, with lung transplant recipients presenting with a more severe clinical course and complications.[29,32] Viral shedding is usually prolonged and seen even with the use of antivirals.[29,32] Transplant recipients are at higher risk of infectious complications, including fungal and bacterial pneumonia. Respiratory viral infections appear to be a risk factor for both acute and chronic rejection, especially in lung transplant recipients.[29,33–36] Diagnostic workup should consist of a nasopharyngeal swab, wash, or aspirate. If upper tract samples fail to document the cause or if there is clinical or radiological evidence of lower tract involvement, bronchoalveolar lavage (BAL) should be considered. Polymerase chain reaction (PCR)-based assays are commercially available with many centers adopting them because they are the most preferred mode of testing given the high sensitivity along with most allowing for simultaneously detecting a broad range of respiratory pathogens from a single sample. Treatment, as is outlined in **Fig. 2**, includes supportive care and reduction in immunosuppression.

Adenovirus is a nonenveloped, lytic double-stranded DNA virus that can be acquired de novo, through reactivation of a latent infection of the recipient, or from transplant organ. Transmission occurs by respiratory route, person-to-person contact, or fecal-oral route. The true incidence among SOT recipients is unknown, with most infections occurring within the first year after transplantation.[37] Clinical manifestations can vary; however, when affecting lung transplant recipients, it can produce a range of clinical manifestations, including acute flulike illness, diffuse alveolar damage, or

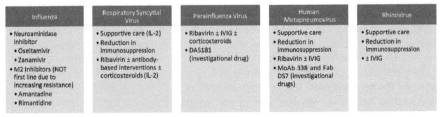

Fig. 2. Treatment recommendations for RNA respiratory viruses in SOT recipients. IL-2, interleukin-2; IVIG, intravenous immunoglobulin; MoAb, monoclonal antibody. (*Data from* Manuel O, Estabrook M. RNA respiratory viruses in solid organ transplantation. Am J Transplant 2013;13(s4):212–9; and Abbas S, Raybould JE, Sastry S, et al. Respiratory viruses in transplant recipients: more than just a cold. Clinical syndromes and infection prevention principles. Int J Infect Dis 2017;62:86–93.)

necrotizing pneumonia along with chronic changes, such as bronchiolitis obliterans, interstitial fibrosis, or bronchiectasis.[38–41] Viral culture, direct antigen detection, molecular methods, and histopathology are available for diagnosis with histopathologic evaluation, as the gold standard for the diagnosis of invasive disease. Rapid antigen detection kits, in particular, immunofluorescence assays when processing respiratory specimens, are commercially available, which yield rapid and specific results. PCR, qualitative and quantitative, has emerged as a widely used tool for detection because it is highly sensitive and rapid. Recovery of adenovirus from respiratory samples does not necessarily confirm disease because patients can shed asymptomatically for a prolonged period of time; therefore, it is essential to correlate with clinical findings along with detection of virus from other sites and histopathological findings. Cidofovir has the best evidence to support its use in the treatment of adenoviral infections. Brincidofovir, the lipid conjugate of cidofovir, has also demonstrated in vitro susceptibility and appears to be promising in vivo with regards to SOT recipients; however, further studies are warranted.[42]

CMV is a major pathogen in SOT recipients, with the ability to cause end-organ disease. The immunomodulatory effects of CMV, impaired T-cell and phagocytic function, and cytokine dysregulation can lead to opportunistic infections, rejection, graft loss, and reduced survival.[43,44] The transplant recipients who are at highest risk are seronegative recipients of seropositive organ, D+/R−, because they have no preexisting immunity, and seropositive recipients, D−/R+, are at intermediate risk. There is little difference between D+/R+ and D−/R− groups, with potentially worse outcomes in D+/R+ (**Fig. 3**).[43] Clinical presentation consists of dyspnea, fever, and malaise with the identification of characteristic CMV cells in lung tissue. Radiographic changes are nonspecific and include diffuse haziness, focal haziness, focal lobar consolidation, and no change.[20] Diagnosis is made via cell culture viral isolation; however, this can be time consuming. Therefore, the detection of CMV DNA by PCR in the peripheral blood leukocytes, providing a sensitivity of 92% and specificity of 76% for CMV pneumonitis, along with the BAL CMV DNA PCR, is an alternative means to diagnosis.[20,45] However, with regards to the BAL findings, it would be imperative to differentiate between infections versus shedding; hence, the concomitant peripheral blood leukocyte PCR along with the clinical picture is necessary to help determine the diagnosis. Treatment consists of ganciclovir or the oral alternative, valganciclovir. Foscarnet and cidofovir are alternative options; however, they are primarily reserved when there is a concern for resistance or documented resistance because their side-effect

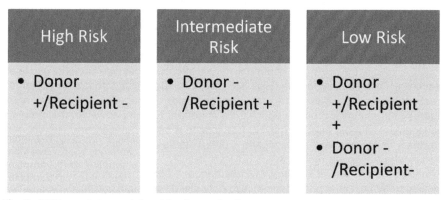

High Risk	Intermediate Risk	Low Risk
• Donor +/Recipient -	• Donor - /Recipient +	• Donor +/Recipient + • Donor - /Recipient-

Fig. 3. CMV serostatus and the risk of complications.

profiles are less desirable.[20] CMV immunoglobulin in conjunction with treatment offers limited efficacy.[43] Maribavir, brincidofovir, and letermovir are novel agents that may provide alternative options for treatment; however, further studies are warranted.

Candida is a frequent colonizer of lung transplant recipients, but less than 10% of patients colonized develop invasive disease.[20,46] Bronchial anastomotic infections may occur early in the postoperative setting, which can lead to anastomotic failure, parenchymal lung infection, and mediastinitis.[47–52] Artificial bronchial stents can serve as a potential site for infection.[47,48] *Candida* tracheobronchitis is based on visual inspection and histologic confirmation along with positive cultures from an appropriate specimen.[47]

Aspergillus species, a saprophytic organism, has higher rates of mortality, up to 54%, and an incidence of 3% in lung, 2.4% in heart, 2% in liver, and 0.2% in kidney transplant recipients.[47] Infection may be due to reactivation or de novo infection following inhalation of the mold. Renal failure, hemodialysis, repeated bacterial infections, leukopenia, CMV disease, high levels of immunosuppression, retransplantation, chronic exposure of the transplanted lung to the environment, and abnormal anatomic and physiologic function of the transplanted and, if still present, the native lung, airway ischemia, hypogammaglobulinemia, cystic fibrosis, and bronchial stent are all risk factors for invasive aspergillosis.[47,53–56] In lung transplant recipients, 20% to 40% are colonized with *Aspergillus* with complicated infections affecting up to 13% of all patients.[20,57–60] Colonization can also lead to bronchiolitis obliterans syndrome after lung transplantation.[47,61] Clinical manifestations can range from asymptomatic colonization to tracheobronchitis, invasive pulmonary aspergillosis, empyema, and disseminated disease,[47,62] with symptoms including purulent sputum, fever, malaise, respiratory distress, and hemoptysis.[20,63] *Aspergillus* tracheobronchitis can cause airway obstruction, ulcerations, and pseudomembrane formation.[47]

Nonaspergillus mycelial fungi are also increasing with frequency, as high as 30%, and an overall mortality of 55%[20,64]; however, zygomycosis (*rhizopus* and *mucor* species) and non–aspergillus hyalohyphomycosis (*scedosporium apiospermum* and *fusarium* species) have an even higher mortality of up to 100%.[20] Endemic fungi, *Coccidioides immitis*, *Histoplasma capsulatum*, *Blastomyces dermatitidis*, and *cryptococcus* are additional pathogens that may need to be considered.

Radiological findings may demonstrate nodules, cavitary lesions, focal consolidation or patchy densities, wedge-shaped pleural-based lesions, air-filled bronchi with an intraluminal lesion, "air crescent" sign, and halo of decreased density. Tissue invasion by fungal organisms is the gold standard for diagnosis of invasive fungal pneumonia. However, this may be difficult to obtain; therefore, International Society for Heart and Lung Transplantation developed guidelines, A 2010 Working Formulation for the Standardization of Definitions of Infections in Cardiothoracic Transplant Recipients, to assist in the diagnosis of not only fungal infections but also bacterial and viral infections. These definitions may also be applied to abdominal transplant recipients. Treatment is as follows in **Fig. 4**; however, be aware of drug-drug interactions with regards to immunosuppressive agents. It is important to note, however, that empiric management of mold infections in SOT recipients is seldom necessary. The optimal approach is to pursue the diagnostic workup aggressively and treat accordingly even in lung transplant recipients.

Pneumocystis jirovecii, *T gondii*, *Mycobacterium tuberculosis*, and nontuberculosis mycobacteria are other pathogens to also consider as possible causes of respiratory tract infections along with the other pathogens listed in **Fig. 5**.

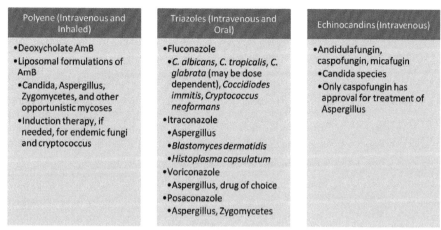

Fig. 4. Treatment of invasive fungal infections in SOT recipients.

NEUROLOGIC INFECTIONS

Central nervous system (CNS) infections can account for approximately 5% to 10% of CNS lesions in transplant recipients.[20,64] Routine prophylaxis aimed at opportunistic infections along with a more conservative approach regarding immunosuppression has led to noticeable trends in infections in transplant recipients. For example, routine administration of trimethoprim-sulfamethoxazole for *P jirovecii* has likely contributed to the reduction in infections owing to *T gondii*, *Nocardia*, and *Listeria monocytogenes* along with acyclovir and valganciclovir attributing to the likely decline in herpesviridae-related infections.[65,66]

Clinical presentation will vary and may include fever, headache, meningismus, Kernig and Brudzinski signs, new-onset seizure, papilledema, altered sensorium, and/or focal neurologic deficits; however, because of their underlying immunosuppression, these may be subtle or absent.[65,67] As listed in **Fig. 6**, possible causes range from

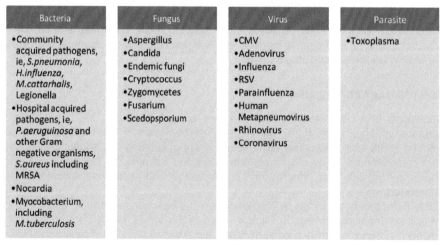

Fig. 5. Infectious causes of pulmonary complications in SOT recipients. RSV, respiratory syncytial virus.

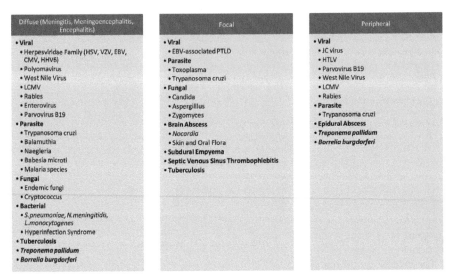

Diffuse (Meningitis, Meningoencephalitis, Encephalitis)	Focal	Peripheral

• Viral
  • Herpesviridae Family (HSV, VZV, EBV, CMV, HHV6)
  • Polyomavirus
  • West Nile Virus
  • LCMV
  • Rabies
  • Enterovirus
  • Parvovirus B19
• Parasite
  • Trypanosoma cruzi
  • Balamuthia
  • Naegleria
  • Babesia microti
  • Malaria species
• Fungal
  • Endemic fungi
  • Cryptococcus
• Bacterial
  • S.pneumoniae, N.meningitidis, L.monocytogenes
  • Hyperinfection Syndrome
• Tuberculosis
• Treponema pallidum
• Borrelia burgdorferi
	• Viral
	  • EBV-associated PTLD
	• Parasite
	  • Toxoplasma
	  • Trypanosoma cruzi
	• Fungal
	  • Candida
	  • Aspergilllus
	  • Zygomyces
	• Brain Abscess
	  • Nocardia
	  • Skin and Oral Flora
	• Subdural Empyema
	• Septic Venous Sinus Thrombophlebitis
	• Tuberculosis
		• Viral
		  • JC virus
		  • HTLV
		  • Parvovirus B19
		  • West Nile Virus
		  • LCMV
		  • Rabies
		• Parasite
		  • Trypanosoma cruzi
		• Epidural Abscess
		• Treponema pallidum
		• Borrelia burgdorferi

Fig. 6. Infectious causes of CNS and peripheral nervous system infections in SOT recipients. EBV, Epstein-Barr virus; LCMV, lymphocytic choriomeningitis virus; PTLD, posttransplant lymphoproliferative disease.

community-acquired organisms, donor-derived infections, reactivation, to opportunistic pathogens. Metastatic or direct lesions along with "pulmonary-brain" syndrome are also considerations in such organisms as Cryptococcus, Nocardia, Aspergillus, Zygomycetes, Strongyloides, and Toxoplasma; therefore, further investigations are warranted (eg, computed tomography of sinus and computed tomography of chest).[2,67]

Evaluation should include neuroimaging along with lumbar puncture as soon as possible if no contraindication exists. Cerebral spinal fluid examination should always include cell counts and differential, glucose, protein; routine smears; and cultures for bacteria, fungi, and mycobacteria.[65,67] Additional specialized testing, such as viral PCR, antigen or antibody, and 16S ribosomal RNA, may be required depending on the clinical scenario.[65,67] However, brain biopsy with appropriate staining may be the definitive diagnosis if findings are inconclusive. Empiric treatment should cover common bacterial and viral pathogens; however, additional agents may be needed depending on the epidemiologic history.

HEPATOBILIARY INFECTIONS

Cholangitis is a common infection after liver transplant, and in fact, is the most common infection more than 1 year after liver transplant.[68] Most cases occurred within 5 years and were associated with primary sclerosing cholangitis and Roux-en-Y anastomosis.[68] The most frequently identified bacteria are Enterococcus spp and E coli[68,69]; however, other gram-negative bacilli and anaerobes should also be considered.[68,69]

Bile leaks can occur in 2% to 25% of cases after liver transplantation, especially in living liver donor transplants.[70] Clinical presentation varies with extent of the leak; however, symptoms can include abdominal pain, fever, or any sign of peritonitis. However, because of underlying immunosuppression, they can also be asymptomatic.[70] In these cases, elevations in serum bilirubin, fluctuations in cyclosporine, or bilious ascites should raise suspicion for a bile leak.[70] Biliary strictures at the site of anastomosis can also present with fever, abdominal pain, but also jaundice and asymptomatic biochemical cholestasis.[70] Bilomas can represent an additional source of infection.[41,70]

Hepatic artery thrombosis, although more common in living donor liver transplants (LDLTs), is uncommon with deceased donor liver transplant (DDLT) with an overall incidence up to 9% and can lead to complications, including hepatic abscesses, necrosis, sepsis, and graft loss.[71] Vancomycin-resistant *Enterococcus faecium* (VREF) is of particular concern in liver transplant. Pretransplant colonization increases rates of intra-abdominal and BSIs after transplantation.[72,73] In fact, hospital and intensive care unit stays are longer for patients with VREF versus vancomycin-sensitive *E faecium* infections.[72] Liver, pancreas, and intestinal recipients are at particular risk for fungal infections, most often caused by *Candida* species.[41,74,75]

Regarding DDLT versus LDLT, there are variations with infectious complications. The rate of infection appears to be similar to DDLT; however, because of the more complex nature of the surgery, there are observable difference and specific concerns as detailed in **Box 1**.[76–78]

The clinical syndrome of hepatic dysfunction can range from mild elevated liver enzymes to hepatitis to fulminant hepatic failure. Hepatic dysfunction can present in any SOT recipient; however, of utmost concern would be liver transplant recipients. Causes can range from infectious to noninfectious with noninfectious causes primarily an issue with liver transplant recipients regarding postoperative complications, recurrence of primary disease, drug-induced complications, and rejection.[79] The infectious causes listed in **Fig. 7** can range from donor-derived infections, postoperative complications, community-acquired organisms, reactivation, to opportunistic pathogens. Evaluation should include imaging (eg, ultrasound, computed tomography, or MRI) along with the appropriate infectious workup (eg, blood cultures, serum PCR, serology, antigen, and/or antibodies). If the diagnosis remains inconclusive, a liver biopsy may need to be pursued with appropriate staining obtained.

ENTEROCOLITIS

Diarrhea following transplantation is frequently observed and is estimated to occur in 22% to 52% of patients.[80–84] It can be associated with allograft loss and increased

---

Box 1
Observable differences and specific concerns regarding living donor liver transplant

- Higher incidence of biliary strictures
- Roux-en-Y choledochojejunostomy
- Increased risk of blood product transfusions
- Biliary leakage leading to bilomas
- Prolonged cholestasis and coagulopathy known as small-for-size liver syndrome
- BSI related to intra-abdominal sources (vs catheter related in DDLT)
- Contamination in abdominal cavity
- Poor premorbid host condition

Data from Abad CL, Lahr BD, Razonable RR. Epidemiology and risk factors for infection after living donor liver transplantation. Liver Transpl 2017;23(4):465–77.

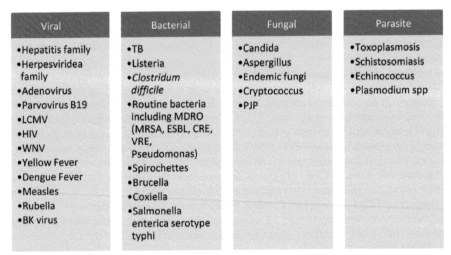

Viral	Bacterial	Fungal	Parasite
•Hepatitis family	•TB	•Candida	•Toxoplasmosis
•Herpesviridea family	•Listeria	•Aspergillus	•Schistosomiasis
•Adenovirus	•*Clostridum difficile*	•Endemic fungi	•Echinococcus
•Parvovirus B19	•Routine bacteria including MDRO (MRSA, ESBL, CRE, VRE, Pseudomonas)	•Cryptococcus	•Plasmodium spp
•LCMV		•PJP	
•HIV	•Spirochettes		
•WNV	•Brucella		
•Yellow Fever	•Coxiella		
•Dengue Fever	•Salmonella enterica serotype typhi		
•Measles			
•Rubella			
•BK virus			

Fig. 7. Infectious causes of hepatitis in SOT recipients. HIV, human immunodeficiency virus; PJP, pneumocystis jirovecii pneumonia; TB, tuberculosis; WNV, West Nile virus. (*Data from* Fedoravicius A, Charlton M. Abnormal liver tests after liver transplantation. Clin Liver Dis 2016;7(4):73–9; and Talwani R, Gilliam BL, Howell C. Infectious diseases and the liver. Clin Liver Dis 2011;15(1):111–30.)

mortality.[80,82,85,86] In fact, it results in 900,000 hospitalizations and 6000 deaths annually.[87,88] The severity and cause of diarrhea can lead to hypovolemia and/or septic shock. Diarrhea is a recognized side effect of some immunosuppressive agents; however, infectious causes should be considered based on the clinical picture. Causes are detailed in **Fig. 8**. Evaluation should include stool culture, ova and parasite and giardia antigen along with appropriate PCR, antigen testing, and/or special staining. Imaging may include a computed tomography to evaluate for bowel wall edema along with

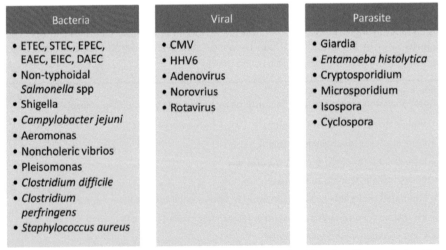

Bacteria	Viral	Parasite
• ETEC, STEC, EPEC, EAEC, EIEC, DAEC	• CMV	• Giardia
• Non-typhoidal *Salmonella* spp	• HHV6	• *Entamoeba histolytica*
• Shigella	• Adenovirus	• Cryptosporidium
• *Campylobacter jejuni*	• Norovrius	• Microsporidium
• Aeromonas	• Rotavirus	• Isospora
• Noncholeric vibrios		• Cyclospora
• Pleisomonas		
• *Clostridium difficile*		
• *Clostridium perfringens*		
• *Staphylococcus aureus*		

Fig. 8. Infectious causes of diarrhea in SOT recipients. DAEC, Diffusely adherent Escherichia coli; EAEC, Enteroaggregative Escherichia coli; EIEC, Enteroinvasive Escherichia coli; EPEC, Enteropathogenic Escherichia coli; ETEC, Enterotoxigenic Escherichia coli; HHV6, Human Herpesvirus 6; STEC, Shiga toxin-producing E. coli.

colonic wall thickening and dilation.[87] Esophagogastroduodenoscopy (EGD) and/or colonoscopy along with biopsy may also be warranted. CMV colitis is diagnosed via histopathology obtained during a biopsy. Serum PCR can be low to undetectable in this setting. If there is a clinical suspicion (eg, elevated serum PCR along with diarrhea, however the patient is unable to undergo colonoscopy), this may warrant empiric treatment.

Clostridium difficile infection (CDI) is among the most common health care–associated pathogen and is the most common cause of nosocomial infectious diarrhea.[89] The highest incidence of CDI in SOT occurs within the first 3 months following the transplant and is likely related to frequent exposure to antimicrobials, health care settings, and immunosuppressants.[89] Proton pump inhibitors (PPIs) are known to be a risk for CDI and may still be used in the setting of mechanical ventilation, versus H2 blockers.[90] Hospitalized patients who use PPIs are twice as likely to develop CDI.[89,91] Fulminant colitis develops in up to 13% of SOT recipients with CDI.[89,92] Relapsing disease is common, and protracted courses of therapy are often essential.[74,93,94] IDSA and Society for Healthcare Epidemiology of America recently updated the Clinical Practice Guidelines for Clostridium difficile Infection in Adults and Children for 2017, and although this is for immunocompetent patients, these guidelines can be applied to SOT recipients because there have been limited studies into the treatment of CDI in SOT patients.

GENITOURINARY INFECTIONS

The most common infectious complication in SOT is UTI, accounting for 45% to 72% of all infections, and 30% of all hospitalizations for sepsis in KTRs.[19,95–99] Most UTI are seen within the first 6 months after transplant; however, it can occur any time after transplantation.[96,100,101] Empirical treatment is imperative, as it has been demonstrated that inappropriate antibiotic therapy is associated with an increase in mortality.[100,102,103] To guide empirical therapy, local epidemiologic data, patient's microbiological history, and prior antibiotic use need to be taken into account.[95,100] The most frequent organisms causing UTIs are gram-negative bacilli[100,104]; however, when a urinary catheter is involved, *Enterococci* and *S aureus* should also be considered. The duration of treatment varies from 7–21 days depending on the clinical syndrome. Recurrent UTI, defined as 3 or more episodes of symptomatic UTIs over a 12-month period or 2 in the previous 6 months, should prompt further investigation regarding anatomic and functional abnormalities along with behavioral modifications (eg, postcoital voiding) and may need a prolonged course of antibiotics, possibly 4 to 6 weeks.[95,100,101] Asymptomatic bacteriuria should only be treated during the early postoperative period and up to 1 month after transplant in renal transplant patients.[100]

The data on UTI related to *Candida* spp in SOT are limited and mostly include KTR. In KTR, *Candida* spp are the most frequently isolated fungal cause of UTI. Unfortunately, there are no clinical trials in the management of *Candida* UTI in SOT.[100] Candiduria is frequent, occurring in up to 11% of KTR; however, it is mostly asymptomatic.[95] Asymptomatic candiduria is usually treated as there is concern regarding the allograft and potential for complications regarding the upper urinary tract; however, it should only be treated if the patient is neutropenic, or undergoing a urologic procedure.[95,100] Candiduria should be classified based on risk factors for disseminated candidiasis. Urinary catheters should be removed or exchanged, and candiduria should be confirmed with a second, clean voided urine culture. Disseminated candidiasis may be considered if clinical manifestations are consistent (eg, positive blood cultures, a second urine culture after removal or replacement of the urinary catheter, funduscopic examination, cultures from any other significant site, and kidney imaging). Persistent candiduria along with

---

Box 2
Duration of antibiotic therapy for urinary tract infections

- Fluconazole is the treatment of choice for cystitis and pyelonephritis

- Alternative options:
  - Single dose of parenteral AMB deoxycholate with or without 5-flucytosine for cystitis; d-AMB can also be used for pyelonephritis
  - AMB deoxycholate bladder irrigation for cystitis
  - Liposomal AMB with or without 5-flucytosine for pyelonephritis (low concentrations in urine therefore relapse may occur)
  - Echinocandins, drug of choice in unstable patients with systemic candidiasis for pyelonephritis (low concentrations in urinary tract and therefore relapse may occur)

Abbreviations: AMB, Amphotericin B; d-AMB, Amphotericin B deoxycholate.
   Data from Vidal E, Cervera C, Cordero E, et al. Management of urinary tract infection in solid organ transplant recipients: consensus statement of the Group for the Study of Infection in Transplant Recipients (GESITRA) of the Spanish Society of Infectious Diseases and Clinical Microbiology (SEIMC) and the Spanish Network for Research in Infectious Diseases (REIPI). Enferm Infecc Microbiol Clin 2015;33(10):679.e1–21.

---

no indwelling catheters should prompt imaging of the kidneys and collecting system to exclude renal abscess, fungus balls, or other urologic abnormalities. Treatment options can range from fluconazole treatment of choice, to echinocandins, amphotericin B, and flucytosine depending on the clinical situation and organism sensitivities with durations from at least 14 days for UTI to 2 to 4 weeks for pyelonephritis (**Box 2**).[100]

SUMMARY

SOT recipients are a complex group of patients with diverse causes given the underlying immunosuppression. As with all infectious processes, rapid identification of the

---

Box 3
Summary of the considerations in the management of infections in solid organ transplant recipients

Bloodstream infections/sepsis

- Always consider previous microbiological data and local epidemiology with regards to empiric antibiotics

- If an intravascular catheter is involved, consider broad gram-positive cocci, including MRSA, coverage in addition to broad gram-negative coverage, including ESBLs and CREs, if warranted

- Empiric antifungal is not needed, unless there is a high index of suspicion

Respiratory tract infections

- Always consider previous microbiological data and local epidemiology with regards to empiric antibiotics

- CAP should include empiric coverage for atypicals along with community-associated organisms

- HAP and VAP should include broad gram-positive coverage, especially MRSA, along with broad gram-negative coverage, including ESBLs and CREs if warranted

- Influenza is the only virus with approved treatment, oseltamivir; therefore, this should be started empirically if there is a concern

- Antifungals should not be started empirically, even in lung transplant recipients; however, fungal infections should be worked up thoroughly

CNS infections

- Empiric therapy should consist of ceftriaxone and vancomycin ± acyclovir

Hepatobiliary and gastrointestinal infections

- Always consider previous microbiological data and local epidemiology with regards to empiric antibiotics
- If VRE positive, will need to consider coverage using high-dose daptomycin or linezolid along with broad gram-negative coverage, including ESBLs and CREs, if warranted
- Regarding *C difficile* infections, oral vancomycin should be initiated empirically, if suspected, as first-line therapy

Genitourinary infections

- Always consider previous microbiological data along with local epidemiology with regards to empiric antibiotic decisions
- Asymptomatic bacteriuria should only be treated in renal transplant patients during the first month posttransplantation
- Antimicrobials should be tailored to the causative agent, with durations that generally range from 7 to 21 days depending on the clinical context
- Fluconazole is the treatment of choice for cystitis and pyelonephritis if *Candida* is the causative organism

Abbreviations: CRE, carbapenem-resistant enterobacteriaceae; ESBL, extended spectrum beta-lactamase inhibitors; VAP, ventilator-associated pneumonia.

pathogen, source control, and adjustment of immunosuppression is the hallmark of treatment. There is a summary of the management of infections in SOT recipients included in **Box 3**.

REFERENCES

1. Fernández-Ruiz M, Kumar D, Humar A. Clinical immune-monitoring strategies for predicting infection risk in solid organ transplantation. Clin Transl Immunology 2014;3(2):e12.
2. Fishman JA. From the classic concepts to modern practice. Clin Microbiol Infect 2014;20(Suppl 7):4–9.
3. Berenger BM, Doucette K, Smith SW. Epidemiology and risk factors for nosocomial bloodstream infections in solid organ transplants over a 10-year period. Transpl Infect Dis 2016;18(2):183–90.
4. Moreno A, Cervera C, Gavalda J, et al. Bloodstream infections among transplant recipients: results of a nationwide surveillance in Spain. Am J Transplant 2007; 7(11):2579–86.
5. Sanroman Budino B, Vazquez Martul E, Pertega Diaz S, et al. Autopsy-determined causes of death in solid organ transplant recipients. Transplant Proc 2004;36(3):787–9.
6. Camargo LF, Marra AR, Pignatari AC, et al. Nosocomial bloodstream infections in a nationwide study: comparison between solid organ transplant patients and the general population. Transpl Infect Dis 2015;17(2):308–13.
7. Silva M Jr, Marra AR, Pereira CA, et al. Bloodstream infection after kidney transplantation: epidemiology, microbiology, associated risk factors, and outcome. Transplantation 2010;90(5):581–7.

8. Candel FJ, Grima E, Matesanz M, et al. Bacteremia and septic shock after solid-organ transplantation. Transplant Proc 2005;37(9):4097–9.

9. Kalil AC, Syed A, Rupp ME, et al. Is bacteremic sepsis associated with higher mortality in transplant recipients than in nontransplant patients? A matched case-control propensity-adjusted study. Clin Infect Dis 2015;60(2):216–22.

10. Kalil AC, Opal SM. Sepsis in the severely immunocompromised patient. Curr Infect Dis Rep 2015;17(6):487.

11. Kalil AC, Dakroub H, Freifeld AG. Sepsis and solid organ transplantation. Curr Drug Targets 2007;8(4):533–41.

12. Hsu J, Andes DR, Knasinski V, et al. Statins are associated with improved outcomes of bloodstream infection in solid-organ transplant recipients. Eur J Clin Microbiol Infect Dis 2009;28(11):1343–51.

13. Bodro M, Sabe N, Tubau F, et al. Risk factors and outcomes of bacteremia caused by drug-resistant ESKAPE pathogens in solid-organ transplant recipients. Transplantation 2013;96(9):843–9.

14. Ruttmann E, Bonatti H, Legit C, et al. Severe endocarditis in transplant recipients–an epidemiologic study. Transpl Int 2005;18(6):690–6.

15. Paterson DL, Dominguez EA, Chang F-Y, et al. Infective endocarditis in solid organ transplant recipients. Clin Infect Dis 1998;26(3):689–94.

16. Schuster MG, Edwards JE Jr, Sobel JD, et al. Empirical fluconazole versus placebo for intensive care unit patients: a randomized trial. Ann Intern Med 2008;149(2):83–90.

17. Timsit JF, Azoulay E, Schwebel C, et al. Empirical micafungin treatment and survival without invasive fungal infection in adults with ICU-acquired sepsis, Candida colonization, and multiple organ failure: the EMPIRICUS randomized clinical trial. JAMA 2016;316(15):1555–64.

18. Singh N, Gayowski T, Wagener M, et al. Pulmonary infections in liver transplant recipients receiving tacrolimus. Changing pattern of microbial etiologies. Transplantation 1996;61(3):396–401.

19. Alangaden GJ, Thyagarajan R, Gruber SA, et al. Infectious complications after kidney transplantation: current epidemiology and associated risk factors. Clin Transplant 2006;20(4):401–9.

20. Singh. N CKM, Garrison. G,. Pneumonia Infection In Organ Transplant Recipients. 2017. Available at: http://www.antimicrobe.org/t35.asp. Accessed April 11, 2018.

21. Bonatti H, Pruett TL, Brandacher G, et al. Pneumonia in solid organ recipients: spectrum of pathogens in 217 episodes. Transplant Proc 2009;41(1):371–4.

22. Cervera C, Agusti C, Angeles Marcos M, et al. Microbiologic features and outcome of pneumonia in transplanted patients. Diagn Microbiol Infect Dis 2006;55(1):47–54.

23. Chan KM, Allen SA. Infectious pulmonary complications in lung transplant recipients. Semin Respir Infect 2002;17(4):291–302.

24. Sileri P, Pursell KJ, Coady NT, et al. A standardized protocol for the treatment of severe pneumonia in kidney transplant recipients. Clin Transplant 2002;16(6):450–4.

25. Giannella M, Munoz P, Alarcon JM, et al. Pneumonia in solid organ transplant recipients: a prospective multicenter study. Transpl Infect Dis 2014;16(2):232–41.

26. Chang GC, Wu CL, Pan SH, et al. The diagnosis of pneumonia in renal transplant recipients using invasive and noninvasive procedures. Chest 2004;125(2):541–7.

27. Lenner R, Padilla ML, Teirstein AS, et al. Pulmonary complications in cardiac transplant recipients. Chest 2001;120(2):508–13.

28. Wiesmayr S, Stelzmueller I, Tabarelli W, et al. Nocardiosis following solid organ transplantation: a single-centre experience. Transpl Int 2005;18(9):1048–53.

29. Manuel O, Estabrook M. RNA respiratory viruses in solid organ transplantation. Am J Transplant 2013;13(s4):212–9.

30. Couch RB, Englund JA, Whimbey E. Respiratory viral infections in immunocompetent and immunocompromised persons. Am J Med 1997;102(3a):2–9 [discussion: 25–6].

31. Lopez-Medrano F, Aguado JM, Lizasoain M, et al. Clinical implications of respiratory virus infections in solid organ transplant recipients: a prospective study. Transplantation 2007;84(7):851–6.

32. Ison MG. Respiratory viral infections in transplant recipients. Antivir Ther 2007; 12(4 Pt B):627–38.

33. Billings JL, Hertz MI, Savik K, et al. Respiratory viruses and chronic rejection in lung transplant recipients. J Heart Lung Transplant 2002;21(5):559–66.

34. Khalifah AP, Hachem RR, Chakinala MM, et al. Respiratory viral infections are a distinct risk for bronchiolitis obliterans syndrome and death. Am J Respir Crit Care Med 2004;170(2):181–7.

35. Kumar D, Erdman D, Keshavjee S, et al. Clinical impact of community-acquired respiratory viruses on bronchiolitis obliterans after lung transplant. Am J Transplant 2005;5(8):2031–6.

36. Milstone A, Brumble L, Barnes J, et al. A single-season prospective study of respiratory viral infections in lung transplant recipients. Eur Respir J 2006;28(1): 131–7.

37. Abbas S, Raybould JE, Sastry S, et al. Respiratory viruses in transplant recipients: more than just a cold. Clinical syndromes and infection prevention principles. Int J Infect Dis 2017;62:86–93.

38. Florescu DF, Hoffman JA. Adenovirus in solid organ transplantation. Am J Transplant 2013;13(s4):206–11.

39. Ohori NP, Michaels MG, Jaffe R, et al. Adenovirus pneumonia in lung transplant recipients. Hum Pathol 1995;26(10):1073–9.

40. Bridges ND, Spray TL, Collins MH, et al. Adenovirus infection in the lung results in graft failure after lung transplantation. J Thorac Cardiovasc Surg 1998;116(4): 617–23.

41. Humar A, Doucette K, Kumar D, et al. Assessment of adenovirus infection in adult lung transplant recipients using molecular surveillance. J Heart Lung Transplant 2006;25(12):1441–6.

42. Hirsch HH, Martino R, Ward KN, et al. Fourth European Conference on Infections in Leukaemia (ECIL-4): guidelines for diagnosis and treatment of human respiratory syncytial virus, parainfluenza virus, metapneumovirus, rhinovirus, and coronavirus. Clin Infect Dis 2013;56(2):258–66.

43. Haidar G, Singh N. Viral infections in solid organ transplant recipients: novel updates and a review of the classics. Curr Opin Infect Dis 2017;30(6):579–88.

44. Singh N. Late-onset cytomegalovirus disease as a significant complication in solid organ transplant recipients receiving antiviral prophylaxis: a call to heed the mounting evidence. Clin Infect Dis 2005;40(5):704–8.

45. Michaelides A, Liolios L, Glare EM, et al. Increased human cytomegalovirus (HCMV) DNA load in peripheral blood leukocytes after lung transplantation correlates with HCMV pneumonitis. Transplantation 2001;72(1):141–7.

46. Flume PA, Egan TM, Paradowski LJ, et al. Infectious complications of lung transplantation. Impact of cystic fibrosis. Am J Respir Crit Care Med 1994;149(6): 1601–7.

47. Shoham S, Marr KA. Invasive fungal infections in solid organ transplant recipients. Future Microbiol 2012;7(5):639–55.

48. Kubak BM. Fungal infection in lung transplantation. Transpl Infect Dis 2002; 4(Suppl 3):24–31.

49. Wahidi MM, Willner DA, Snyder LD, et al. Diagnosis and outcome of early pleural space infection following lung transplantation. Chest 2009;135(2):484–91.

50. Schaenman JM, Rosso F, Austin JM, et al. Trends in invasive disease due to Candida species following heart and lung transplantation. Transpl Infect Dis 2009;11(2):112–21.

51. Horvath J, Dummer S, Loyd J, et al. Infection in the transplanted and native lung after single lung transplantation. Chest 1993;104(3):681–5.

52. Hadjiliadis D, Howell DN, Davis RD, et al. Anastomotic infections in lung transplant recipients. Ann Transplant 2000;5(3):13–9.

53. Gavalda J, Len O, San Juan R, et al. Risk factors for invasive aspergillosis in solid-organ transplant recipients: a case-control study. Clin Infect Dis 2005; 41(1):52–9.

54. Rosenhagen M, Feldhues R, Schmidt J, et al. A risk profile for invasive aspergillosis in liver transplant recipients. Infection 2009;37(4):313–9.

55. Singh N, Pruett TL, Houston S, et al. Invasive aspergillosis in the recipients of liver retransplantation. Liver Transpl 2006;12(8):1205–9.

56. Fortún J, Martín-Dávila P, Moreno S, et al. Risk factors for invasive aspergillosis in liver transplant recipients. Liver Transpl 2002;8(11):1065–70.

57. Iversen M, Burton CM, Vand S, et al. Aspergillus infection in lung transplant patients: incidence and prognosis. Eur J Clin Microbiol Infect Dis 2007;26(12): 879–86.

58. Kotloff RM, Ahya VN, Crawford SW. Pulmonary complications of solid organ and hematopoietic stem cell transplantation. Am J Respir Crit Care Med 2004; 170(1):22–48.

59. Mehrad B, Paciocco G, Martinez FJ, et al. Spectrum of Aspergillus infection in lung transplant recipients: case series and review of the literature. Chest 2001;119(1):169–75.

60. Monforte V, Roman A, Gavalda J, et al. Nebulized amphotericin B prophylaxis for Aspergillus infection in lung transplantation: study of risk factors. J Heart Lung Transplant 2001;20(12):1274–81.

61. Weigt SS, Elashoff RM, Huang C, et al. Aspergillus colonization of the lung allograft is a risk factor for bronchiolitis obliterans syndrome. Am J Transplant 2009; 9(8):1903–11.

62. Grossi P, Farina C, Fiocchi R, et al. Prevalence and outcome of invasive fungal infections in 1,963 thoracic organ transplant recipients: a multicenter retrospective study. Italian Study Group of Fungal Infections in Thoracic Organ Transplant Recipients. Transplantation 2000;70(1):112–6.

63. Westney GE, Kesten S, De Hoyos A, et al. Aspergillus infection in single and double lung transplant recipients. Transplantation 1996;61(6):915–9.

64. Husain S, Alexander BD, Munoz P, et al. Opportunistic mycelial fungal infections in organ transplant recipients: emerging importance of non-Aspergillus mycelial fungi. Clin Infect Dis 2003;37(2):221–9.

65. Smith JA. CNS infections in solid organ transplant recipients. Hospital Physician Neurology Board manual 2005;9(3):1–15.

66. Singh N, Husain S. Infections of the central nervous system in transplant recipients. Transpl Infect Dis 2000;2(3):101–11.
67. Wright AJ, Fishman JA. Central nervous system syndromes in solid organ transplant recipients. Clin Infect Dis 2014;59(7):1001–11.
68. Aberg F, Makisalo H, Hockerstedt K, et al. Infectious complications more than 1 year after liver transplantation: a 3-decade nationwide experience. Am J Transplant 2011;11(2):287–95.
69. Raakow R, Bechstein WO, Kling N, et al. The importance of late infections for the long-term outcome after liver transplantation. Berlin (Germany): Springer Berlin Heidelberg; 1996. p. 155–6.
70. Kochhar G, Parungao JM, Hanouneh IA, et al. Biliary complications following liver transplantation. World J Gastroenterol 2013;19(19):2841–6.
71. Mourad MM, Liossis C, Gunson BK, et al. Etiology and management of hepatic artery thrombosis after adult liver transplantation. Liver Transpl 2014;20(6): 713–23.
72. Singh N. Infections in solid-organ transplant recipients. Am J Infect Control 1997;25(5):409–17.
73. Pessoa MG, Terrault NA, Ferrell LD, et al. Hepatitis G virus in patients with cryptogenic liver disease undergoing liver transplantation. Hepatology 1997;25(5): 1266–70.
74. O'Shea DT, Humar A. Life-threatening infection in transplant recipients. Crit Care Clin 2013;29(4):953–73.
75. Person AK, Kontoyiannis DP, Alexander BD. Fungal infections in transplant and oncology patients. Infect Dis Clin North Am 2010;24(2):439–59.
76. Abad CL, Lahr BD, Razonable RR. Epidemiology and risk factors for infection after living donor liver transplantation. Liver Transpl 2017;23(4):465–77.
77. Kim JE, Oh SH, Kim KM, et al. Infections after living donor liver transplantation in children. J Korean Med Sci 2010;25(4):527–31.
78. Kim YJ, Kim SI, Wie SH, et al. Infectious complications in living-donor liver transplant recipients: a 9-year single-center experience. Transpl Infect Dis 2008; 10(5):316–24.
79. Fedoravicius A, Charlton M. Abnormal liver tests after liver transplantation. Clin Liver Dis 2016;7(4):73–9.
80. Echenique IA, Penugonda S, Stosor V, et al. Diagnostic yields in solid organ transplant recipients admitted with diarrhea. Clin Infect Dis 2015;60(5):729–37.
81. Maes B, Hadaya K, de Moor B, et al. Severe diarrhea in renal transplant patients: results of the DIDACT study. Am J Transplant 2006;6(6):1466–72.
82. Bunnapradist S, Neri L, Wong W, et al. Incidence and risk factors for diarrhea following kidney transplantation and association with graft loss and mortality. Am J Kidney Dis 2008;51(3):478–86.
83. Herrero JI, Benlloch S, Bernardos A, et al. Gastrointestinal complications in liver transplant recipients: MITOS study. Transplant Proc 2007;39(7):2311–3.
84. Gil-Vernet S, Amado A, Ortega F, et al. Gastrointestinal complications in renal transplant recipients: MITOS study. Transplant Proc 2007;39(7):2190–3.
85. Nagaraj N, Kahan B, Adler DG. Gastrointestinal complications in renal transplant patients: a large, single-center experience. Dig Dis Sci 2007;52(12): 3394–5.
86. Altiparmak MR, Trablus S, Pamuk ON, et al. Diarrhoea following renal transplantation. Clin Transplant 2002;16(3):212–6.
87. Subramanian A. Diarrhea in organ transplant recipients. 2010. Available at: http://www.antimicrobe.org/new/t12_dw.html. Accessed April 11, 2018.

88. Thielman NM, Guerrant RL. Clinical practice. Acute infectious diarrhea. N Engl J Med 2004;350(1):38–47.

89. Ward SD, ER. Clostridium difficile Infection in Solid Organ Transplant Patients. 2017. Available at: http://www.antimicrobe.org/t40.asp. Accessed April 2018.

90. MacLaren R, Reynolds PM, Allen RR. Histamine-2 receptor antagonists vs proton pump inhibitors on gastrointestinal tract hemorrhage and infectious complications in the intensive care unit. JAMA Intern Med 2014;174(4):564–74.

91. Dubberke ER, Gerding DN, Classen D, et al. Strategies to prevent clostridium difficile infections in acute care hospitals. Infect Control Hosp Epidemiol 2008; 29(Suppl 1):S81–92.

92. Dallal RM, Harbrecht BG, Boujoukas AJ, et al. Fulminant Clostridium difficile: an underappreciated and increasing cause of death and complications. Ann Surg 2002;235(3):363–72.

93. Riddle DJ, Dubberke ER. Clostridium difficile infection in solid organ transplant recipients. Curr Opin Organ Transplant 2008;13(6):592–600.

94. Albright JB, Bonatti H, Mendez J, et al. Early and late onset Clostridium difficile-associated colitis following liver transplantation. Transpl Int 2007;20(10):856–66.

95. Parasuraman R, Julian K. Urinary tract infections in solid organ transplantation. Am J Transplant 2013;13(s4):327–36.

96. Alangaden G. Urinary tract infections in renal transplant recipients. Curr Infect Dis Rep 2007;9(6):475–9.

97. Abbott KC, Oliver JD 3rd, Hypolite I, et al. Hospitalizations for bacterial septicemia after renal transplantation in the United States. Am J Nephrol 2001; 21(2):120–7.

98. Veroux M, Giuffrida G, Corona D, et al. Infective complications in renal allograft recipients: epidemiology and outcome. Transplant Proc 2008;40(6):1873–6.

99. Pelle G, Vimont S, Levy PP, et al. Acute pyelonephritis represents a risk factor impairing long-term kidney graft function. Am J Transplant 2007;7(4):899–907.

100. Vidal E, Cervera C, Cordero E, et al. Management of urinary tract infection in solid organ transplant recipients: Consensus statement of the Group for the Study of Infection in Transplant Recipients (GESITRA) of the Spanish Society of Infectious Diseases and Clinical Microbiology (SEIMC) and the Spanish Network for Research in Infectious Diseases (REIPI). Enferm Infecc Microbiol Clin 2015;33(10):679.e1-e21.

101. Munoz P. Management of urinary tract infections and lymphocele in renal transplant recipients. Clin Infect Dis 2001;33(Suppl 1):S53–7.

102. Kang CI, Kim SH, Park WB, et al. Bloodstream infections caused by antibiotic-resistant gram-negative bacilli: risk factors for mortality and impact of inappropriate initial antimicrobial therapy on outcome. Antimicrob Agents Chemother 2005;49(2):760–6.

103. Schwaber MJ, Carmeli Y. Mortality and delay in effective therapy associated with extended-spectrum beta-lactamase production in Enterobacteriaceae bacteraemia: a systematic review and meta-analysis. J Antimicrob Chemother 2007; 60(5):913–20.

104. Cervera C, Linares L, Bou G, et al. Multidrug-resistant bacterial infection in solid organ transplant recipients. Enferm Infecc Microbiol Clin 2012;30(Suppl 2): 40–8.

Complications of Solid Organ Transplantation
Cardiovascular, Neurologic, Renal, and Gastrointestinal

Ayan Sen, MD, MSc*, Hannelisa Callisen, PA-C, Stacy Libricz, PA-C,
Bhavesh Patel, MD

KEYWORDS

- Solid organ transplant • Hypertension
- New-onset diabetes mellitus after transplantation (NODAT) • Acute kidney injury
- Calcineurin inhibitors • Posterior reversible encephalopathy syndrome
- Posttransplant lymphoproliferative disorder

KEY POINTS

- Despite improvements in overall graft function and patient survival rates after solid organ transplantation (SOT), complications related to cardiovascular, renal, neurologic, and gastrointestinal systems can lead to significant morbidity and mortality in this population.
- Common cardiovascular complications include hypertension, dyslipidemia, coronary artery disease from new-onset diabetes mellitus and renal failure, left ventricular hypertrophy, arrhythmias, and heart failure.
- Neurologic complications will occur in approximately one-third of patients with SOT and can be categorized into stroke and posterior reversible encephalopathy syndrome, central nervous system infections, neuromuscular disease, seizure disorders, and neoplastic disease.
- Clinicians should be aware of the risk of acute kidney injury (AKI), understand both preoperative demographics and patient characteristics predisposing patients at risk for AKI, intraoperative risk factors, and importance of prompt treatment on not only the kidney, but its downstream effect on all organ systems.
- Gastrointestinal (GI) complications occur in almost 40% of SOT recipients and include infection, malignancy (posttransplant lymphoproliferative disorder), mucosal injury, mucosal ulceration, perforation, biliary tract disease, pancreatitis, and diverticular disease. These can manifest as diarrhea, nausea, vomiting, abdominal pain, and GI bleeding.

Disclosure Statement: The authors do not have any relationship with a commercial company that has a direct financial interest in subject matter or materials discussed in article or with a company making a competing product.
Department of Critical Care Medicine, Mayo Clinic Arizona, 5777 East Mayo Boulevard, Phoenix, AZ 85054, USA
* Corresponding author.
E-mail address: Sen.Ayan@mayo.edu

BACKGROUND

Over the past 6 decades, solid organ transplantation (SOT) has evolved from an experimental procedure to a standard-of-care, lifesaving procedure, and survival rates have improved in a relatively short time frame.[1] The field has come a long way since the first documented successful kidney transplantation was performed between living identical twins by Joseph Murray and John Merrill in 1954.[2,3] Data indicate that more than 2 million life-years were saved to date by SOTs during a 25-year study period, a mean of 4.3 life-years per SOT recipient.[4] Despite improvements in overall graft function and patient survival rates, complications related to cardiovascular, renal, neurologic, and gastrointestinal (GI) systems can lead to significant morbidity and mortality in this population. This is attributed to end-stage organ disease processes and exacerbation of these with immunosuppression as well as the added risk of infection and rejection with transplantation.

CARDIOVASCULAR COMPLICATIONS

Cardiovascular complications are common after SOT.[5,6] These depend on the type of organ transplantation, premorbid cardiac risk, and effect of immunosuppressive medications. Cardiovascular disease is the commonest cause of death and graft loss in patients with kidney transplantation. The incidence is 3 to 5 times higher than age-matched patients in the general population but much lower than those on hemodialysis.[7] There is greater risk of sudden death, likely due to arrhythmia, and heart failure, rather than coronary artery disease. The Patient Outcomes in Renal Transplantation (PORT) study showed a cumulative incidence of cardiovascular events of 3.1%, 5.2%, and 7.6% at 1, 3, and 5 years posttransplantation.[8] Risk factors include immunosuppressive therapies, reduced glomerular filtration rate, dyslipidemias, hypertension, new-onset diabetes mellitus, and left ventricular hypertrophy from hypertension (**Table 1**). Approximately 11.1% of kidney transplant recipients have acute

---

Table 1
Risk factors contributing to cardiovascular mortality in solid organ transplant recipients

Recipient (Pretransplant) Risk Factors	Transplant Surgery–Related Risk Factors
• Hypertension	• Immunosuppression
• Diabetes mellitus	• Graft dysfunction
• Dyslipidemia	• Rejection
• Peripheral vascular disease	• Infection
• Smoking	• Anemia
• Obesity or metabolic syndrome	• Transplant renal artery stenosis (kidney transplant recipients)
• Advanced age	

Donor-Related Risk Factors	Additional Risk Factors
• Smoking history	• Hyperhomocysteinemia
• Age of donor	• Decreased renal function
• Quality of donor organ	• Proteinemia
• Organ ischemic time	• Left ventricular hypertrophy
	• Elevated C-reactive protein
	• Inflammation
	• Prothrombotic state

myocardial infarction in 1 series within 3 years.[9,10] Liver transplant patients are also at increased risk of cardiovascular disease with high risk of mortality as a result of it. Major risk factors include age, male gender, primary cardiac disease, hypertension, alcohol cirrhosis history, and posttransplant renal impairment.[7] Cirrhosis-associated cardiomyopathy has been seen in the pretransplant patients and autonomic dysfunction can occur in the perioperative period. Coronary artery disease is underdiagnosed, with approximately 25% of patients demonstrating obstructive coronary artery disease on angiography in 1 cohort.[11] Pancreas transplantation is associated with improved markers of cardiovascular disease. A 5-year retrospective analysis of 71 pancreas transplant recipients found improved HbA1c and serum glucose, lipid profile, and blood pressure in transplant recipients, as well as greater left ventricular function.[12,13] However, if renal failure occurs, it leads to worsening of their cardiovascular morbidities. Long-term cardiovascular event rates in lung transplantation are reduced due to high incidence of graft loss leading to patient death.[14] Cardiovascular causes of death account for only 11.4% of deaths within 30 days of transplantation, and 4.6% of deaths after 5 years, with chronic rejection and infection being the commonest causes of mortality.[15]

Hypertension

Hypertension is common in SOT recipients after renal transplantation due to pretransplant hypertension, delayed and poor allograft function, and immunosuppressants like steroids and calcineurin inhibitors (CNIs).[6,7] CNIs lead to tubular sodium retention and nephrotoxicity, whereas corticosteroids increase salt and water retention and activate the sympathetic nervous system. Hypertension can lead to left ventricular hypertrophy, which is an independent risk factor for death. Blood pressure may be reduced in kidney transplant recipients by alterations to immunosuppressive therapy, such as withdrawal or avoidance of corticosteroids, minimization of CNI, conversion from cyclosporine to tacrolimus, or the use of CNI-free immunosuppressive strategies.[6] Use of costimulation blocker belatacept, or mammalian target of rapamycin inhibitors (mTORi; sirolimus or everolimus) is associated with blood pressure levels lower than CNI-containing regimens.[11,16,17] Calcium channel blockers are effective at reducing blood pressure, may reduce the nephrotoxic effects of CNI, and lead to improvement of left ventricular hypertrophy after renal transplantation.[18] In a retrospective study by the Austrian transplant registry, use of angiotensin-converting enzyme (ACE) inhibitors and angiotensin receptor blockers (ARBs) was associated with improved patient and graft survival,[19] although a similar study by Opelz and colleagues[20] in the Collaborative Transplant Study dataset, failed to confirm this. The SECRET study assessing the role of candesartan after renal transplantation was abandoned due to low event rate of hypertension but was noted to be safe and led to decreased urine proteinuria.[21] The observational dataset of Opelz and Dohler[22] in the Collaborative Transplant Study showed a progressive benefit with systolic blood pressure as low as 120 mm Hg. In addition, with data from the Kidney Disease: Improving Global Outcomes guidelines suggest a target blood pressure of 130/80. Use of beta-blockers and ACE/ARBs in patients with proteinuria (above 1 g/d) or diabetes is recommended.[23]

Avoiding CNI agents and steroid withdrawal and minimization leads to lower blood pressures,[24,25] but the trend has been mostly toward using all classes of antihypertensive agents. Other approaches like posttransplant native nephrectomy or embolization, or percutaneous renal sympathectomy have not yet shown significant benefit for resistant hypertension.[26]

Hypertension is also a problem in heart transplant recipients. Antihypertensive therapy has benefits similar to the general population and similar therapeutic targets have been established in these patients. Calcium channel blockers are commonly used, but polypharmacy is often necessary and inhibitors of the renin-angiotensin system may be preferable in patients with diabetes or renal impairment.[27] Similar challenges are noted in heart, liver, and lung transplant recipients. A list of immunosuppressive medications and their side effects is provided in **Table 2**.

Dyslipidemia

Dyslipidemia is common after renal transplantation, affecting 60% of patients.[28,29] All lipid fractions increase in 3 to 6 months due to the immunosuppression, including total cholesterol, low-density lipoprotein (LDL), high-density lipoprotein (HDL), triglycerides, apolipoprotein B, and lipoprotein A.[30] Glucocorticoids cause hyperglycemia, hyperinsulinemia, and in turn a reduction in lipoprotein lipase activity with concomitant increase in triglyceride levels and secretion of very low density lipoprotein.[31] CNIs lead to reduced lipoprotein lipase activity, alter bile acid metabolism, and also reduce LDL receptor expression. Cyclosporine has a higher effect on increasing LDL cholesterol; mTOR inhibitors like sirolimus and everolimus are associated with significant hyperlipidemia, with unknown mechanisms.[32] However, they do benefit regression of atherosclerosis as evident through the coronary artery stent literature. Belatacept, with reduced CNI use or avoidance, causes lower lipid levels posttransplantation.[17] Large randomized trials have supported the use of statins in the renal transplant cohort. The ALERT study showed fluvastatin reduced LDL cholesterol by a mean of 1.0 mmol/L and 35% reduction in the composite endpoint of cardiac death or nonfatal myocardial infarction.[33] The SHARP study (Study of Heart and Renal Protection), which included a large number of patients who received transplantation, showed cardiovascular risk reduction (RR 0.83, confidence interval 0.74–0.94) with a combination of simvastatin and ezetimibe.[34] Cyclosporine and tacrolimus inhibit CYP3A4, which can lead to high statin levels and side effects from them. Atorvastatin, fluvastatin, and rosuvastatin use different mechanisms and are therefore more beneficial in these patients. Other agents, like ezetimibe, which inhibits small intestinal lipid absorption, may affect absorption of other fat-soluble drugs, whereas cholestyramine interferes with CNI absorption, fibrates cause myopathy, and niacin leads to hepatotoxicity. These drugs should be avoided in transplant recipients. Dyslipidemia is also common in liver transplant recipients due to immunosuppression, and statin therapy has been used with success to improve lipid profile, although, no long-term outcomes are known. Lipid targets are based on studies in the general population

Table 2
Immunosuppressive agents and cardiovascular risk

| | Immunosuppressive Agents | | | |
	Corticosteroids	Cyclosporine A	Tacrolimus	mTORi (Sirolimus, Everolimus)
Hypertension	↑↑	↑↑	↑	↔
New-onset diabetes (posttransplant)	↑↑	↑	↑↑	↑
Dyslipidemia	↑↑	↑↑	↑	↑↑↑
Weight gain	↑↑	↔	↔	↔
↓ Glomerular filtration rate	↔	↑	↑	↑ (+proteinuria)

Abbreviation: Arrows, indicate severity of risk; mTORi, mammalian target of rapamycin inhibitors.

(triglycerides <5.65 mmol/L [500 mg/dL], LDL cholesterol <2.59 mmol/L [100 mg/dL], and non-HDL cholesterol <3.35 mmol/L [130 mg/dL]) due to the scarcity of data in transplant recipients.

Endothelial Dysfunction

Endothelial dysfunction is noted to occur in renal transplant recipients.[7] Statins may reduce mitochondrial production of reactive oxygen species and caveolin in lipid-rich areas of cell membrane that binds and inactivates NO synthase (reduced NO production leads to oxidative stress and vasoconstriction); however, antioxidants, like vitamin B or folic acid, have not shown any benefit in the FAVORIT trial.[35]

Renal Impairment

Renal impairment is a major cause of cardiovascular risk in renal transplant patients. ALERT and FAVORIT trials showed a progressive linear relationship between estimated glomerular filtration rate (eGFR) and cardiovascular risk.[33,35] Although CNI-minimizing regimens are associated with improved graft function and cardiovascular outcome, incidence of acute rejection increases. mTOR inhibitors used as a part of CNI minimization are also associated with significant side effects. Belatacept, the costimulation blocker, showed better graft function in the BENEFIT-ext trial, but increased risks of lymphoma in early clinical trials and cost have limited its use.[17] Renal failure occurs after lung and heart transplantation due to CNI and 3% to 10% progress to end-stage renal disease (ESRD). This leads to incremental increase in cardiovascular risk.[36]

New-Onset Diabetes Mellitus

Posttransplant diabetes mellitus (also called NODAT: new-onset diabetes mellitus after transplantation) is similar to type 2 diabetes mellitus and occurs at peak in the first few months after transplantation due to doses of steroids and tacrolimus. NODAT has greater impact to graft and patient survival in the first year, with risk being higher than acute rejection.[37–39] Age, obesity, preexisting diabetes, and family histories are all risk factors. NODAT occurs due to insulin resistance and reduced insulin secretion.[40] Both cyclosporine and tacrolimus can cause it. In vitro, sirolimus enhances insulin function and glucose utilization through its action with FKB-12 binding protein. But in vivo, it induces pancreatic beta-cell apoptosis, reduced pancreatic B-cell function, and enhanced hepatic gluconeogenesis. Tacrolimus has a 70% higher incidence of NODAT compared with other agents.[41] Insulin resistance is also associated with corticosteroids in a dose-dependent manner.[42] NODAT leads to higher cardiovascular risk. A meta-analysis by Montori and colleagues[43] found the incidence of NODAT to range widely between 2% and 50%, with many studies not using routine oral glucose tolerance testing. The risk may be underestimated.

Management of NODAT is similar to type 2 diabetes mellitus; exercise, weight loss, and lifestyle changes are important. Metformin should be avoided due to high prevalence of renal impairment posttransplantation. Sulfonylureas and thiazolidinediones are usually first-line agents.[44] Dipeptidyl peptidase-4 (DPP-4) inhibitors are also recommended for second-line therapy, alone or in combination. Werzowa and colleagues[45] found that both pioglitazone and vildagliptin improved glucose tolerance in patients with stable renal transplant with newly diagnosed impaired glucose tolerance. Insulin is recommended only if glycemic targets are not met, when NODAT develops early in the posttransplant period, or when glucose levels are very high[46] Based on ACCORD[47] and ADVANCE[47] trials, HbA1c of 6.5% to 7.5% is recommended after renal transplantation. CNI and glucocorticoids lead to NODAT in liver transplants and the incidence has been reported to be from 41.2% at 6 months to 35.9% at 12 months.[48] Hepatitis C, autoimmune hepatitis, hemochromatosis, alcohol cirrhosis, obesity, and older age are risk factors.[49] Insulin therapy is common posttransplantation and can be withdrawn as steroid dose gets reduced. Sulfonylureas and pioglitazone should be avoided due to hepatic metabolism.

Obesity

Fifty percent of patients receiving transplantation may be classified as obese or morbidly obese.[50] Weight gain after transplantation is common and may be related to the use of high-dose glucocorticoids in the peritransplant period, long-term use of maintenance doses of glucocorticoids, improved appetite with reversal of uremia, and physical inactivity.[6] Diet and exercise are the mainstays in lifestyle modification for obese renal transplant recipients. If safe, the dose of glucocorticoids can be reduced, although there is little evidence that reducing chronically administered glucocorticoid doses will result in weight loss, and late glucocorticoid withdrawal may be associated with development of subclinical rejection. Antidepressants, like paroxetine, sertraline, herbal remedies (St John wort) and oral weight loss medication (orlistat) may interact with the cytochrome P450 pathway and reduce efficacy of CNIs. These should not be used in transplant recipients.

Bariatric surgery, including laparoscopic sleeve gastrectomy and Roux-en-Y bypass surgery, may reduce obesity-related morbidity in renal transplant recipients.[51,52] Complications of bariatric surgery include vitamin deficiencies and oxalate nephropathy in renal transplant recipients from enteric hyperoxaluria.

Rejection

The risk for developing rejection is the highest in the first 6 months following heart transplantation, with a decrease as the time from transplantation increases.[53] Sex and age are both linked to rejection risk, with female and younger individuals being at higher risk. Rejection can be due to acute cellular rejection and antibody-mediated rejection. Twenty percent to 40% of patients will experience acute cellular rejection between 6 and 12 months after transplantation, although most patients are asymptomatic.[27] It involves recipient T cells recognizing donor HLA molecules by means of antigen-presenting cells. Antibody-mediated rejection has an incidence of 10% to 20% in the first year posttransplantation.[54] This involves antibody-driven immune response to vascular endothelial antigens involving both B and T cells. A United Network for Organ Sharing/Organ Procurement and Transplantation Network (UNOS/OPTN) database study reported that patients with a most recent pretransplant panel reactive antibody (PRA) greater than 25% had a higher risk of treated rejection in their first year posttransplantation when compared with patients with a 0% PRA.[55]

Donor-specific antibodies are also associated with rejection and they develop after transplantation. The presence of donor-specific antibodies was also significantly associated with the development of biopsy-proven rejection episodes in the first year posttransplantation.[56]

Rejection can lead to diastolic allograft dysfunction due to myocardial edema.[53] Clinical presentation may consist of no symptoms, to general malaise, arrhythmias, pericardial effusions, exertional dyspnea, fatigue, hypotension, and cardiogenic shock.[57] Rejection may also result in sudden cardiac death. The ISHLT (International Society of Heart and Lung Transplantation) registry reports that acute rejection caused up to 11% of deaths between 1 and 3 years posttransplantation.[58] Rejection is diagnosed by endomyocardial biopsy. Immunotherapy is used both to prevent and treat rejection. The widely used regimen consists of immunosuppression (IS) involving corticosteroids and CNIs. Severe rejection may require antithymocyte globulin or OKT3. Rebound rejection can occur shortly after OKT3 or antithymocyte globulin; these episodes can be treated with corticosteroids. Alternative approaches include photopheresis, total lymphoid irradiation, plasmapheresis, and changes in the maintenance immunosuppressive regimen.

Cardiac Allograft Vasculopathy

Cardiac allograft vasculopathy is an accelerated form of intimal hyperplasia that occurs in the coronaries of the transplanted heart.[27] According to the 2015 ISHLT report, cardiac allograft vasculopathy was detectable by angiography in 8% of survivors within the first year, 30% by 5 years, and 50% by 10 years after transplantation.[59] Allograft vasculopathy occurs due to endothelial damage initiated as a result of immune and nonimmune mechanisms.[60] Risk factors include donor age, ischemic heart failure, cytomegalovirus infection, HLA antigen matching, and number of rejection episodes at 1 year. The most widely used cardiac allograft vasculopathy screening test is coronary angiography. The recent ISHLT guidelines on cardiac allograft vasculopathy nomenclature classifies cardiac allograft vasculopathy into 4 categories: 0 (nonsignificant), 1 (mild disease), 2 (severe), and 3 (severe cardiac allograft vasculopathy associated with graft dysfunction).[61] Dobutamine stress echocardiography is the noninvasive test of choice, with specificities of up to 88% and negative predictive value of 92% to 100% when referenced to intravascular ultrasound.[62] Cardiac MRI has also been safe and noted to have high diagnostic accuracy. Fludeoxyglucose (FDG)-PET is investigational and shows promise. Denervation of the transplanted heart limits the usefulness of typical symptoms of coronary disease, such as angina, leading to more serious late clinical presentations, heart failure, and sudden death. In a report from the UNOS database, 6% of patients with cardiac allograft vasculopathy experienced sudden cardiac death, with 45% of all sudden cardiac deaths being attributed to cardiac allograft vasculopathy.[63] Statin therapy posttransplant has been shown to reduce the risk of cardiac allograft vasculopathy.[64] mTOR inhibitors like sirolimus or everolimus slow progression of allograft vasculopathy.[65,66] Percutaneous coronary intervention and coronary artery bypass graft have been attempted in observational studies. For select patients, retransplantation remains the best option.

NEUROLOGIC COMPLICATIONS AFTER SOLID ORGAN TRANSPLANTATION

Neurologic complications will occur in approximately one-third of patients with SOT.[67] The type of complication seen may be related to several factors that include the timeline after transplantation, the type of solid organ transplanted, and the immunosuppressive regimen used. Most neurologic complications can be subcategorized into cerebrovascular events including stroke and posterior reversible encephalopathy syndrome (PRES), central nervous system (CNS) infections, neuromuscular disease, seizure disorders, neoplastic disease, and a few other disorders that include encephalopathy, myelopathy, headache, movement disorders, and visual as well as auditory disturbances.[68,69]

Encephalopathy

Although the term encephalopathy is frequently used as a diagnosis, it more appropriately refers to a general state of brain dysfunction or structural damage that can be related to metabolism, chemistry, toxins, trauma, infections, anoxia, tumor, and several other factors. The result is a change in mentation and/or consciousness that spans from confusion or delirium to coma.[69] Encephalopathy, particularly within the first 30 days of SOT, may be related to the initiation of immunosuppressive medications.[69] Several categories including monoclonal antibodies and CNIs have been associated with symptoms of encephalopathy. Although occasionally related to infection or seizure, the encephalopathy may also be a primary side effect of the medication itself. Although supra-therapeutic serum levels of CNIs are a common cause, it is important to recognize that these symptoms also may occur within therapeutic ranges.[70–72] The use of corticosteroids and non-CNIs, such as sirolimus and everolimus, also have been recognized as a cause of delirium, confusion, tremors, and insomnia.[73]

Another cause of early encephalopathy posttransplantation may be related to metabolic derangements such as hyperammonemia, which is frequently seen with liver transplantation and rarely in lung transplantation.[68] The encephalopathy in this case results from multiple mechanisms that include astrocyte edema from glutamine synthesis, impairment of the blood-brain barrier, changes in neurotransmission, and oxidative stress.[74] Patients who have pretransplant hepatic encephalopathy and those who receive a cadaveric graft as opposed to a living donor transplant have higher rates of neurologic complications postoperatively.[75] Although rare in lung transplant patients, severe hyperammonemia within the first 30 days has been associated with a significantly high mortality rate.[76] Other causes of metabolic encephalopathy in the SOT population include hypoglycemia, hyponatremia, hypernatremia, hypercalcemia, and hypermagnesemia.[67] Uremic encephalopathy may also be seen, particularly in renal transplant patients.[3] In general, "encephalopathy," whether caused by drug toxicity or other derangements, has been recognized as one of the most common neurologic complications posttransplantation.[70,72,77]

Infection

CNS infection is also not uncommon in the postoperative state of patients with SOT, with a prevalence of approximately 1% to 2%.[68] The type of organ transplanted, degree of immunosuppression, and time out from transplantation will impact the likelihood of CNS infection being the result of reactivation of prior disease or transmission of infection from the community, nosocomially, or from donor to recipient. The presence of CNS infection may result in altered mentation, headache, and fever, although these symptoms may be blunted by the patient's impaired ability to induce an inflammatory reaction in the setting of immunosuppression.[70,78,79] Further detailed description of infectious complications is provided in another article in this series.[71–78]

Other Neurologic Complications

Many of the comorbidities that are frequently seen in patients who undergo SOT put them at risk of cerebrovascular complications postoperatively. The most common etiologies include PRES and stroke, both ischemic and hemorrhagic. Concomitant hypertension, hyperlipidemia, and diabetes, as well as hypercoagulability and arrhythmias are more often seen in the heart and kidney transplant population, putting them at highest risk of stroke, with an incidence of 2% to 10% and 5% to 10%, respectively.[80,81] In heart transplant patients, almost 20% of cerebrovascular events occur within 2 weeks posttransplantation, with most being ischemic.[81] Patients with liver transplantation have a much lower rate of ischemic strokes; however, due to peritransplant coagulopathy and thrombocytopenia have a higher incidence of intracranial hemorrhage (ICH). Other risk factors for ICH in the SOT population include polycystic kidney disease, hypertension, diabetes, left ventricular hypertrophy, and certain infections, such as aspergillosis.[68] PRES is a condition manifested primarily by headache, vision changes, paresis, hemianopia, nausea, and altered mentation over several days. It is accompanied by a uniquely atypical MRI pattern consistent with white matter edema that is posterior hemisphere predominant. PRES has most commonly been associated with calcineurin-inhibitor use, hypertension, and hypomagnesemia.[68] With treatment or removal of the precipitating factor as well as management of brain edema, PRES may be reversible.[82]

Seizures are a common postoperative neurologic complication, recognized in approximately 5% to 10% of all transplant patients. The causes are related to many of the problems already addressed, including immunosuppression toxicity, metabolic derangements, infections, stroke, and malignancy.[70,83] Seizures due to CNIs have been described and are usually generalized.[84] Additionally, patients who have fulminant liver failure have an incidence of seizure near 30%, which may impact risk in the postoperative state.[85] Tremors and myoclonus also have been identified in this general population and are most commonly related to metabolic abnormalities or medication side effects. When treating with antiepileptic drugs, it is important to consider how they are metabolized and potential interactions they may have with immunosuppressive agents.

A unique risk for central pontine myelinolysis occurs particularly in the liver transplant population, with an incidence of nearly 17%. Although incompletely understood, the pathophysiology is suggested to be related to an often chronic hypo-osmolar pre-transplantation state and rapid volume replacements and sodium correction perioperatively.[86,87] The result is osmotic demyelination and oligodendroglial apoptosis.[86]

Ultimately, the neurologic complications that can occur in patients who have undergone SOT are vast and can have significant impact on outcome, making recognition and management critical.

RENAL COMPLICATIONS AFTER SOLID ORGAN TRANSPLANTATION

With the increase in number of SOTs, there is a temporal trend toward an increase in acute kidney injury (AKI) and chronic kidney disease (CKD) in the SOT patient.[88,89] CKD occurs despite advancements in immunosuppression and perioperative management, as well as attention to cardiovascular risk factors and infectious complications.[90] In patients with cardiac and liver transplantation, AKI complicating hospitalizations tripled between 2002 and 2013, 9.7% to 32.7% and 8.5% to 28.5%, respectively.[91] The data in post isolated pancreas transplant patients and renal failure is scarce. There does exist, however, a positive trend in delayed development of nephropathy in diabetic patients who receive a pancreas transplant compared with patients who do not receive a transplant. In lung transplantation, acute renal failure is a known complication in the postoperative period. In a study, 25% to 62% of recipients developed AKI and 5.5% required renal replacement therapy, which was associated with decreased survival.[91,92]

Postoperative AKI is a known consequence that has significant impact on mortality and morbidity.[93] Older age, preexisting AKI, existing comorbidities of systemic disease, like diabetes, and extent of organ-specific disease are all factors that contribute to the development of AKI postoperatively.[94] Intraoperative factors include intraoperative blood loss, length of ischemic time, (arguably) cardiopulmonary bypass (CPB) time, and hemodynamic instability. CPB is associated with proinflammatory mediation, reduced kidney perfusion, and generation of microemboli.[95] Patients with liver transplantation are at increased risk for AKI in relation to HIRI (hepatic ischemia reperfusion injury), which is an unavoidable injury to the transplanted organ during resection and reperfusion.[96] The HIRI takes into account both warm ischemia and cold ischemia time, and its pathophysiological mechanisms are not well understood.

CNIs are a significant risk factor for posttransplant AKI.[97] The effect of CNI consists of vascular obliteration, focal hyalinosis of small renal arteries and arterioles, global or segmental glomerulosclerosis, tubular atrophy, and interstitial fibrosis.[97,98] Additional factors include mTOR inhibitors, reactivation of hepatitis C in liver transplants, and surgical issues.

AKI in non–renal transplant recipients has a similar workup to AKI in other conditions. Defining the etiology of the AKI will help guide treatment. Workup should consist of obtaining general laboratory work along with imaging if indicated. Cystatin C can be considered in underweight patients.[93] Laboratory work to ensure adequate resuscitation, a urinalysis to define the injury (ie, acute tubular necrosis, prerenal process), tacrolimus levels, and renal ultrasound with Doppler to ensure no hydronephrosis and patent vessels should be done.[93]

In the immediate postoperative period, the focus of the clinician in treating AKI should be recognition, correction of acidosis and electrolytes, obtaining hemodynamic stability with resuscitation, and ensuring adequate oxygen delivery.[93] Ensuring target mean arterial pressure ensures that the kidney receives adequate flow and oxygen delivery. Pulmonary edema and volume overload should be corrected not only for management of hypoxia but also to ensure there is no increasing venous pressure on the kidney. Increased venous pressure can affect cardiac, hepatic, and pancreas total venous pressure and impairing oxygen exchange within the organ itself leading to graft dysfunction.[99] The use of therapeutic modalities to reduce degree of proteinuria may delay progression of renal failure. Use of ACE inhibitors or ARBs slows the progression of renal insufficiency.[100] Tight control of diabetes and hyperlipidemia is important. Tacrolimus causes less renal vasoconstriction than cyclosporine. mTOR inhibitors have been used to delay CNI initiation to reduce renal effects but it comes at the cost of compromised immunosuppressive efficacy and patient outcomes.[101] They should be avoided in patients with eGFR less than 40 or proteinuria, as they can accelerate renal dysfunction. Initiation of hemodialysis can be required if medical management fails. For nonrenal transplant recipients who develop ESRD, kidney transplantation results in superior survival than dialysis.[102] Timely referral of medically appropriate patients for kidney transplantation, early discussion about live-donor kidney transplantation, and low threshold to recommend use of nonstandard criteria deceased-donor kidneys is recommended due to high risk of dying or being delisted while awaiting a kidney.[102]

GASTROINTESTINAL COMPLICATIONS AFTER SOLID ORGAN TRANSPLANTATION

Gastrointestinal (GI) complications occur in almost 40% of SOT recipients.[103,104] These include infection, malignancy (posttransplant lymphoproliferative disorder), mucosal injury, mucosal ulceration, perforation, biliary tract disease, pancreatitis, and diverticular disease. These can manifest as diarrhea, nausea, vomiting, abdominal pain, and GI bleeding. Immunosuppressive drugs have frequent side effects and also predispose to infections and malignancies.

Infections

GI infections can be categorized by the time from transplantation-perioperative, early (1–6 months), or late (beyond 6 months).[104] Perioperative infections usually occur due to preexisting pathogens in recipient, donor-derived infections, or as a consequence of the transplant surgery. Viral and opportunistic infections occur in the early period, but the incidence is less with chemoprophylaxis.[105] Risk factors include poor graft function, exposure in the community or nosocomial, and intense immunosuppression.

Typical signs and symptoms of GI infection may not exist due to immunosuppression.[106–109] Further detailed discussion on GI infections post-SOT is provided in a different article in this series.

Immunosuppression-Related

Immunosuppressive agents have significant GI side effects. Cyclosporine, a CNI derived from a fungus, causes gingival hyperplasia by inducing collagenolytic activity in gums.[104] Gingival hyperplasia may necessitate a substitution with tacrolimus or sirolimus. Tacrolimus, another CNI, as well as cyclosporine, can cause nausea, abdominal pain, diarrhea, anorexia, and weight loss.

At high levels, both cyclosporine and tacrolimus can cause cholestasis. Sirolimus can lead to dose-dependent elevation in serum aminotransferases. A black box warning exists in the liver transplant setting for association with hepatic artery thrombosis. Mycophenolate mofetil has a number of GI side effects, including oral ulcerations, nausea, vomiting, and diarrhea. Dose reduction often improves symptoms.

General Gastrointestinal Complications

Peptic ulcer disease is common in the transplant population, particularly in kidney recipients.[110] In a series of patients with renal transplantation with peptic ulcer disease, 20% experiences significant bleeding.[110] Peptic ulcer prophylaxis is common post-transplantation. Corticosteroids and immunosuppressive medications can lead to genesis of peptic ulcers. Symptomatic peptic ulcer disease should incorporate evaluation for *Helicobacter pylori* infection and upper GI endoscopy.

Acute biliary tract disease is a complication in the transplant recipient, with mortality as high as 29% in some series.[104] Hepatic artery thrombosis post liver transplantation can lead to significant biliary complications with multiple strictures.[103] Hepatic artery thrombosis presents as fulminant liver failure. In the late period, strictures, cholangitis, and intrahepatic abscess can occur. Acute portal vein thrombosis also can cause hepatic ischemia and severe graft dysfunction if it occurs early.[103] Colonic perforation has an incidence of 1% to 2% after transplantation and a mortality rate of 20% to 38%.[111] Possible etiologies include diverticular disease, ischemia, and cytomegalovirus colitis. Kidney transplant recipients are at particularly high risk for ischemic gut because they often possess underlying vascular disease. Diarrhea in transplant recipients is common, with a variety of etiologies (**Table 3**).

Gastrointestinal Malignancies

Posttransplant malignancies are an important cause of morbidity and mortality, with increased probability of GI malignancy over longer follow-up duration. Immunosuppression can facilitate posttransplant malignancy by creating an environment for oncogenic viruses to thrive. Immunosuppressive medications, such as CNIs, also could play a role, having pro-oncogenic effects,[112] where other agents, such as sirolimus, are thought to have antiproliferative properties. Infections can lead to malignancies of the GI tract, like Epstein-Barr virus (EBV) causing lymphoproliferative diseases, human herpesvirus 8 causing Kaposi sarcoma, hepatitis C virus and hepatitis B virus causing hepatocellular carcinoma, and *H pylori* causing gastric cancer.[103] EBV is also linked to nasopharyngeal and oral cancer, and transplant recipients have a sixfold higher risk for oral cancer. Anal cancer, linked to human papilloma virus, also occurs at a 10-fold to 20-fold higher frequency in transplant recipients.[104] Liver transplant recipients secondary to primary sclerosing cholangitis can develop colonic dysplasia and diffuse colon cancer related to underlying ulcerative colitis. If severe

Table 3
Causes of diarrhea in solid organ transplantation

Infection	Medication	Other
• *Clostridium difficile*	• Antibiotics	• Ischemia
• *Campylobacter, Salmonella, Shigella, Escherichia coli, Yersinia, Vibrio parahemolyticus*	• Mycophenolate mofetil	• Inflammatory bowel disease
	• Sirolimus	• Celiac disease
	• Cyclosporine	• Graft-versus-host disease
• Rotavirus, adenovirus, Norwalk virus, *Giardia*	• Tacrolimus	• Posttransplant lymphoproliferative disease
• *Cryptosporidium, Cyclospora*		• Overflow diarrhea
• *Entamoeba histolytica*		• Colorectal cancer

colonic dysplasia is discovered, colectomy can be performed safely as early as 10 to 12 weeks following transplant.

Posttransplant Lymphoproliferative Disorder

Posttransplant lymphoproliferative disorder (PTLD) is a well-known complication of chronic immunosuppression in solid organ recipients. PTLD can involve the GI tract because the gut has an abundance of lymphoid tissue. The overall incidence of PTLD is approximately 1% to 3% in recipients of SOT.[103] The intensity of the immunosuppressive regimen is directly associated with the risk for PTLD. The pathogenesis is partly related to B-cell proliferation induced by EBV, but EBV-negative disease can also occur.

Patients with PTLD can present with nonspecific symptoms like fever, malaise, respiratory symptoms, or localized lymphoproliferation involving a variety of organs. GI involvement may cause obstruction, bleeding, or perforation. A biopsy is needed for a definitive diagnosis. An early detection strategy (a rise in the titer of EBV DNA after periodic measurements) should trigger a reduction in immunosuppression and careful surveillance. Imaging modalities with computed tomography scan and PET scan can help in diagnosis and staging of disease. Reduction of immunosuppression and rituximab, an anti-CD20 antibody, is usually the first-line therapy.

REFERENCES

1. Kellar CA. Solid organ transplantation overview and delection criteria. Am J Manag Care 2015;21(1 Suppl):S4–11.
2. Bloom RD, Goldberg LR, Wang AY, et al. An overview of solid organ transplantation. Clin Chest Med 2005;26(4):529–43, v.
3. Linden PK. History of solid organ transplantation and organ donation. Crit Care Clin 2009;25(1):165–84, ix.
4. Rana A, Gruessner A, Agopian VG, et al. Survival benefit of solid-organ transplant in the United States. JAMA Surg 2015;150(3):252–9.
5. Foley RN, Parfrey PS, Sarnak MJ. Clinical epidemiology of cardiovascular disease in chronic renal disease. Am J Kidney Dis 1998;32(5 Suppl 3):S112–9.
6. Munagala MR, Phancao A. Managing cardiovascular risk in the post solid organ transplant recipient. Med Clin North Am 2016;100(3):519–33.
7. Gillis KA, Patel RK, Jardine AG. Cardiovascular complications after transplantation: treatment options in solid organ recipients. Transplant Rev (Orlando) 2014; 28(2):47–55.

8. Israni AK, Snyder JJ, Skeans MA, et al. Predicting coronary heart disease after kidney transplantation: patient outcomes in renal transplantation (PORT) study. Am J Transplant 2010;10(2):338–53.

9. Kasiske BL, Maclean JR, Snyder JJ. Acute myocardial infarction and kidney transplantation. J Am Soc Nephrol 2006;17(3):900–7.

10. Lentine KL, Brennan DC, Schnitzler MA. Incidence and predictors of myocardial infarction after kidney transplantation. J Am Soc Nephrol 2005;16(2):496–506.

11. Tiukinhoy-Laing SD, Rossi JS, Bayram M, et al. Cardiac hemodynamic and coronary angiographic characteristics of patients being evaluated for liver transplantation. Am J Cardiol 2006;98(2):178–81.

12. Boggi U, Vistoli F, Amorese G, et al. Long-term (5 years) efficacy and safety of pancreas transplantation alone in type 1 diabetic patients. Transplantation 2012; 93(8):842–6.

13. Larsen JL, Colling CW, Ratanasuwan T, et al. Pancreas transplantation improves vascular disease in patients with type 1 diabetes. Diabetes Care 2004;27(7): 1706–11.

14. Studer SM, Levy RD, McNeil K, et al. Lung transplant outcomes: a review of survival, graft function, physiology, health-related quality of life and cost-effectiveness. Eur Respir J 2004;24(4):674–85.

15. Hertz MI, Taylor DO, Trulock EP, et al. The registry of the International Society for Heart and Lung Transplantation: nineteenth official report-2002. J Heart Lung Transplant 2002;21(9):950–70.

16. Oberbauer R, Segoloni G, Campistol JM, et al. Early cyclosporine withdrawal from a sirolimus-based regimen results in better renal allograft survival and renal function at 48 months after transplantation. Transpl Int 2005;18(1):22–8.

17. Vanrenterghem Y, Bresnahan B, Campistol J, et al. Belatacept-based regimens are associated with improved cardiovascular and metabolic risk factors compared with cyclosporine in kidney transplant recipients (BENEFIT and BENEFIT-EXT studies). Transplantation 2011;91(9):976–83.

18. Midtvedt K, Ihlen H, Hartmann A, et al. Reduction of left ventricular mass by lisinopril and nifedipine in hypertensive renal transplant recipients: a prospective randomized double-blind study. Transplantation 2001;72(1):107–11.

19. Heinze G, Mitterbauer C, Regele H, et al. Angiotensin-converting enzyme inhibitor or angiotensin II type 1 receptor antagonist therapy is associated with prolonged patient and graft survival after renal transplantation. J Am Soc Nephrol 2006;17(3):889–99.

20. Opelz G, Zeier M, Laux G, et al. No improvement of patient or graft survival in transplant recipients treated with angiotensin-converting enzyme inhibitors or angiotensin II type 1 receptor blockers: a collaborative transplant study report. J Am Soc Nephrol 2006;17(11):3257–62.

21. Philipp T, Martinez F, Geiger H, et al. Candesartan improves blood pressure control and reduces proteinuria in renal transplant recipients: results from SECRET. Nephrol Dial Transplant 2010;25(3):967–76.

22. Opelz G, Dohler B, Collaborative Transplant S. Improved long-term outcomes after renal transplantation associated with blood pressure control. Am J Transplant 2005;5(11):2725–31.

23. Kidney Disease: Improving Global Outcomes Transplant Work Group. KDIGO clinical practice guideline for the care of kidney transplant recipients. Am J Transplant 2009;9(Suppl 3):S1–155.

24. Pascual J, Zamora J, Galeano C, et al. Steroid avoidance or withdrawal for kidney transplant recipients. Cochrane Database Syst Rev 2009;(1):CD005632.

25. Pestana JO, Grinyo JM, Vanrenterghem Y, et al. Three-year outcomes from BENEFIT-EXT: a phase III study of belatacept versus cyclosporine in recipients of extended criteria donor kidneys. Am J Transplant 2012;12(3):630–9.

26. Symplicity HTNI, Esler MD, Krum H, et al. Renal sympathetic denervation in patients with treatment-resistant hypertension (The Symplicity HTN-2 Trial): a randomised controlled trial. Lancet 2010;376(9756):1903–9.

27. Alba C, Bain E, Ng N, et al. Complications after heart transplantation: hope for the best, but prepare for the worst. Int J Transplant Res Med 2016;2:022.

28. Ballantyne C. Clinical lipidology: a companion to Braunwald's heart disease; special populations: transplant recipients. Saunders; 2009.

29. Tse KC, Lam MF, Yip PS, et al. A long-term study on hyperlipidemia in stable renal transplant recipients. Clin Transplant 2004;18(3):274–80.

30. Ghanem H, van den Dorpel MA, Weimar W, et al. Increased low density lipoprotein oxidation in stable kidney transplant recipients. Kidney Int 1996;49(2):488–93.

31. Kasiske BL. Hyperlipidemia in patients with chronic renal disease. Am J Kidney Dis 1998;32(5 Suppl 3):S142–56.

32. Blum CB. Effects of sirolimus on lipids in renal allograft recipients: an analysis using the Framingham risk model. Am J Transplant 2002;2(6):551–9.

33. Holdaas H, Fellstrom B, Cole E, et al. Long-term cardiac outcomes in renal transplant recipients receiving fluvastatin: the ALERT extension study. Am J Transplant 2005;5(12):2929–36.

34. Baigent C, Landray MJ, Reith C, et al. The effects of lowering LDL cholesterol with simvastatin plus ezetimibe in patients with chronic kidney disease (Study of Heart and Renal Protection): a randomised placebo-controlled trial. Lancet 2011;377(9784):2181–92.

35. Weiner DE, Carpenter MA, Levey AS, et al. Kidney function and risk of cardiovascular disease and mortality in kidney transplant recipients: the FAVORIT trial. Am J Transplant 2012;12(9):2437–45.

36. Bloom RD, Doyle AM. Kidney disease after heart and lung transplantation. Am J Transplant 2006;6(4):671–9.

37. Cole EH, Johnston O, Rose CL, et al. Impact of acute rejection and new-onset diabetes on long-term transplant graft and patient survival. Clin J Am Soc Nephrol 2008;3(3):814–21.

38. Cosio FG, Pesavento TE, Osei K, et al. Post-transplant diabetes mellitus: increasing incidence in renal allograft recipients transplanted in recent years. Kidney Int 2001;59(2):732–7.

39. Rakel A, Karelis AD. New-onset diabetes after transplantation: risk factors and clinical impact. Diabetes Metab 2011;37(1):1–14.

40. Vincenti F, Friman S, Scheuermann E, et al. Results of an international, randomized trial comparing glucose metabolism disorders and outcome with cyclosporine versus tacrolimus. Am J Transplant 2007;7(6):1506–14.

41. Kasiske BL, Guijarro C, Massy ZA, et al. Cardiovascular disease after renal transplantation. J Am Soc Nephrol 1996;7(1):158–65.

42. Hjelmesaeth J, Hartmann A, Kofstad J, et al. Glucose intolerance after renal transplantation depends upon prednisolone dose and recipient age. Transplantation 1997;64(7):979–83.

43. Montori VM, Basu A, Erwin PJ, et al. Posttransplantation diabetes: a systematic review of the literature. Diabetes Care 2002;25(3):583–92.

44. Nissen SE, Wolski K. Effect of rosiglitazone on the risk of myocardial infarction and death from cardiovascular causes. N Engl J Med 2007;356(24):2457–71.

45. Werzowa J, Hecking M, Haidinger M, et al. Vildagliptin and pioglitazone in patients with impaired glucose tolerance after kidney transplantation: a randomized, placebo-controlled clinical trial. Transplantation 2013;95(3):456–62.

46. Wilkinson A, Davidson J, Dotta F, et al. Guidelines for the treatment and management of new-onset diabetes after transplantation. Clin Transplant 2005; 19(3):291–8.

47. Action to Control Cardiovascular Risk in Diabetes Study Group, Gerstein HC, Miller ME, Byington RP, et al. Effects of intensive glucose lowering in type 2 diabetes. N Engl J Med 2008;358(24):2545–59.

48. Oufroukhi L, Kamar N, Muscari F, et al. Predictive factors for posttransplant diabetes mellitus within one-year of liver transplantation. Transplantation 2008; 85(10):1436–42.

49. Laish I, Braun M, Mor E, et al. Metabolic syndrome in liver transplant recipients: prevalence, risk factors, and association with cardiovascular events. Liver Transpl 2011;17(1):15–22.

50. Vincenti F, Charpentier B, Vanrenterghem Y, et al. A phase III study of belatacept-based immunosuppression regimens versus cyclosporine in renal transplant recipients (BENEFIT study). Am J Transplant 2010;10(3):535–46.

51. Modanlou KA, Muthyala U, Xiao H, et al. Bariatric surgery among kidney transplant candidates and recipients: analysis of the United States renal data system and literature review. Transplantation 2009;87(8):1167–73.

52. Golomb I, Winkler J, Ben-Yakov A, et al. Laparoscopic sleeve gastrectomy as a weight reduction strategy in obese patients after kidney transplantation. Am J Transplant 2014;14(10):2384–90.

53. Costanzo MR, Dipchand A, Starling R, et al. The International Society of Heart and Lung Transplantation guidelines for the care of heart transplant recipients. J Heart Lung Transplant 2010;29(8):914–56.

54. Kobashigawa J, Crespo-Leiro MG, Ensminger SM, et al. Report from a consensus conference on antibody-mediated rejection in heart transplantation. J Heart Lung Transplant 2011;30(3):252–69.

55. Nwakanma LU, Williams JA, Weiss ES, et al. Influence of pretransplant panel-reactive antibody on outcomes in 8,160 heart transplant recipients in recent era. Ann Thorac Surg 2007;84(5):1556–62 [discussion: 62–3].

56. Smith JD, Banner NR, Hamour IM, et al. De novo donor HLA-specific antibodies after heart transplantation are an independent predictor of poor patient survival. Am J Transplant 2011;11(2):312–9.

57. Fishbein MC, Kobashigawa J. Biopsy-negative cardiac transplant rejection: etiology, diagnosis, and therapy. Curr Opin Cardiol 2004;19(2):166–9.

58. Lund LH, Edwards LB, Kucheryavaya AY, et al. The registry of the International Society for Heart and Lung Transplantation: thirtieth official adult heart transplant report—2013; focus theme: age. J Heart Lung Transplant 2013;32(10): 951–64.

59. Yusen RD, Edwards LB, Kucheryavaya AY, et al. The registry of the International Society for Heart and Lung Transplantation: thirty-second official adult lung and heart-lung transplantation report–2015; focus theme: early graft failure. J Heart Lung Transplant 2015;34(10):1264–77.

60. Ramzy D, Rao V, Brahm J, et al. Cardiac allograft vasculopathy: a review. Can J Surg 2005;48(4):319–27.

61. Mehra MR, Crespo-Leiro MG, Dipchand A, et al. International Society for Heart and Lung Transplantation working formulation of a standardized nomenclature

for cardiac allograft vasculopathy—2010. J Heart Lung Transplant 2010;29(7): 717–27.

62. Akosah KO, Mohanty PK, Funai JT, et al. Noninvasive detection of transplant coronary artery disease by dobutamine stress echocardiography. J Heart Lung Transplant 1994;13(6):1024–38.

63. Vakil K, Taimeh Z, Sharma A, et al. Incidence, predictors, and temporal trends of sudden cardiac death after heart transplantation. Heart Rhythm 2014;11(10): 1684–90.

64. Kobashigawa JA, Moriguchi JD, Laks H, et al. Ten-year follow-up of a randomized trial of pravastatin in heart transplant patients. J Heart Lung Transplant 2005;24(11):1736–40.

65. Arora S, Andreassen AK, Andersson B, et al. The effect of everolimus initiation and calcineurin inhibitor elimination on cardiac allograft vasculopathy in de novo recipients: one-year results of a Scandinavian randomized trial. Am J Transplant 2015;15(7):1967–75.

66. Kobashigawa JA, Pauly DF, Starling RC, et al. Cardiac allograft vasculopathy by intravascular ultrasound in heart transplant patients: substudy from the everolimus versus mycophenolate mofetil randomized, multicenter trial. JACC Heart Fail 2013;1(5):389–99.

67. Senzolo M, Ferronato C, Burra P. Neurologic complications after solid organ transplantation. Transpl Int 2009;22(3):269–78.

68. Pizzi M, Ng L. Neurologic complications of solid organ transplantation. Neurol Clin 2017;35(4):809–23.

69. Pedroso JL, Dutra LA, Braga-Neto P, et al. Neurological complications of solid organ transplantation. Arq Neuropsiquiatr 2017;75(10):736–47.

70. Dhar R, Human T. Central nervous system complications after transplantation. Neurol Clin 2011;29(4):943–72.

71. Wijdicks EF, Wiesner RH, Krom RA. Neurotoxicity in liver transplant recipients with cyclosporine immunosuppression. Neurology 1995;45(11):1962–4.

72. Bronster DJ, Emre S, Boccagni P, et al. Central nervous system complications in liver transplant recipients–incidence, timing, and long-term follow-up. Clin Transplant 2000;14(1):1–7.

73. Anghel D, Tanasescu R, Campeanu A, et al. Neurotoxicity of immunosuppressive therapies in organ transplantation. Maedica (Buchar) 2013;8(2):170–5.

74. Ciecko-Michalska I, Szczepanek M, Slowik A, et al. Pathogenesis of hepatic encephalopathy. Gastroenterol Res Pract 2012;2012:642108.

75. Lewis MB, Howdle PD. Neurologic complications of liver transplantation in adults. Neurology 2003;61(9):1174–8.

76. Shigemura N, Sclabassi RJ, Bhama JK, et al. Early major neurologic complications after lung transplantation: incidence, risk factors, and outcome. Transplantation 2013;95(6):866–71.

77. Kim JM, Jung KH, Lee ST, et al. Central nervous system complications after liver transplantation. J Clin Neurosci 2015;22(8):1355–9.

78. Conti DJ, Rubin RH. Infection of the central nervous system in organ transplant recipients. Neurol Clin 1988;6(2):241–60.

79. van de Beek D, Patel R, Daly RC, et al. Central nervous system infections in heart transplant recipients. Arch Neurol 2007;64(12):1715–20.

80. Pustavoitau A, Bhardwaj A, Stevens R. Neurological complications of transplantation. J Intensive Care Med 2011;26(4):209–22.

81. Alejaldre A, Delgado-Mederos R, Santos MA, et al. Cerebrovascular complications after heart transplantation. Curr Cardiol Rev 2010;6(3):214–7.

82. Fugate JE, Rabinstein AA. Posterior reversible encephalopathy syndrome: clinical and radiological manifestations, pathophysiology, and outstanding questions. Lancet Neurol 2015;14(9):914–25.

83. Gilmore RL. Seizures and antiepileptic drug use in transplant patients. Neurol Clin 1988;6(2):279–96.

84. Patchell RA. Neurological complications of organ transplantation. Ann Neurol 1994;36(5):688–703.

85. Frontera JA, Kalb T. Neurological management of fulminant hepatic failure. Neurocrit Care 2011;14(2):318–27.

86. Fukazawa K, Nishida S, Aguina L, et al. Central pontine myelinolysis (CPM) associated with tacrolimus (FK506) after liver transplantation. Ann Transplant 2011;16(3):139–42.

87. Fryer JP, Fortier MV, Metrakos P, et al. Central pontine myelinolysis and cyclosporine neurotoxicity following liver transplantation. Transplantation 1996; 61(4):658–61.

88. Miller BW. Chronic kidney disease in solid-organ transplantation. Adv Chronic Kidney Dis 2006;13(1):29–34.

89. Srinivas TR, Stephany BR, Budev M, et al. An emerging population: kidney transplant candidates who are placed on the waiting list after liver, heart, and lung transplantation. Clin J Am Soc Nephrol 2010;5(10):1881–6.

90. O'Riordan A, Wong V, McCormick PA, et al. Chronic kidney disease post-liver transplantation. Nephrol Dial Transplant 2006;21(9):2630–6.

91. Nadkarni GN, Chauhan K, Patel A, et al. Temporal trends of dialysis requiring acute kidney injury after orthotopic cardiac and liver transplant hospitalizations. BMC Nephrol 2017;18(1):244.

92. Arnaoutakis GJ, George TJ, Robinson CW, et al. Severe acute kidney injury according to the RIFLE (risk, injury, failure, loss, end stage) criteria affects mortality in lung transplantation. J Heart Lung Transplant 2011;30(10):1161–8.

93. Bloom RD. Renal function and nonrenal solid organ transplantation. The Netherlands: Wolters Kulwer Health; 2016. Available at: https://www.uptodate.com/contents/renal-function-and-nonrenal-solid-organ-transplantation?search=acute%20kidney%20injury%20post%20solid%20organ%20transplant&source=search_result&selectedTitle=1~150&usage_type=default&display_rank=1.

94. De Santo LS, Romano G, Amarelli C, et al. Implications of acute kidney injury after heart transplantation: what a surgeon should know. Eur J Cardiothorac Surg 2011;40(6):1355–61 [discussion: 61].

95. Schiferer A, Zuckermann A, Dunkler D, et al. Acute kidney injury and outcome after heart transplantation: large differences in performance of scoring systems. Transplantation 2016;100(11):2439–46.

96. Jochmans I, Meurisse N, Neyrinck A, et al. Hepatic ischemia/reperfusion injury associates with acute kidney injury in liver transplantation: prospective cohort study. Liver Transpl 2017;23(5):634–44.

97. Puschett JB, Greenberg A, Holley J, et al. The spectrum of ciclosporin nephrotoxicity. Am J Nephrol 1990;10(4):296–309.

98. Xia T, Zhu S, Wen Y, et al. Risk factors for calcineurin inhibitor nephrotoxicity after renal transplantation: a systematic review and meta-analysis. Drug Des Devel Ther 2018;12:417–28.

99. Bacchi G, Buscaroli A, Fusari M, et al. The influence of intraoperative central venous pressure on delayed graft function in renal transplantation: a single-center experience. Transplant Proc 2010;42(9):3387–91.

100. Stigant CE, Cohen J, Vivera M, et al. ACE inhibitors and angiotensin II antagonists in renal transplantation: an analysis of safety and efficacy. Am J Kidney Dis 2000;35(1):58–63.
101. Asrani SK, Wiesner RH, Trotter JF, et al. De novo sirolimus and reduced-dose tacrolimus versus standard-dose tacrolimus after liver transplantation: the 2000-2003 phase II prospective randomized trial. Am J Transplant 2014;14(2): 356–66.
102. Cassuto JR, Reese PP, Sonnad S, et al. Wait list death and survival benefit of kidney transplantation among nonrenal transplant recipients. Am J Transplant 2010;10(11):2502–11.
103. Chandok N, Wyat K. Gastrointestinal complications of solid organ and hematopoietic cell transplantation. In: Talley NJ, Kane SV, Wallace MB, et al, editors. Practical gastroenterology and hepatology board review toolkit. 2nd edition. Hoboken (NJ): John Wiley and Sons Ltd; 2016. p. 419–24.
104. Gautam A. Gastrointestinal complications following transplantation. Surg Clin North Am 2006;86(5):1195–206, vii.
105. Fischer SA. Infections complicating solid organ transplantation. Surg Clin North Am 2006;86(5):1127–45, v-vi.
106. Snydman DR. Infection in solid organ transplantation. Transpl Infect Dis 1999; 1(1):21–8.
107. Lowance D, Neumayer HH, Legendre CM, et al. Valacyclovir for the prevention of cytomegalovirus disease after renal transplantation. International Valacyclovir Cytomegalovirus Prophylaxis Transplantation Study Group. N Engl J Med 1999; 340(19):1462–70.
108. Mitchell O, Gurakar A. Management of hepatitis C post-liver transplantation: a comprehensive review. J Clin Transl Hepatol 2015;3(2):140–8.
109. Veldt BJ, Poterucha JJ, Watt KD, et al. Impact of pegylated interferon and ribavirin treatment on graft survival in liver transplant patients with recurrent hepatitis C infection. Am J Transplant 2008;8(11):2426–33.
110. Reese J, Burton F, Lingle D, et al. Peptic ulcer disease following renal transplantation in the cyclosporine era. Am J Surg 1991;162(6):558–62.
111. Stelzner M, Vlahakos DV, Milford EL, et al. Colonic perforations after renal transplantation. J Am Coll Surg 1997;184(1):63–9.
112. Gutierrez-Dalmau A, Campistol JM. Immunosuppressive therapy and malignancy in organ transplant recipients: a systematic review. Drugs 2007;67(8): 1167–98.

Moving?

Make sure your subscription moves with you!

To notify us of your new address, find your **Clinics Account Number** (located on your mailing label above your name), and contact customer service at:

Email: journalscustomerservice-usa@elsevier.com

800-654-2452 (subscribers in the U.S. & Canada)
314-447-8871 (subscribers outside of the U.S. & Canada)

Fax number: 314-447-8029

Elsevier Health Sciences Division
Subscription Customer Service
3251 Riverport Lane
Maryland Heights, MO 63043

*To ensure uninterrupted delivery of your subscription, please notify us at least 4 weeks in advance of move.

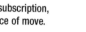

Printed and bound by CPI Group (UK) Ltd, Croydon, CR0 4YY

07/10/2024

01040503-0018